DENTOFACIAL DEFORMITIES

SURGICAL-ORTHODONTIC CORRECTION

DENTOFACIAL DEFORMITIES
SURGICAL-ORTHODONTIC CORRECTION

Bruce N. Epker, D.D.S., Ph.D.

Director, Oral and Maxillofacial Surgery,
Director, Center for Correction Dentofacial Deformities,
John Peter Smith Hospital,
Fort Worth, Texas

Larry M. Wolford, D.D.S.

Assistant Director, Oral and Maxillofacial Surgery,
Assistant Director, Center for Correction Dentofacial Deformities,
John Peter Smith Hospital,
Fort Worth, Texas

with 691 illustrations

The C. V. Mosby Company

ST. LOUIS • TORONTO • LONDON   1980

Printed in the United States of America

The C. V. Mosby Company
11830 Westline Industrial Drive, St. Louis, Missouri 63141

Library of Congress Cataloging in Publication Data
Epker, Bruce N
 Dentofacial deformities.

 Bibliography: p.
 1. Teeth—Abnormalities—Surgery. 2. Jaws—
Surgery. 3. Face—Surgery. 4. Orthodontics,
Corrective. I. Wolford, Larry, joint author. II. Title.
[DNLM: 1. Face—Surgery—Atlases. 2. Jaw
abnormalities—Surgery—Atlases. 3. Face—
Abnormalities—Atlases. WU17 E63d]
RK529.E64   617′.52059   80-12405
ISBN 0-8016-1606-9

C/CB/B 9 8 7 6 5 4 3 2 1   01/B/080

Preface

During the last decade the progress of knowledge in the correction of dentofacial and craniofacial deformities has been immense. Diagnostic acumen, surgical possibilities, surgical-orthodontic interaction, treatment results, and patient acceptance have undergone a remarkable transformation. Much of the art in this area is fast becoming a science. It has been challenging, exciting, and engrossing for those of us deeply involved in this area of patient care.

This text assimilates current knowledge in this rapidly developing field. Many distinguished oral and maxillofacial surgeons and orthodontists have made important contributions that we have drawn on in presenting the material herein. Their contributions are numerous and invaluable; without the works of these pioneers this text would not have been possible. As Einstein expressed so forcefully: "A hundred times every day I remind myself that my inner and outer life depend on the labours of other men, living and dead, and that I must exert myself in order to give in the same measure as I have received and am still receiving."

As this historical, technical, and scientific metamorphosis has occurred in the correction of dentofacial deformities, innumerable surgical-orthodontic techniques have been proposed, modified, tested, and accepted, while others have been discarded. The primary intent of this text is to discuss and illustrate the surgical-orthodontic techniques that we have utilized with good success for the correction of dentofacial deformities.

The illustrated presurgical orthodontics are of special note in that they differ with the various dentofacial deformities. In this regard the orthodontic-surgical interaction for each of the various deformities is specific and of notable importance in order to achieve the most expedient and stable result.

The specific surgical techniques discussed, and masterfully illustrated by William M. Winn, are those that we have developed, modified, or simply employed and found to be reliable and safe. No attempt is made in this text to describe all the available surgical-orthodontic techniques. Some of the procedures omitted may be as reliable as those described and illustrated, but we have found many to be less reliable, less safe, and more difficult technically. Finally, the surgical-orthodontic procedures covered are those that are within the scope and capabilities of the well-trained oral and maxillofacial surgeon and orthodontist. Similarly, the surgical techniques described cover the entire scope of those available, which permits the correction of virtually all dentofacial deformities.

This text has been divided into three major parts: Part One, Mandibular Surgery; Part Two, Maxillary Surgery; and Part Three, Midface Surgery. Within these parts chapters are devoted to each of the various types of operative procedures available for use in the correction of different types of dentofacial deformities involving that anatomic region (e.g., segmental mandibular surgery, mandibular ramus surgery, mandibular body surgery, genioplasty, mandibular augmentation, and condyle surgery). Further, within each chapter the various specific operative procedures are discussed in the context of the specific deformity that lends itself best to correction via the described surgical procedure. This organization, according to procedure rather than deformity, was chosen to avoid repetition. Our intent is that the text be complete and precise but not redundant.

The ultimate objective of our profession is betterment of patient care. Inasmuch as this text contributes to this end, it will be worthy of the time, energy, and effort put forth in its development.

Finally, we owe a special thanks to Walter Lorenz Surgical Instruments, Inc., for their help in developing many of the special instruments that have greatly simplified many of the procedures illustrated and for their financial assistance that helped make this text possible.

Bruce N. Epker, D.D.S., Ph.D.

The authors wish to acknowledge the following orthodontists for their treatments of the patients included in the text on the pages indicated.

Leward C. Fish, D.D.S., M.S.	4, 67, 96, 103, 121, 150, 194, 239, 307, 321, 334, 383
Jerry Mills, D.D.S.	43, 267
Peter J. Paulus, D.D.S., M.S.	141, 212
John L. Gerloff, Jr., D.D.S.	160
Charles R. Sullivan, D.D.S.	227
Quentin M. Ringenberg, D.D.S.	291
Burdette Warner, D.D.S.	357
Harold J. Koppel, D.D.S., M.S.D.	377
John P. Bolthouse, D.D.S.	407
Charles Van Dyken, D.D.S.	448
Thomas P. Weirich, D.D.S.	458

Contents

PART ONE
Mandibular surgery

4 Genioplasties, 119

5 Alloplastic augmentation of mandible, 149

6 Temporomandibular joint surgery, 157

PART TWO
Maxillary surgery

7 Segmental maxillary surgery, 191

PART THREE
Midface surgery

12 Midface osteotomies, 412

DENTOFACIAL DEFORMITIES
SURGICAL-ORTHODONTIC CORRECTION

MANDIBULAR SURGERY

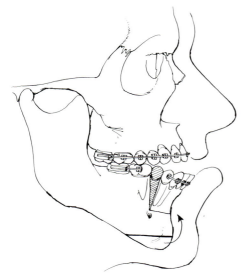

**ANTERIOR SUBAPICAL
MANDIBULAR SURGERY**

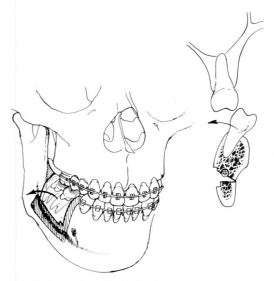

**POSTERIOR SUBAPICAL
MANDIBULAR SURGERY**

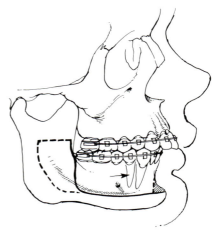

**TOTAL SUBAPICAL
MANDIBULAR SURGERY**

CHAPTER 1

Segmental mandibular surgery

Mandibular subapical surgery techniques can be utilized to reposition the anterior, posterior, or entire mandibular dentoalveolus. A number of technical variations have been proposed for the various types of segmental mandibular surgical procedures. The specific operative techniques to be described here have been developed or used by us with good clinical success. In this regard they are predicated on the following basic orthognathic surgical principles:

1. To provide optimal exposure for technical ease in performing surgery
2. To maintain optimal vascularity to any mobilized segments
3. To preserve the inferior alveolar and mental neurovascular bundles
4. To maintain optimal periodontal health

The anterior, posterior, and total subapical mandibular osteotomies are sequentially described in this chapter.

Anterior subapical mandibular surgery

The anterior mandibular segmental osteotomy or ostectomy is a commonly used procedure. The basic indications for its use are:

1. To correct mandibular dentoalveolar protrusion
2. To close certain types of open bites
3. To level an excessive curve of Spee
4. To correct mandibular dental arch asymmetry

In many instances anterior mandibular subapical surgery is done as an adjunctive procedure concurrent with other surgical procedures (e.g., with an anterior maxillary ostectomy to correct bimaxillary protrusion; with mandibular advancement to level the curve of Spee). Often a given case presents two or three of the basic indications for utilizing an anterior mandibular subapical procedure, as in closure of a class III open bite where the mandibular anterior segment is moved posteriorly and superiorly, thereby not only closing the open bite but leveling the curve of Spee and correcting dentoalveolar protrusion.

Regardless of the specific problem to be corrected by the anterior mandibular subapical osteotomy, the same basic surgical technique is used, as illustrated.

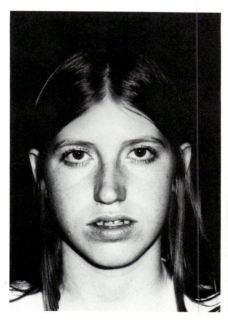 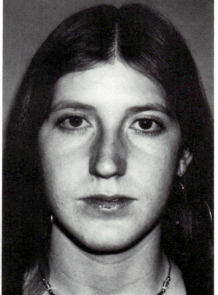

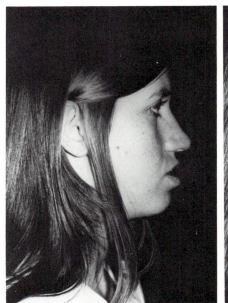
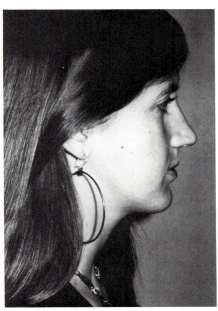

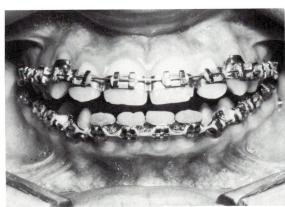
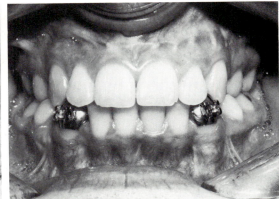

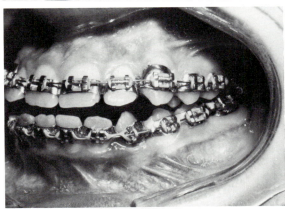
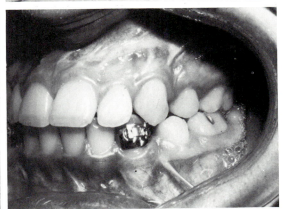

5

ANTERIOR SUBAPICAL MANDIBULAR SURGERY
Plate 1-1

A. The deformity illustrated is a class III open bite with a reverse curve of Spee, mandibular dentoalveolar protrusion, and a long lower third face. The upper incisor tooth-to-lip relationship is within normal limits. The open bite extends from the second premolars forward. Presurgical segmental orthodontics have been done in the mandibular arch. Continuous arch orthodontics have been done in the upper arch because *no major leveling was required,* which would tend to close the bite. This deformity will be corrected surgically by extracting the mandibular second premolars and performing a mandibular anterior subapical osteotomy with posterior and superior repositioning. The bone defect created secondary to the superior movement of the segment will be grafted with the inferior border of the mandibular symphysis. The precise amount of bone to be removed in the second premolar extraction site is determined from accurately done definitive model surgery. In this case a triangular section of bone is indicated for removal. If a rectangle is removed as a result of poor planning, a periodontal defect will result and stability may be affected.

B. Following extraction of the second premolars a circumvestibular incision is made with a diathermy knife from one cuspid area to the opposite cuspid area, well out into the vestibule. This incision is made in the lip (approximately 15 mm anterior to the depth of the vestibule) and is carried tangentially down to the bone *(insert)*. While making this incision it is helpful to place a finger on the cutaneous side of the lip to appreciate the depth of the incision and avoid incising through the entire lip. By extending this initial incision just distal to the cuspid area, possible injury to the mental nerves is avoided and an optimum buccal pedicle to the segment to be mobilized is provided. A subperiosteal dissection is carried to the inferior border of the mandible, and the symphysis is degloved. If a simultaneous genioplasty is not to be performed, this dissection is carried inferiorly only far enough to adequately expose the mandible below the apices of the teeth. The dissection is then carried subperiosteally, posteriorly along the inferior border until the mental foramina and existing neurovascular bundles are identified. After identification of the mental neurovascular bundles the primary mucosal incision can safely be extended posteriorly above the bundle to the area where the interdental ostectomy is to be done.

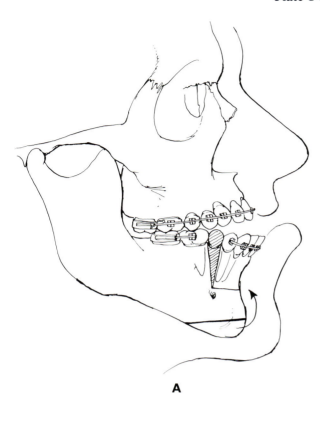

A

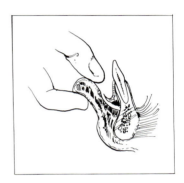

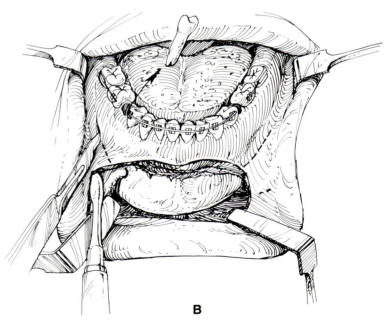

B

Plate 1-1

C. Incising and releasing the periosteum surrounding the mental neurovascular bundle provides increased exposure with less possible nerve damage secondary to stretching. This is best done with a linear incision through the periosteum around the exiting neurovascular bundle and then delicately releasing the periosteum with a hemostat.

The mucoperiosteum and attached gingiva overlying the second premolar extraction sites are then undermined to the crestal bone. When doing so an attempt is made to maintain the maximum amount of soft tissue attached to the anterior segment, that segment which is to be mobilized, at the expense of a more liberal reflection of the soft tissue distally from the stable segment.

D. The horizontal subapical osteotomy is made about 5 mm below the teeth apices. The mandibular cuspid is approximately 27 mm in length, and because the tooth root apices per se are seldom clinically visible, measurement with calipers of the level at which the cut is to be made ensures that the subapical osteotomy will be at the proper level. In this case the mental foramen is sufficiently below the premolar apices, so that the horizontal osteotomy can be done above it. When the mental foramen is close to the premolar apices it may be necessary to inferiorly reposition the neurovascular bundle, as illustrated in (Plate 1-2). When making the horizontal cut a finger is placed lingually to determine when the cut is completed through the lingual cortex.

E. After completion of the horizontal osteotomy a periosteal elevator is judiciously inserted subperiosteally lingually through the extraction site. This elevates the attached gingiva and periosteum adjacent to the extraction site and protects the lingual soft tissues while the interdental ostectomy is performed. No attempt is made to elevate excessive mucoperiosteum. The greater the amount of soft tissue left attached to the segment to be mobilized the better its vascular pedicle. When the vertical interdental cut is to be made without extractions the osteotomy is accomplished from the buccal totally, as described and illustrated in Plate 1-3. The buccal flap is gently retracted superiorly and the vertical interdental ostectomy completed through the extraction site. It is important that *excessive interdental bone is not removed,* especially in the crestal area, as this will create a serious periodontal problem.

ANTERIOR SUBAPICAL MANDIBULAR SURGERY

Plate 1-1

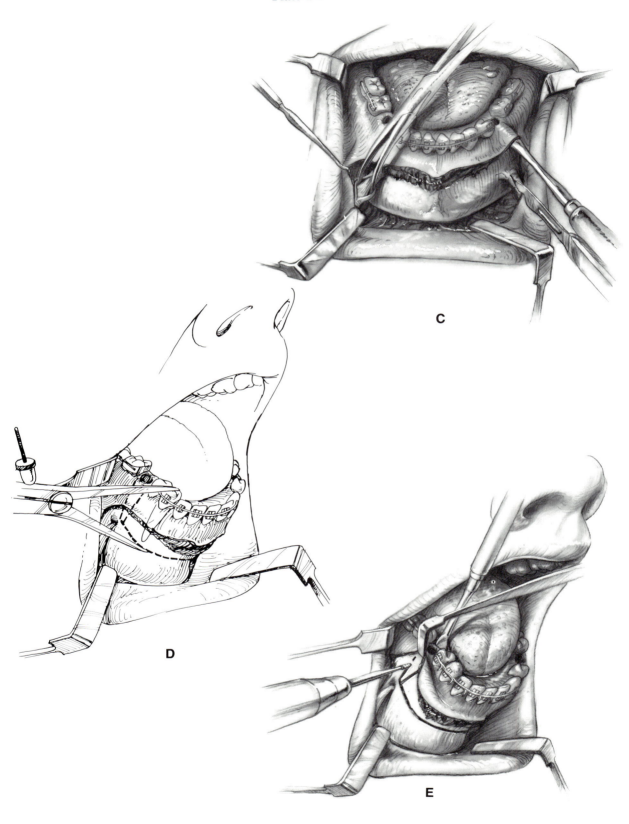

C

D

E

F. A midsymphysis osteotomy is sometimes necessary to narrow or widen the intercuspid distance. The midline split is done following completion of the horizontal subapical osteotomy and the vertical ostectomy *on one side*. It is easier to accomplish the midsymphysis osteotomy prior to mobilization of the entire anterior segment, because it is generally necessary to use a mallet and osteotome to complete the midline osteotomy. The labial mucogingival flap is incised vertically between the incisors to the level of the attached gingiva and minimally reflected. A vertical osteotomy through the outer cortex is done with a fine fissure bur. The bur cut *does not* extend superiorly to the crestal bone, which would result in a permanent periodontal defect. Moreover, attempts to complete this cut through the lingual cortex superiorly with a bur may result in damage to the incisor roots when they are in close proximity. Inferiorly, where the tooth roots are more divergent, the cut can be extended through the lingual cortex with the bur, and a fine osteotome is used to complete the superior aspect of the lingual cut. In making this cut the osteotome is angled so that the corner of the osteotome initiates the cut. Pathologic fracturing of the lingual cortex often occurs when this is not done.

G. On completion of the vertical midsymphysis osteotomy, one half of the anterior segment will be mobile. Completion of the remaining vertical interdental ostectomy through the extraction site on the opposite side completes the osseous cuts.

   The segments are mobilized and an attempt is made to place the teeth into the preformed occlusal splint. At this stage in the surgery there may be small areas of bony interference in the vertical ostectomy sites that prevent precise positioning of the segments. These are generally on the lingual cortex, and direct observation of the ostectomy sites while attempting to fit the splint will reveal their exact location. *It is preferable to remove additional interdental bone at this time rather than initially removing an excessive amount, which will result in either a periodontal defect* (if superior) *or a poor bone interface* (inferiorly) *that delays healing and can adversely affect stability.*

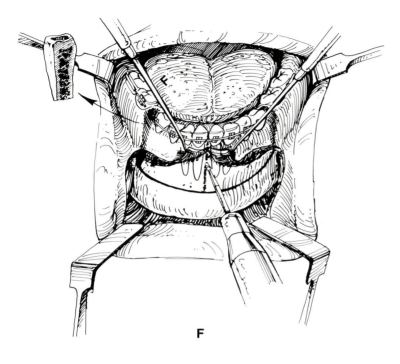

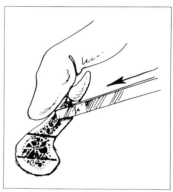

F

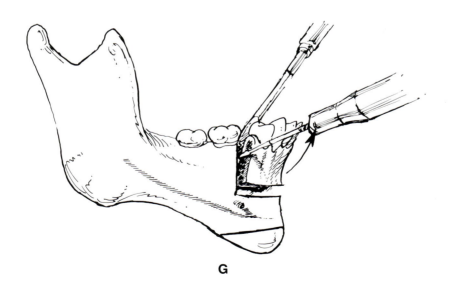

G

H. When all areas of bony interferences have been removed and the anterior segment can be passively positioned in the splint, the splint is wired to the mandibular orthodontic brackets. Intermaxillary fixation (IMF) is generally not necessary; however, when IMF is not utilized it is important that the splint has been constructed on an anatomic articulator so that its superior surface functionally occludes with the maxillary teeth. A bone graft is generally inserted into the osseous gap created inferiorly. Bank bone, autogenous hip, or the inferior border of the symphysis can be utilized for this purpose. In the case illustrated the symphysis is long vertically and well suited to serve as the donor site. Wiring of the graft is not necessary, however, additional stabilization of the graft and anterior segment can be achieved with circummandibular or direct wiring. If the vertical defect created is small (less than 5 mm) and good approximation of the vertical interdental bone has been achieved, a graft is not essential for either healing or stability.

I. The incision is closed in two layers, a muscle and a mucosal layer, and a pressure dressing is applied. In closure it is best to place a midline tacking suture in both layers prior to a running suture closure so as to prevent pulling the lip to one side. It is important that the pressure dressing be applied so that it elevates the chin and lower lip soft tissues superiorly so that healing does not occur with the lower lip retracted inferiorly. The dressing is maintained for 5 to 7 days.

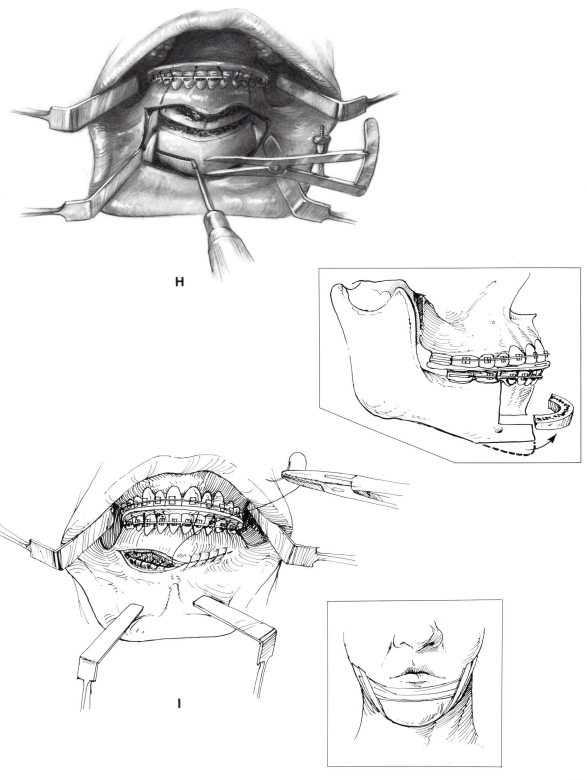

H

I

ANTERIOR SUBAPICAL MANDIBULAR SURGERY

Lowering mental nerve (Plate 1-2)

Repositioning of the mental neurovascular bundle is occasionally indicated in order to perform the necessary osseous cuts and avoid injury to the premolar root apices. The mental neurovascular bundle branches from the inferior alveolar neurovascular bundle and courses in a superior, posterior, and lateral direction in most adults. A bony window is therefore made through the outer cortex anterior and inferior to the mental foramen to allow the nerve to be identified within the mandible and repositioned inferiorly. This bone cut is carried into the mental foramen while the small end of a periosteal elevator is gently inserted into the foramen to protect the neurovascular bundle. The window is then created by removing the lateral cortex and carefully dissecting out the nerve from the surrounding trabecular bone with a curet. The incisive branch will be observed in this dissection continuing forward and can be transected if necessary.

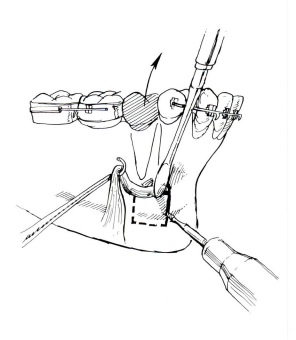

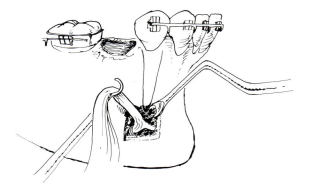

SPECIAL CONSIDERATION
ANTERIOR SUBAPICAL MANDIBULAR SURGERY

Leveling curve of Spee without removal of teeth (Plate 1-3)

When vertical interdental osteotomies are indicated without removal of teeth the osteotomy between adjacent teeth is made through the lateral cortical bone with a fine fissure bur, ending 2 to 3 mm below the crestal bone. Depending on the proximity of the adjacent tooth roots to the vertical osteotomy, as determined by periapical radiographs, some of the lingual cortex may be cut through at the inferior aspect of the vertical osteotomy with a bur from the buccal approach. However, most of the lingual cortex will need to be cut with an osteotome. A thin, sharp osteotome is directed at about a 45° angle to complete the cut through the lingual cortex. Thus the lingual cortex is cut with the sharp corner of the instrument. A finger is placed lingually to detect completion of the lingual cortical cut and minimize injury to the lingual mucoperiosteum.

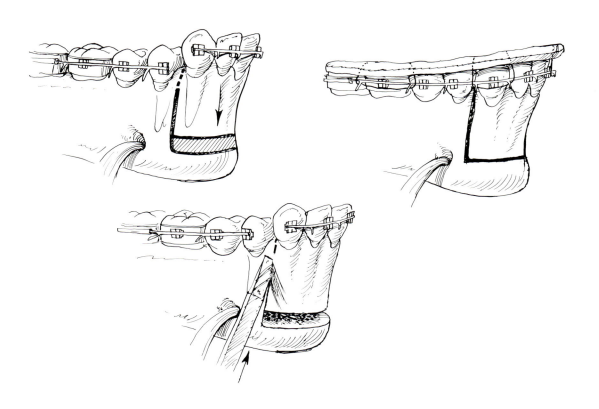

Posterior subapical mandibular surgery

Posterior subapical mandibular surgery has been less commonly utilized than other segmental procedures in the mandible for several reasons: it is technically difficult, there is a high risk of injury to the inferior alveolar neurovascular bundle with resultant dysesthesia of the ipsilateral lower lip, and maintenance of a good vascular supply to the segment is more difficult. Despite these legitimate considerations, this surgical procedure can be done successfully and is useful in several instances:

1. To upright posterior mandibular teeth in severe linguoversion or buccoversion
2. To upright posterior teeth in severe mesioversion
3. To close a premolar or molar space
4. To level supererupted posterior teeth

The feasibility of accomplishing these objectives with conventional orthodontics must be considered; however, in many adult patients orthodontic resolution of these problems may be impossible, inordinately difficult, or at best unpredictable. When such is the case a posterior subapical mandibular ostectomy must be considered.

Despite the aforementioned reasons for due respect for this operative approach, it can be successfully employed to resolve the listed occlusal deformities. Further, the potential problems encountered with its use are primarily technical and can be eliminated with a properly designed and executed surgical technique. The technique described has been employed with good success by us and is intended to minimize the potential problems incumbent with this procedure.

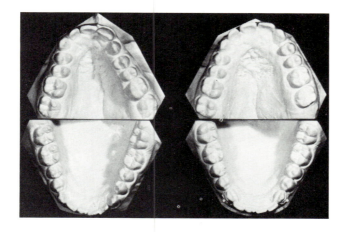

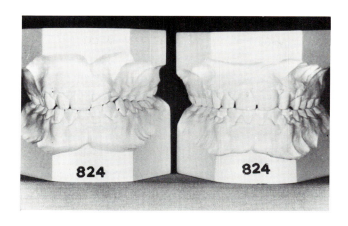

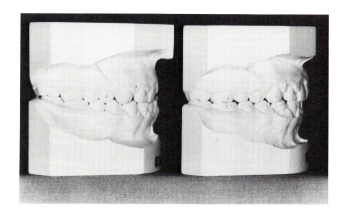

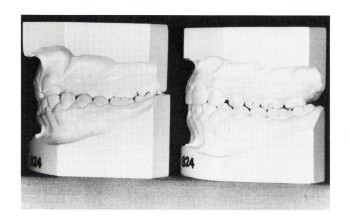

17

POSTERIOR SUBAPICAL MANDIBULAR SURGERY

Plate 1-4

A. The surgical technique is illustrated in a case where the mandibular posterior teeth are in linguoversion and supererupted, with the second premolar missing. The maxillary arch form is normal, and the right second molar is missing. The surgery will be designed to upright the mandibular first and second molars and close the second premolar space. The position of the inferior alveolar neurovascular canal, as determined radiographically, dictates whether the horizontal portion of the posterior osteotomy will be performed superior or inferior to the canal. When a space of 5 mm or more exists between the apices of the teeth and the inferior alveolar neurovascular bundle, the osteotomy can be done above the canal. However, if the posterior segment is to be lowered and a subapical ostectomy is required, the nerve will generally have to be exposed and dissected out. If such is the case it is easiest to begin the dissection with deliberate exposure of the neurovascular bundle.

In this case the osteotomy must be done below the level of the inferior alveolar canal.

B. A horizontal vestibular incision is made with a diathermy knife from distal to the second molar anteriorly past the location where the interdental osteotomy or ostectomy is to be done. This incision is made so as to maintain the maximum possible amount of buccal mucoperiosteum attached to the segment to be mobilized. A subperiosteal dissection is done to identify the mental neurovascular bundle. The mental neurovascular bundle can be dissected out if necessary, as illustrated and described in Plate 1-1, C. The tissues are reflected subperiosteally laterally until the inferior border of the mandible is identified. In the edentulous area an incision along the crest of the ridge between the adjacent teeth provides a site for insertion of a periosteal elevator lingually to reflect and protect the lingual mucoperiosteum while performing the vertical interdental ostectomy. This crestal incision also allows for the soft tissues in the area to be displaced lingually and buccally when the posterior segment is moved forward.

18

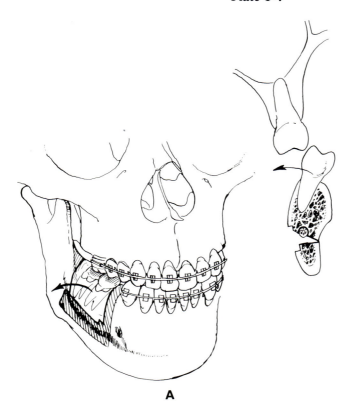

A

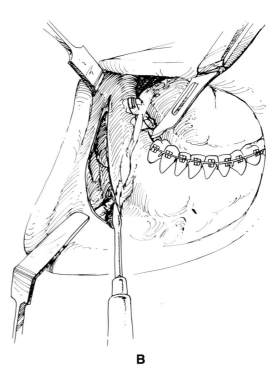

B

POSTERIOR SUBAPICAL MANDIBULAR SURGERY

Plate 1-4

C. *Care is exercised to avoid unnecessary elevation of both the buccal and lingual mucoperiosteum from the segment to be mobilized.* When inserting the periosteal elevator lingually it is important that the lingual mucoperiosteum be elevated almost exclusively from the anterior stable segment. The buccal mucoperiosteum and attached gingiva are elevated to the ridge and retracted superiorly in the second premolar area. Again, this elevation of soft tissues from the bone is done primarily from the anterior segment so as to maintain the best possible buccal pedicle to the segment to be mobilized.

   The proposed osteotomy lines are outlined with calipers as predetermined by model surgery. The vertical interdental ostectomy is carried inferiorly to approximately the level of the teeth apices through both the buccal and lingual cortices. The distance to the tooth apices and inferior alveolar neurovascular bundle is determined by direct measurement with calipers, as extrapolated from the radiographs.

D. Next the portion of lateral cortex that overlies the inferior alveolar neurovascular bundle is removed. Note that this window extends several millimeters posterior to the proposed vertical cut, which is distal to the second molar. This extension of the buccal window improves identification and visualization of the neurovascular bundle during the posterior cut. This is done by carefully cutting through only the lateral cortex with a bur, then removing the cortex with an osteotome. This bone is saved. This ''window'' provides a means of identifying the nerve within the mandible and therefore may be made somewhat larger than the exact size required to reposition (upright) the segment as determined by the model surgery.

   The trabecular bone is carefully removed with a curet until the neurovascular bundle is identified within the mandible.

E. After the neurovascular bundle is identified the lingual cortex is carefully osteotomized. The horizontal osteotomy is completed with a bur below the neurovascular bundle while placing a finger lingually to detect the bur as it perforates the lingual cortex. For technical ease this cut is made more inferiorly on the lingual than buccal cortex, as illustrated in Plate 1-4, *F*. The horizontal osteotomy is extended at least 5 mm posterior to the second molar.

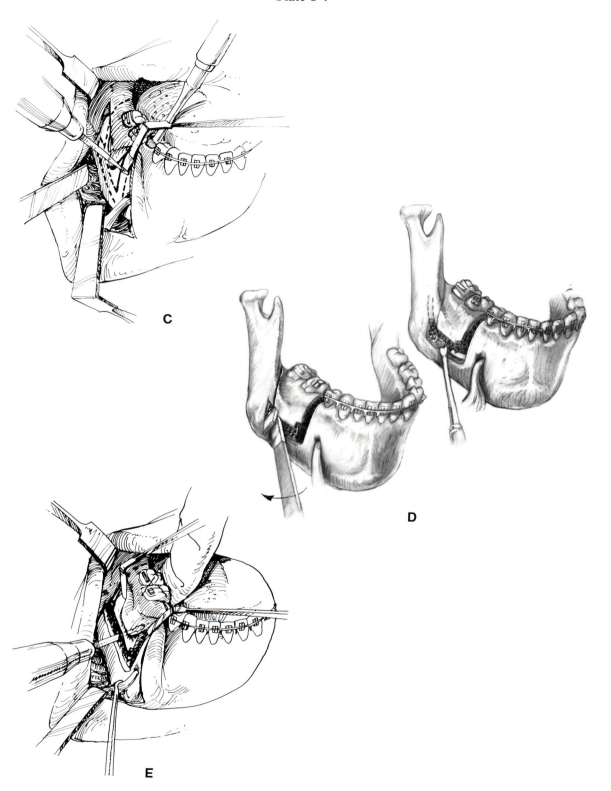

C

D

E

POSTERIOR SUBAPICAL MANDIBULAR SURGERY

Plate 1-4

F. If the inferior alveolar neurovascular bundle, once identified, is located such that it interferes with the making of this lingual cut, it can be more completely mobilized and gently retracted from the mandibular canal and then the lingual portion of the horizontal osteotomy completed.

G. Several technical points are important when performing the posterior vertical cut: (1) it is best to mobilize the soft tissues by subperiosteal dissection as far distally as possible to avoid excessive stripping of the buccal mucoperiosteum from the segment to be mobilized, (2) the buccal bone window is best extended slightly distal to the proposed vertical osteotomy site to permit optimal exposure and lateral retraction of the inferior alveolar neurovascular bundle, and (3) the vertical cut is to be made 4 to 5 mm distal to the last molar to avoid periodontal problems.

   When performing the posterior vertical osteotomy, with gentle retraction of the neurovascular bundle laterally, the medial cut can be easily completed. This cut is also best made tangentially, as noted in Plate 1-4, *I*.

H. The segment is then mobilized by inserting an osteotome in the posterior vertical osteotomy and mobilizing it medially and forward. The segment can then be moved into its new position as determined by the preformed occlusal splint constructed from the model surgery casts. When considerable movement of this segment is required it is helpful to initially depress the segment into the floor of the mouth *to permit judicious elevation of the lingual periosteum from the stable posterior and inferior portion of the mandible*.

I. At this time the splint is wired to the mobilized segment only, and attempts at seating the remainder of the splint into the stable teeth will disclose areas of additional bone interference that require removal.

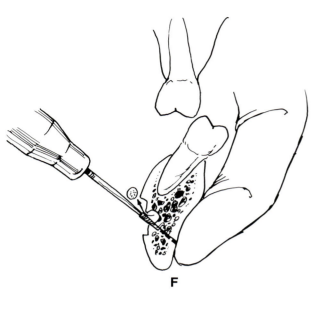

F

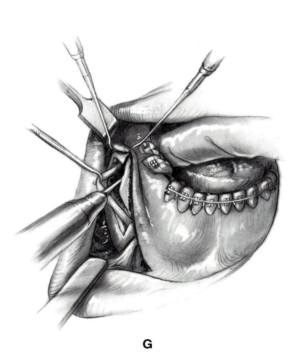

G

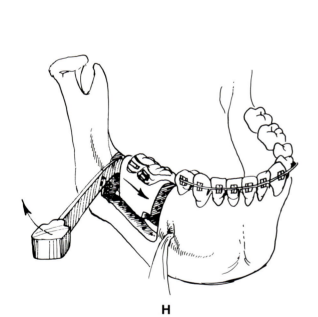

H

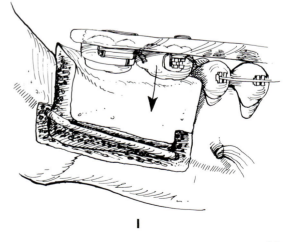

I

J. If additional lingual cortex needs to be removed, it can be readily done at this time. It is best to remove interferences from the inferior stable segment or the inferior aspect of the lingual cortex of the mobilized segment to adjust the vertical position of the segment. Of course, if there are any bony discrepancies in the anterior vertical ostectomy area, they are carefully removed.

K. The segment can then be stabilized by fixing the occlusal splint to the remainder of the teeth and placing a circummandibular wire over the splint in the area of the mobilized segment to improve vertical and transverse stability. These wires should not interfere with the occlusion. The osseous defects at the posterior vertical osteotomy site and along the inferolateral cortical margin may be bone grafted. To do this the lateral cortical plate previously removed can be mulched and reinserted. However, if the posterior vertical cut is made at least 5 mm distal to the last tooth and tangential as described, a periodontal defect is not a concern and bone grafting is not essential.

L. When there is greater than about 4 to 5 mm of bone between the apices of the posterior teeth and the inferior alveolar neurovascular canal and the posterior segment does not need to be lowered, the horizontal osteotomy can be done above the canal. The soft-tissue incisions are made as previously described. The anterior vertical ostectomy is completed down to the level of the planned horizontal osteotomy, as determined with calipers, through the buccal and lingual cortices, and the predetermined amount of vertical interdental bone is removed.

The horizontal osteotomy and posterior vertical osteotomy are completed above the canal. A finger is maintained lingually to detect when the osteotomy is completely through the lingual cortex. The bur is angled from buccal to lingual as parallel to the occlusal plane as possible. The segment is mobilized, repositioned, and stabilized as previously described.

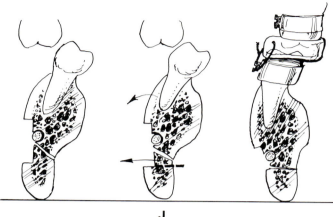

J

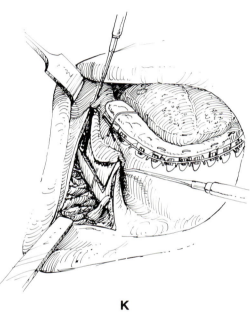

K

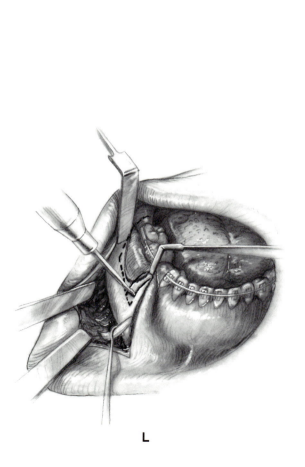

L

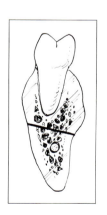

Total subapical mandibular surgery

A single basic technique is described here that can be utilized for any of those conditions that may warrant the use of a total subapical mandibular osteotomy. Those conditions in which a total subapical mandibular osteotomy may be considered are:

1. Class II malocclusion with a low mandibular plane angle and a normal anterior position of pogonion ("prominent pogonion")
2. Simultaneous advancement of the total mandibular dentoalveolus and surgical leveling of an excessive curve of Spee
3. Simultaneous advancement of the total mandibular dentoalveolus and lengthening of the lower third face
4. Closure of an unusual open-bite deformity

The primary indication for the total subapical mandibular osteotomy is in the case of a class II, low mandibular plane angle with a normal anterior position of pogonion. An alternative treatment plan for these types of cases is a modified sagittal ramus osteotomy for mandibular advancement with simultaneous anteroposterior reduction genioplasty, because it is technically easier to perform this surgical approach than the total subapical osteotomy. The mandibular anatomy in most instances of class II, low mandibular plane angle is such that the tooth apices are in close proximity to the inferior alveolar neurovascular bundle, making it impossible to perform the total subapical bone cut between the tooth root apices and the nerve. Moreover, the distance between the inferior alveolar neurovascular bundle and the inferior border of the mandible is not great. These anatomic conditions make the total subapical mandibular osteotomy technically difficult and associated with a higher incidence of postoperative inferior alveolar nerve dysesthesia.

When surgical leveling of the curve of Spee is indicated with simultaneous mandibular advancement, this can generally be most easily achieved via an anterior mandibular subapical osteotomy combined with a sagittal ramus osteotomy. Yet in rare instances independent movement of the anterior and posterior tooth-bearing segments to level, widen, narrow, or tip these segments may warrant the use of the total subapical osteotomy with segmentalization.

In most patients with a low mandibular plane angle and class II malocclusion the lower third face is short. If it is excessively short the total subapical osteotomy for advancement and interpositional grafting can optimize esthetics by increasing lower face height. Finally, in very rare instances this procedure may be utilized to close an unusual open-bite deformity when the open bite is the result of a true mandibular deformity rather than a maxillary deformity.

The basic surgical technique that we currently use for the total subapical mandibular osteotomy is described.

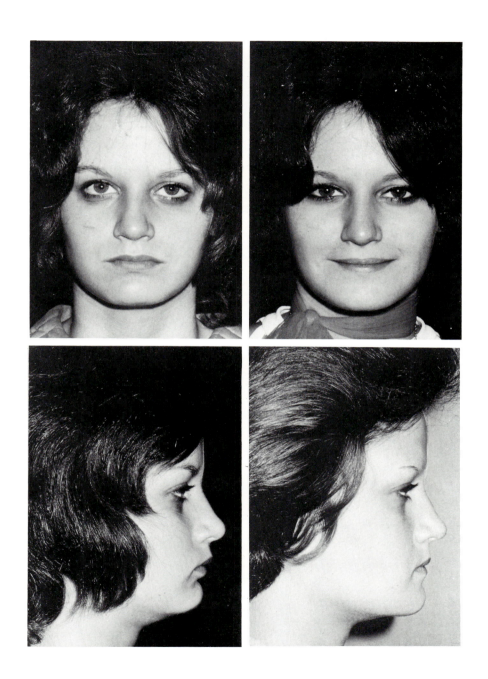

27

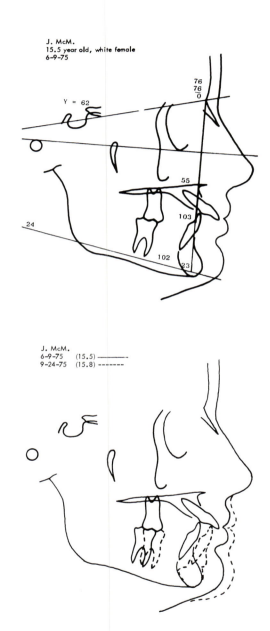

J. McM.
15.5 year old, white female
6-9-75

Y = 62

76
76
0

55

103

24

102

23

J. McM.
6-9-75   (15.5) ————
9-24-75   (15.8) --------

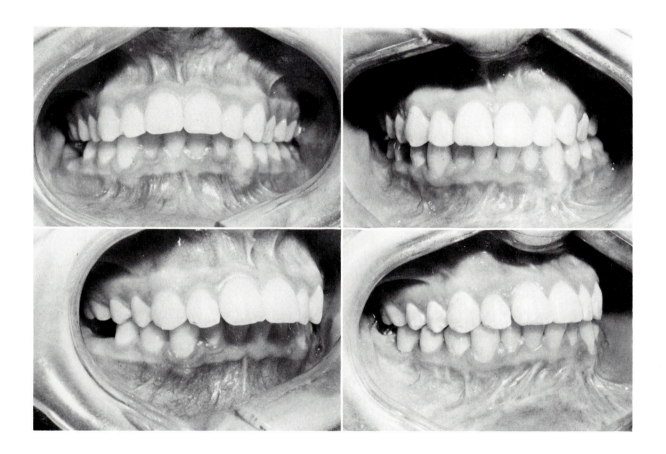

TOTAL SUBAPICAL MANDIBULAR SURGERY
Plate 1-5

A. A total subapical mandibular osteotomy is illustrated and described in a patient with a low mandibular plane angle, normal anterior projection of pogonion, and a class II malocclusion. Characteristically these individuals possess a very deep labiomental fold and often a short lower third face. The object of the procedure is to advance the entire dentoalveolus to a class I occlusal relationship while anatomically maintaining the ascending ramus, inferior border, and pogonion unaltered.

B. A circumvestibular incision is made well out into the buccolabial sulcus with a diathermy knife, extending from the lateral aspect of the ascending ramus on one side to the same area on the opposite side. In the areas overlying the mental nerves the initial incision is made only through the mucosa and is completed to bone after the mental nerves are identified via blunt dissection. Posteriorly the incision lies approximately over the external oblique ridge and extends about one third of the way up the ascending ramus of the mandible. This incision provides the optimum amount of pedicle-attached soft tissues to the segment to be mobilized and permits good surgical access.

   The anterior portion of this incision is made tangentially, beginning on the inner aspect of the lower lip and passing to bone, as described and illustrated in Plate 1-1, *B*. The incision is designed to expose the bone at about the level of the mandibular tooth root apices.

C. A subperiosteal dissection is carried inferiorly, exposing the symphysis and inferior border of the mandible laterally. However, the symphysis and lateral inferior borders are generally not degloved. The mental neurovascular bundles are released from the periosteum and liberally dissected free of the surrounding soft tissues. Distally the tissues are reflected from the anterior border of the ascending ramus well up onto the coronoid process until the coronoid notch can be identified as a superior referent. Then a medial subperiosteal soft-tissue dissection is done in the ascending mandibular ramus to expose the lingula and the inferior alveolar neurovascular bundle where it enters the mandible. This soft-tissue dissection need not extend distal to the area where the inferior alveolar neurovascular bundle enters the mandible.

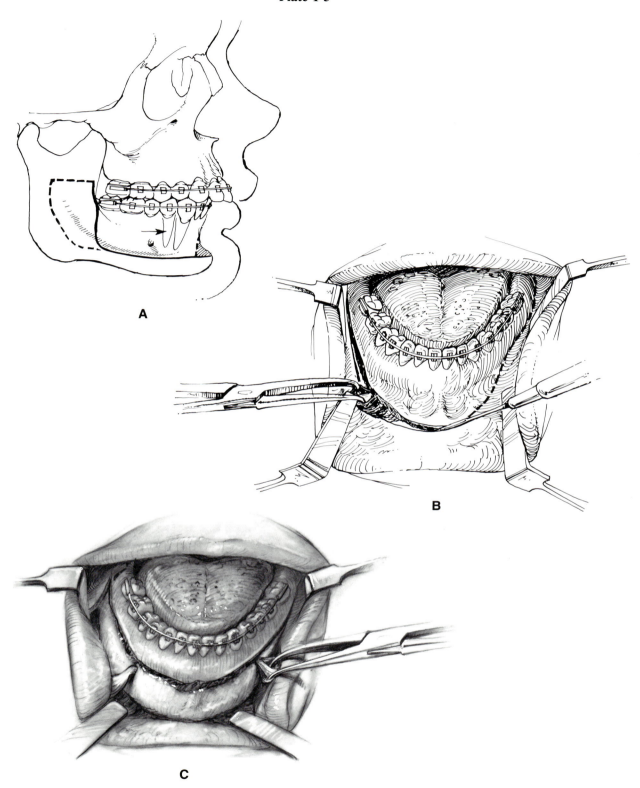

A

B

C

D. The location of the horizontal subapical osteotomy is generally below the level of the inferior alveolar neurovascular bundle, except in some open-bite cases. The proposed level of the horizontal osteotomy is accurately determined from appropriate radiographs, and the actual osteotomy location is marked on the mandible by making direct measurements from the occlusal plane. The horizontal osteotomy is initiated anteriorly in the symphysis and proceeds posteriorly. The mental neurovascular bundles are gently retracted superiorly and posteriorly for the anterior portion of the osteotomy. *The lateral aspect of the horizontal cut* is made with the cutting instrument directed at about a 45° angle inferiorly toward the lingual cortex. A finger is placed in the floor of the mouth adjacent to the area where the cut is being made to detect completion of the cut through the lingual cortex. The horizontal subapical osteotomy is carried just posterior to the last molar.

E. At this point the osteotomy is extended up the lateral border of the mandible and then along the anterior border of the ascending ramus *through the outer cortex only*. This portion of the osteotomy is similar to that used for the sagittal ramus osteotomy. The superior extent of this osteotomy lies just above the level where the inferior alveolar neurovascular bundle enters the mandible.

F. A small retractor is placed subperiosteally just superior and posterior to the inferior alveolar neurovascular bundle where it enters the mandible to protect it and elevate the soft tissues medially. A horizontal osteotomy parallel to the occlusal plane that extends only through the *lingual cortical bone* is completed from the superior extent of the anterior ramus cut to just superior and posterior to the lingula. This cut *must be completed through the lingual cortex, particularly at the most posterior extent of the osteotomy*. Because the mandible is concave in this area and visualization may not be good, this portion of the osteotomy is sometimes difficult to complete. When the osteotomy is not complete, difficulty in completing the split may be encountered.

Plate 1-5

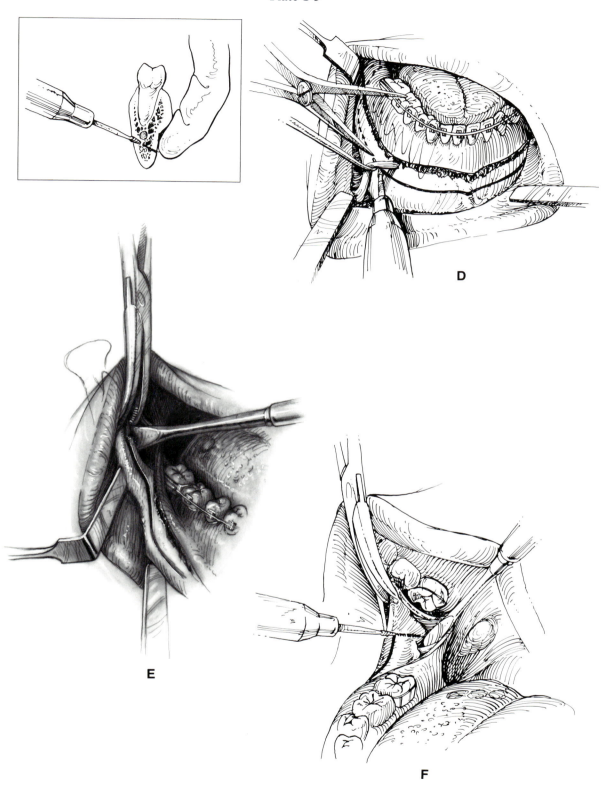

D

E

F

TOTAL SUBAPICAL MANDIBULAR SURGERY

Plate 1-5

G. The identical bone cuts are made on the opposite side, and then all of the bone cuts are checked for completeness with osteotomes. In particular the completeness of the lingual aspect of the subapical cut is carefully checked. Osteotomes are then used to mobilize the total subapical segment by fracturing the medial aspect of the ascending ramus. To do this an osteotome is inserted both in the ascending ramus and in the vertical osteotomy distal to the second molar and levered.

H. The fracture generally occurs lingually just posterior to the location of the mandibular canal, from the posterior aspect of the superior horizontal cut downward to the horizontal aspect of the subapical osteotomy. Once the medial ramus is fractured by torquing with the osteotomes, the entire segment can be mobilized.

I. By inserting the osteotomes in the subapical cut and levering the total subapical segment upward, additional force is achieved to mobilize the segment if necessary. Excessive force during this maneuver can cause pathologic fracturing of the stable inferior border of the mandible. However, sometimes it is necessary to simultaneously lever on the ascending ramus, as illustrated in Plate 1-5, *G,* and in the subapical cut to achieve the medial fracture. Once the segment is initially mobilized, additional firm manual manipulation of the segment is required to achieve complete mobility to allow passive repositioning of the segment into the desired relationship.

J. The occlusal splint is inserted, and the advanced total subapical segment can be stabilized with interosseous wires through the lateral cortices or by circummandibular wires. The inferior aspect of the advanced symphysis area is reduced if protrusive, or the addition of an alloplast to the inferior portion of the symphysis is done, depending on the esthetic requirements of the individual case.

34

TOTAL SUBAPICAL MANDIBULAR SURGERY

Plate 1-5

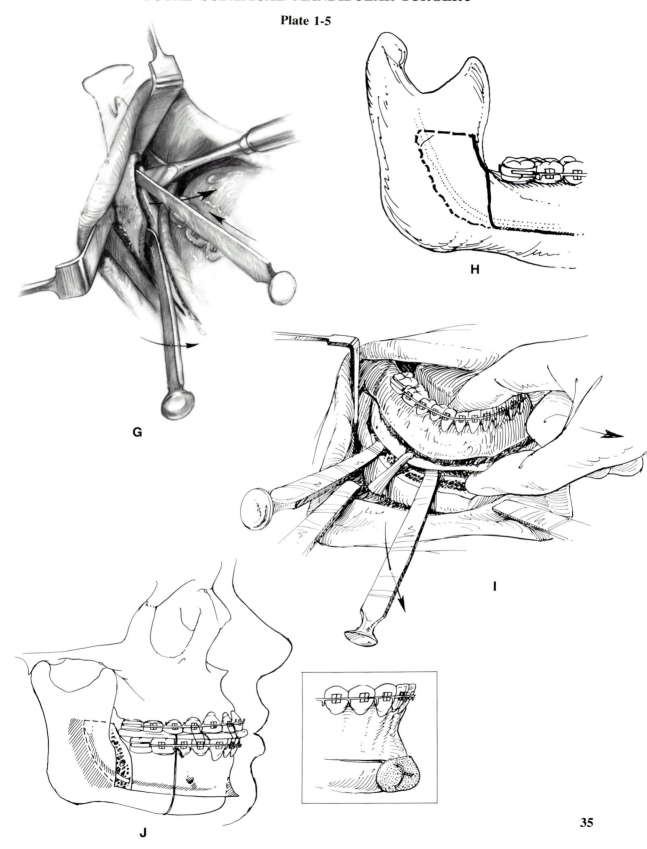

G

H

I

J

35

TOTAL SUBAPICAL MANDIBULAR SURGERY

Simultaneous leveling of curve of Spee (Plate 1-6)

In certain instances when orthodontic treatment is not to be done, or to facilitate orthodontic treatment, or when segmental orthodontics are used, the procedure just described can be combined with surgical leveling of the curve of Spee. After mobilization of the total mandibular subapical segment, osteotomies between the cuspids and premolars are accomplished as previously described in Plate 1-3.

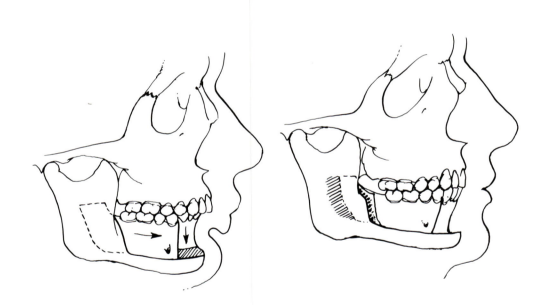

TOTAL SUBAPICAL MANDIBULAR SURGERY

Simultaneous lengthening of lower third face (Plate 1-7)

In some individuals with a class II malocclusion of the low mandibular plane angle type, the lower third face is *excessively* short. Generally both the pre-surgical orthodontic mechanics and the surgery tend to satisfactorily increase the anterior lower third face height in these individuals. However, in selected individuals the lower third anterior face height may be so decreased that it is esthetically desirable to additionally increase it from 5 to 10 mm. In these patients the total subapical mandibular osteotomy can be done in concert with an interpositional autogenous bone graft. Three cortical blocks of bone are wedged at the midline and in each canine area to achieve the desired increase in lower third face height, and the remainder of the defect is packed with *fresh autogenous cancellous* bone from the ilium. This results in a solid bony union in about 2 to 4 weeks.

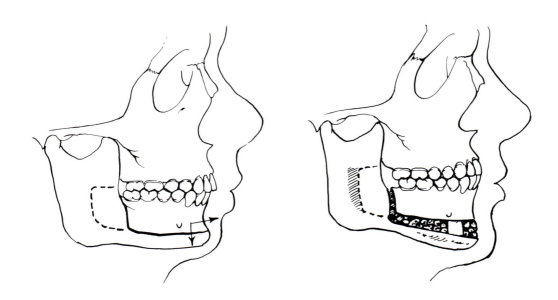

TOTAL SUBAPICAL MANDIBULAR SURGERY

Retromolar osteotomy (Plate 1-8)

A. The difference between the retromolar osteotomy and the total subapical technique described is that with the retromolar osteotomy, only a vertical posterior osteotomy is done without the sagittal split component of the ramus.

In this procedure after the horizontal subapical osteotomy is completed distal to the last tooth, a vertical osteotomy is made approximately 5 mm posterior to the last molar. This cut begins superiorly and is carried through both the buccal and lingual cortices to about the level of the inferior alveolar neurovascular bundle. The buccal cut is then completed through only the lateral cortex, and the remainder of the lingual cortex adjacent to and below the neurovascular bundle is fractured.

B. With advancement of the segment the nerve is stretched, and therefore the possibility of injury to it is increased. In general this nerve can tolerate a moderate amount of stretching (3 to 6 mm) without permanent damage.

TOTAL SUBAPICAL MANDIBULAR SURGERY

Retromolar osteotomy (Plate 1-8)

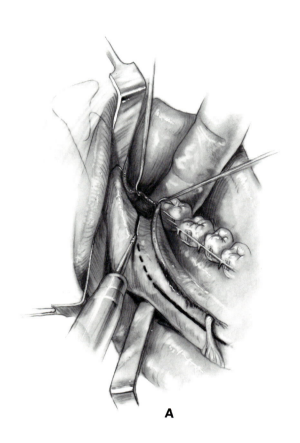

A

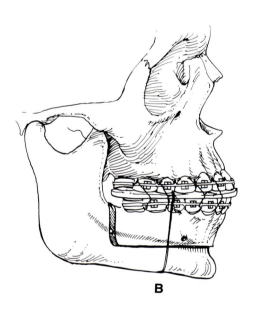

B

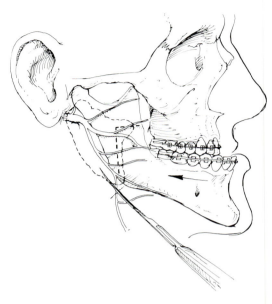

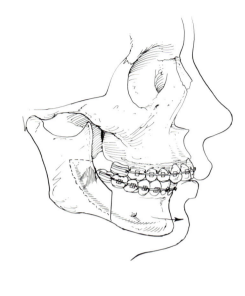

SUBCONDYLAR RAMUS OSTEOTOMY   **MODIFIED SAGITTAL RAMUS OSTEOTOMY**

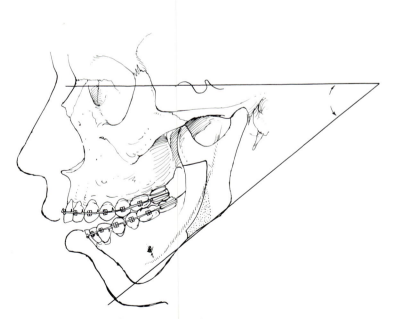

ARCING RAMUS OSTEOTOMY

CHAPTER 2

Mandibular ramus surgery

Surgery in the ramus of the mandible is routinely performed to correct a variety of dentofacial deformities. Numerous surgical procedures, or more often modifications of previously reported procedures, have been proposed for various reasons, some of which are sound, but the majority of which are biologically, biomechanically, and technically without proved advantage over their predecessors. The three basic mandibular ramus procedures illustrated in this chapter are those we have found to be reliable for the correction of any dentofacial deformity that warrants correction via ramus surgery. The procedures are:

1. Subcondylar ramus osteotomy
   a. Extraoral approach
   b. Intraoral approach
2. Modified sagittal ramus osteotomy
3. Arcing ramus osteotomy

These procedures are sequentially discussed and illustrated in detail with regard to their indications and useful modifications.

Subcondylar ramus osteotomy

The subcondylar ramus osteotomy can be performed either extraorally or intraorally. The extraoral approach has advantages over the intraoral approach in that there is better visibility and access to both the lateral and medial aspects of the ramus. This permits a more accurate sectioning of the ramus, complete access to the pterygoid muscle, easier removal of areas of bony interference that can prevent passive positioning of the proximal segment, and more appropriate interosseous wire placement for better positioning of the condyle in its proper position in the glenoid fossa. The extraoral incision, when properly placed and closed, leaves a fine scar in the submandibular area. Even in young patients careful placement and closure of the skin incision results in a fairly inconspicuous scar. The relative indications for the extraoral and intraoral subcondylar ramus osteotomy are:

1. Extraoral subcondylar ramus osteotomy
   a. Major setback of mandible (greater than 10 mm)
   b. Asymmetric mandibular setback
   c. Vertical shortening of mandibular ramus
   d. Reoperation of previously corrected prognathism
   e. Reoperation of malunion or nonunion of mandibular ramus
2. Intraoral subcondylar ramus osteotomy
   a. Minor setback of mandible (less than 10 mm)
   b. Minimal asymmetric mandibular setback
   c. Vertical shortening of mandibular ramus

Because the extraoral procedure affords optimum exposure and versatility, this approach permits the surgeon to modify the "traditional" lines of bone cuts according to the existing anatomic conditions, as in unusual cases, postfracture cases, and previously treated prognathisms. Moreover, in correction of laterognathism or major setbacks it affords excellent access for the removal of bony interferences and assurance of not displacing the condyle from the fossa by arbitrary wiring techniques.

In most "routine" cases of prognathism the intraoral procedure works well. With some modifications, which will be discussed, the intraoral procedure can predictably produce results comparable to those of the extraoral procedure. The primary advantage of the intraoral subcondylar ramus osteotomy is that there are no facial scars. A major disadvantage is difficulty in controlling the condylar position in the glenoid fossa, which results in a tendency for relapse. The extraoral procedure is discussed and illustrated first.

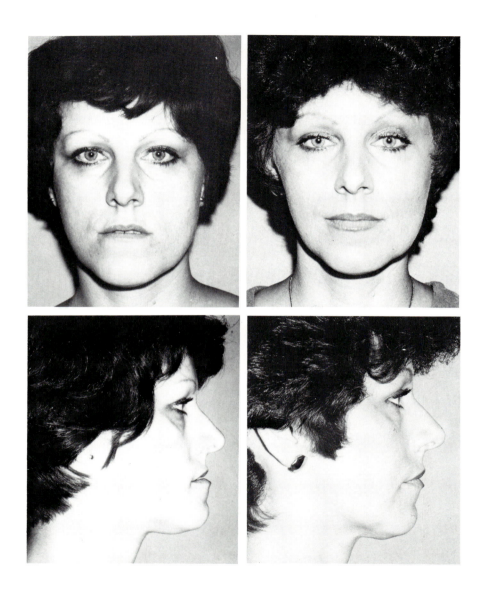

43

SUBCONDYLAR RAMUS OSTEOTOMY

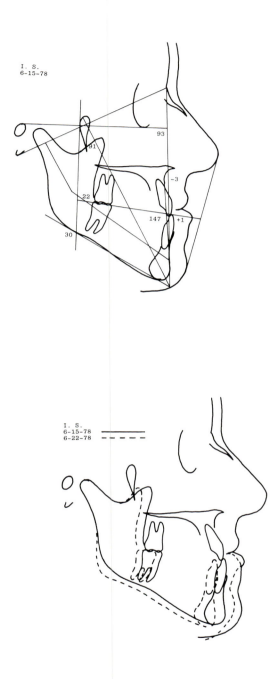

44

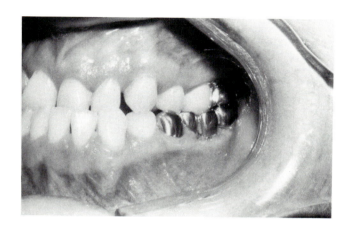

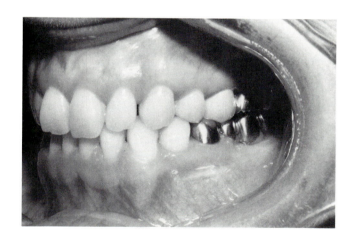

EXTRAORAL SUBCONDYLAR RAMUS OSTEOTOMY
Plate 2-1

A. The illustrated case demonstrates a mandibular prognathism with a 14-mm anteroposterior occlusal discrepancy. The extraoral inverted-L subcondylar ramus osteotomy to be done is outlined and is the preferred technique for correction of major prognathism. This bone cut eliminates the temporalis-coronoid relationship as a source of relapse potential and maintains more normal masticatory muscle function. The line for the proposed incision is marked 2 cm below the inferior border of the mandible in the angle region. It is preferable that the proposed incision lines be marked with the patient's head postured straight forward, because rotation of the head to the side for the actual surgery alters the location of the skin in relation to the mandible. The midpoint of each proposed incision is crosshatched to aid in anatomic closure of the superficial layers. The skin incision is made about 4 cm long and is initially carried to the level of the platysma.

B. The subcutaneous tissues overlying the platysma are undermined. This undermining is not extensive, as it is only to permit identification and reapproximation of the platysma at the time of incision closure.

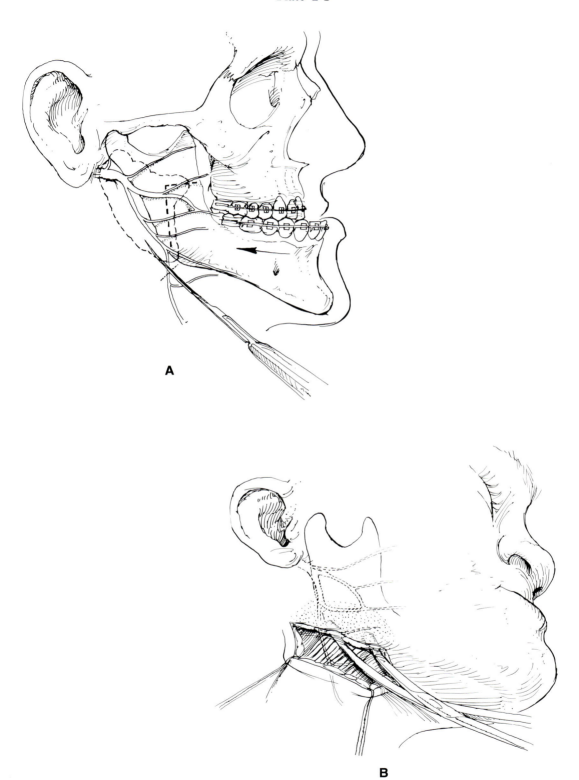

A

B

EXTRAORAL SUBCONDYLAR RAMUS OSTEOTOMY

Plate 2-1

C. An incision is then carefully made just through the platysma to the depth of the underlying superficial layer of the deep cervical fascia. The platysma is again slightly undermined on its deep surface to facilitate layered anatomic closure and to visually inspect the superficial layer of the deep cervical fascia for evidence of an unusually low marginal mandibular branch of the facial nerve. The marginal mandibular branch of the facial nerve passes in this fascial plane and is almost always superior to this level of dissection. If it passes unusually low it will be seen within the superficial layer of the deep cervical fascia. It can be identified by the anterosuperior direction in which it traverses. Communicating branches of the cervical plexus or the cervical branch of the facial nerve often exist at the level of the incision but pass in a more vertical direction and can be incised without consequence. (See Plate 2-1, *A.*)

D. At this time superior and inferior retraction will expose the pterygomasseteric sling and some overlying subcutaneous tissue. Extending the dissection anteriorly with combined sharp and blunt dissection into the gonial notch area will expose the facial vessels as they cross the mandible near the anterior border of the masseter muscle. These can usually be left intact or ligated and cut to provide increased exposure if necessary.

A finger is placed just beneath the inferior border of the mandible at this time to retract the soft tissues and provide orientation to make the incision onto the inferolateral aspect of the mandible from the area of the mandibular angle anteriorly to the region of the facial vessels.

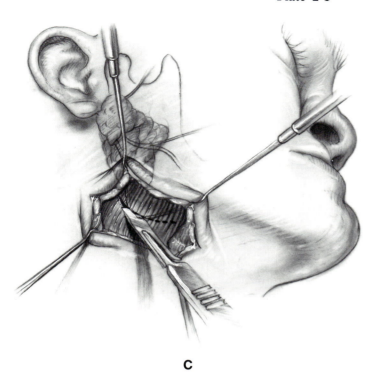

C

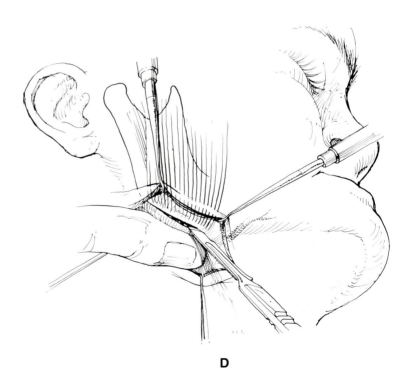

D

EXTRAORAL SUBCONDYLAR RAMUS OSTEOTOMY

Plate 2-1

E. After the incision is made through the pterygomasseteric sling, a periosteal elevator is utilized to subperiosteally reflect all of the tissues from the lateral aspect of the ascending ramus. The inferior, posterior, and lateral aspects of the ascending ramus of the mandible are exposed, including the sigmoid notch and the coronoid process. The temporalis, however, need not be reflected from the coronoid process of the mandible. Following reflection of the lateral tissues, visual exposure is improved by incising the periosteum at the posterolateral aspect of the ramus to provide added soft-tissue relaxation.

F. A view of the medial aspect of the ramus illustrates the interrelationship of the neurovasculature of that area. The anatomic location of the internal maxillary artery, inferior alveolar artery, and retromandibular vein must be appreciated to avoid inadvertent damage to them. A limited medial dissection is accomplished next.

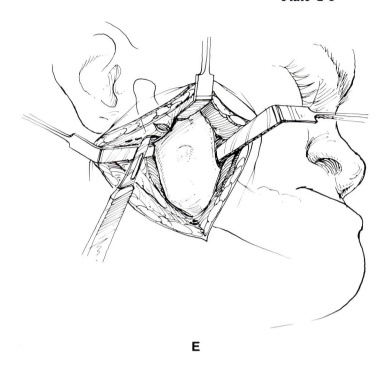

E

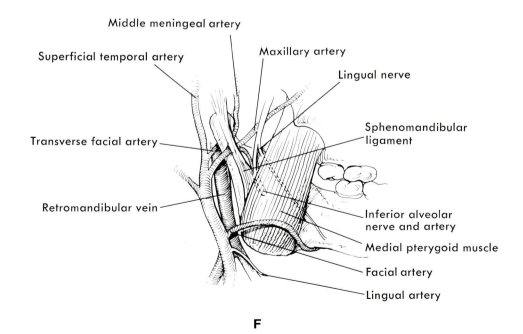

Middle meningeal artery

Superficial temporal artery

Maxillary artery

Lingual nerve

Transverse facial artery

Sphenomandibular ligament

Retromandibular vein

Inferior alveolar nerve and artery

Medial pterygoid muscle

Facial artery

Lingual artery

F

EXTRAORAL SUBCONDYLAR RAMUS OSTEOTOMY
Plate 2-1

G. The medial dissection is done to reflect the medial pterygoid muscle from the mandible and allow insertion of a small malleable retractor medially in the region of the proposed vertical bone cut to protect the medial tissues. Extensive medial dissection is not necessary, because the medial pterygoid muscle attachment is confined to the angle area as illustrated. Care is taken with this dissection and subsequent retractor placement not to damage the inferior alveolar neurovascular bundle where it enters the mandible.

H. With a small malleable retractor in place to protect the medial soft tissues, the vertical component of the bone cut is made beginning just above and posterior to the level of the lingula, which is identifiable about 50% of the time by a slight protuberance on the lateral cortex. This cut is extended through both cortices with the bur angled posteriorly so the resultant tangential osteotomy will facilitate better approximation of the segments following repositioning.

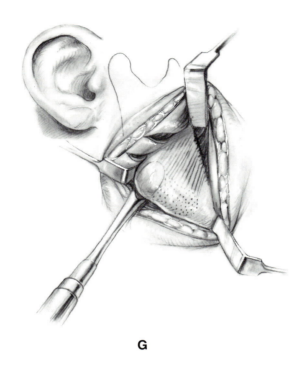

G

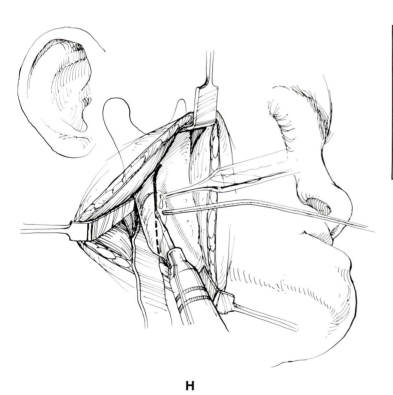

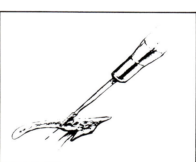

H

EXTRAORAL SUBCONDYLAR RAMUS OSTEOTOMY

Plate 2-1

I. A horizontal bone cut is then made above the level of the entering inferior alveolar neurovascular bundle from the superior extent of the vertical cut to the anterior border of the ramus.

If a vertical osteotomy from the sigmoid notch to the angle of the mandible is used in cases such as this, in which a major posterior repositioning of the mandible is being done, then either the temporalis muscle must be reflected completely off the coronoid process or a coronoidectomy done. Either of these manipulations is less desirable, biologically and biomechanically, than leaving the anatomic relationship of the coronoid-temporalis relatively unchanged, as in the inverted-L osteotomy.

J. The segments are then mobilized. On completion of the osteotomies of both mandibular rami the mandible is placed into the occlusal splint made from the dental model surgery, and intermaxillary fixation is applied. The passive position of the proximal segments is noted. In this case the proximal segment is displaced posteriorly and laterally, and this condition must be corrected before the end of surgery or relapse will occur.

K. If the degree of posterior repositioning, rotational movements, or the flare of the ascending ramus is such that the proximal segment is displaced laterally or posteriorly, as shown, bone is removed from the lateral aspect of the distal segment or the medial aspect of the proximal segment to minimize the displacement. The inferior tip of the proximal segment is often removed, especially if it is flared laterally. Wiring without removal of the bony interferences tends to distract the condyle, usually laterally or inferiorly, from the glenoid fossa and subsequently can result in relapse.

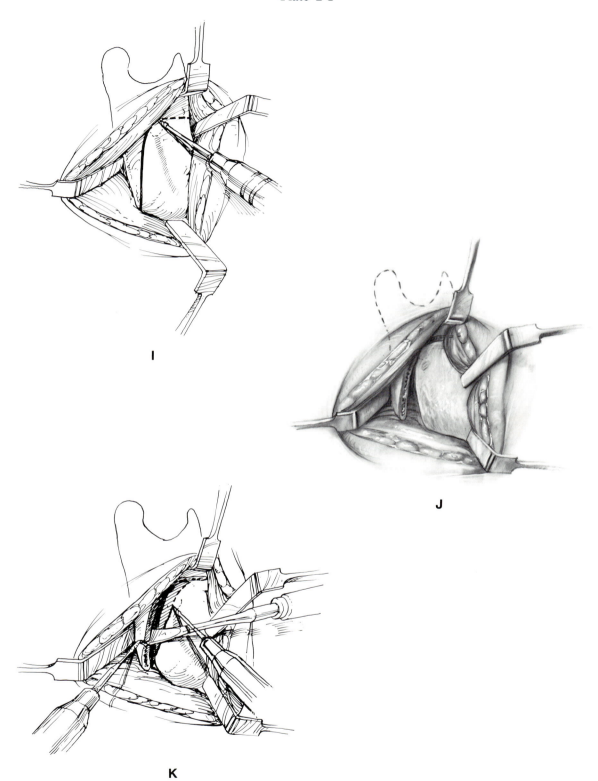

I

J

K

EXTRAORAL SUBCONDYLAR RAMUS OSTEOTOMY

Plate 2-1

L. The proximal segment is manipulated with gentle finger pressure while palpating the glenoid fossa area with the other hand to be certain that the condyle is well seated in the glenoid fossa. A passive wire is placed, creating a very slight superior force vector to prevent condylar sag. This is achieved by placing the interosseous hole more superiorly in the distal segment and more inferiorly in the proximal segment and *lightly* tightening it.

M. The exact location of the wire will vary with the degree of setback, but care is taken not to wire the proximal segment abnormally either distally or proximally. Preoperative cutouts and a cephalometric prediction tracing will help ensure the proper anteroposterior position of the proximal segment at the time of surgery.

N. The masseteric muscle sling, platysma, subcutaneous tissues, and skin are closed in a routine layered fashion. Antibiotic ointment is coated along the incision line, a strip of Telfa layed on this, Steri-Strips placed over it, and a pressure dressing applied. When the skin sutures are removed at 5 days, new Steri-Strips are applied for 1 week to minimize tension on the skin edges and thereby reduce scar formation.

Intermaxillary fixation is usually maintained for approximately 6 weeks, after which appropriate postsurgical jaw physiotherapy is begun. Generally during the 2 to 3 weeks immediately following removal of the intermaxillary fixation, intermaxillary elastics are worn for progressively decreasing duration, and jaw exercises and diet consistency are progressively increased.

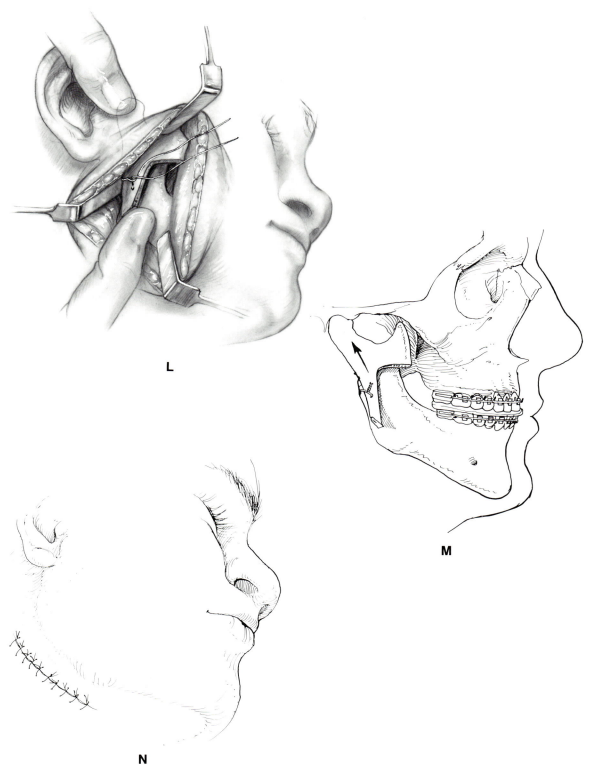

L

M

N

INTRAORAL SUBCONDYLAR RAMUS OSTEOTOMY

Plate 2-2

A. For the routine mandibular setback of up to about 8 mm the intraoral sub-condylar ramus approach must be considered. The procedure can be done rapidly and does not leave facial scars. When properly done it produces a predictably stable result. The illustrated case demonstrates a 6-mm class III malocclusion and mandibular prognathism.

B. The mandible is maximally opened by inserting a bite block between the teeth on the side opposite that to be sectioned first. A soft-tissue incision is made with a diathermy knife over the external oblique ridge from midway up the anterior border of the ascending ramus of the mandible into the vestibule lateral to the mandibular first molar. The incision is made far enough laterally to allow for soft-tissue closure at the completion of the procedure when the jaws are wired into intermaxillary fixation.

C. A subperiosteal reflection of the entire lateral, posterior, and inferior borders of the ascending ramus of the mandible is performed. This includes removal of the entire temporalis muscle from the coronoid for both visual identification of the sigmoid notch superiorly and to prevent relapse. If, however, it is elected to perform an intraoral inverted-L ramus osteotomy, the temporalis muscle need not be removed from the coronoid process. This option is discussed in greater detail later in this section.

   A J periosteal elevator is used to remove the pterygoid-masseteric sling and as much as is possible of the medial pterygoid muscle attachment. Leaving the medial pterygoid attached to the distal segment can contribute to relapse.

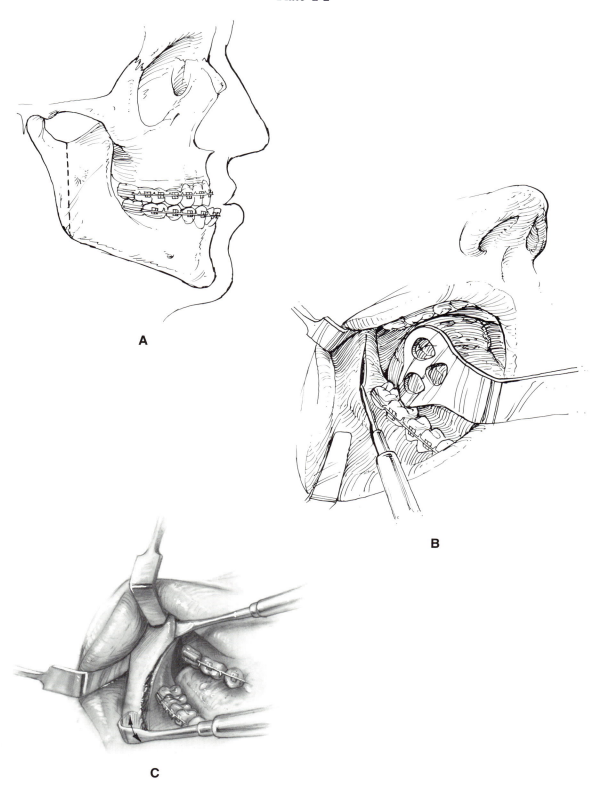

A

B

C

D. Several incisions through the lateral periosteum aid in achieving improved soft-tissue relaxation for retraction and exposure. A special ramus retractor is inserted to provide retraction and protection of adjacent soft tissue. This retractor is curved at the tip to engage the posterior border of the mandible; thus the ramus can be pulled slightly forward, improving access.

E. The bone cut is made from the sigmoid notch area and carried inferiorly to the region of the mandibular angle. This cut is made with a 120° beveled reciprocating saw blade. This beveled blade is especially important in that the angle of the bone cut helps minimize medial displacement of the proximal segment caused by the pull of the medial pterygoid muscle. If a 90° angled blade is used the proximal segment often tends to retract medially, making lateral positioning of it extremely difficult. In addition the proximal segment will be displaced more laterally with the 90° angled blade than with the 120° angled blade. The blade and cut are illustrated in a tangential section through the ramus at the level of the occlusal plane.

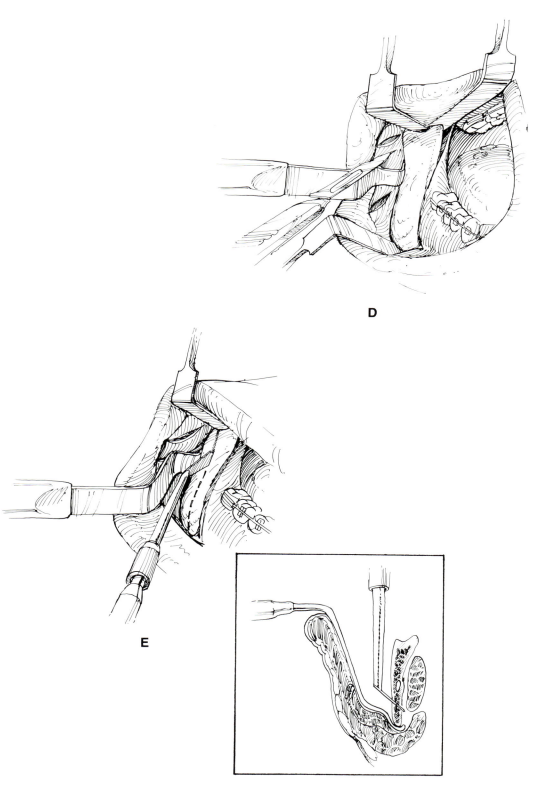

D

E

INTRAORAL SUBCONDYLAR RAMUS OSTEOTOMY

Plate 2-2

F. When a short vertical subcondylar cut is made, medial retraction of the proximal segment does not occur because the medial pterygoid muscle is not attached to it, making it easier to position the proximal segment laterally. However, the more anteriorly on the ramus that the inferior aspect of the vertical cut is made, the less pterygoid muscle there will be *left attached to the distal segment of the mandible* and thus the less effect the pterygoid muscle will have on relapse. Residual muscle attachment to the distal segment becomes progressively more important with increasing magnitudes of mandibular setback.

G. When the bone cut is completed the proximal segment is held medially as a result of the pull of the residual medial pterygoid muscle or the remaining periosteum attached to it. Therefore it must be retracted laterally and the remaining attachment of the medial pterygoid muscle and periosteum removed.

H. The J periosteal elevator can be used again at this time to release additional pterygoid muscle and periosteum attachment on the distal segment. The proximal segment should be freely mobile and remain passively positioned lateral to the ascending ramus.

I. After completion of the osteotomies on both sides and placement of the mandible into the occlusal splint, intermaxillary fixation is applied. The positions of the proximal segments are checked bilaterally. They should rest passively lateral to the distal segment of the ascending mandibular ramus. If the inferior aspect of the proximal segment is protruding excessively laterally, the inferior aspect of the proximal segment can be removed or bone on the superoposterior aspect of the distal segment removed to permit more passive approximation of the segments. This will minimize the problem of distraction of the condyle laterally and inferiorly out of the glenoid fossa that otherwise may occur when the segments are wired.

J. With this procedure it has been advocated that no wire be placed or that a circumramus wire be placed to approximate the proximal and distal segments. When no wire is placed there is a tendency for the mandible to relapse into a slightly class II open bite as a result of the condyle healing slightly anterior and inferior to its normal position. Therefore it is preferable that a wire be placed. By rotating the proximal segment laterally, an interosseous hole can be placed tangentially through it, exiting out the posterior border. On the distal segment the hole is similarly placed, although at a slightly higher level.

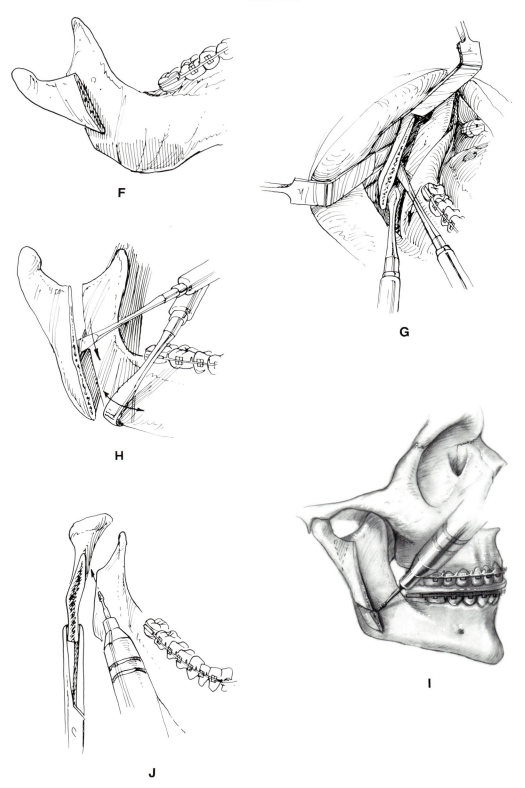

F

G

H

I

J

INTRAORAL SUBCONDYLAR RAMUS OSTEOTOMY

Plate 2-2

K. A wire is passed as illustrated, and when this wire is lightly tightened it will seat the condyle in the fossa. As this wire is tightened a finger is used to palpate externally to be certain the condyle is properly seated in the glenoid fossa.

L. Relapse with this operation occurs for *at least* three reasons related to the technique: (1) temporalis muscle stretch, (2) medial pterygoid muscle stretch, and (3) poorly achieved condylar position. In cases with the minimal posterior movements these factors are less critical than in cases with increasing amounts of posterior movement. When using this procedure to correct more major mandibular prognathisms, consideration must be given to modifying the intraoral subcondylar osteotomy into an inverted L. When this is contemplated, in addition to the dissection already described a medial ramus dissection is done whereby the periosteum is reflected medially until identification of the lingula and entering inferior alveolar neurovascular bundle is achieved. After its identification a periosteal elevator inserted medially protects the soft tissues and neurovascular bundle so that the horizontal bone cut can be made through both lingual and buccal cortices. This cut extends just posterior to the lingula. From the distal extent of this horizontal cut the vertical cut is made from the lateral aspect to the mandibular angle as previously described. This eliminates untoward effects of temporalis muscle pull and function.

Our current approach to performing the intraoral subcondylar ramus osteotomy is to almost routinely utilize the inverted-L bone cut with direct wiring as illustrated in Plate 2-2, *K*.

M. The surgical sites are thoroughly irrigated and suctioned and the incisions sutured with resorbable sutures. No drains are placed. Postsurgical care is the same as outlined for the extraoral subcondylar ramus osteotomy.

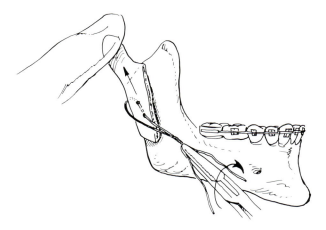

K

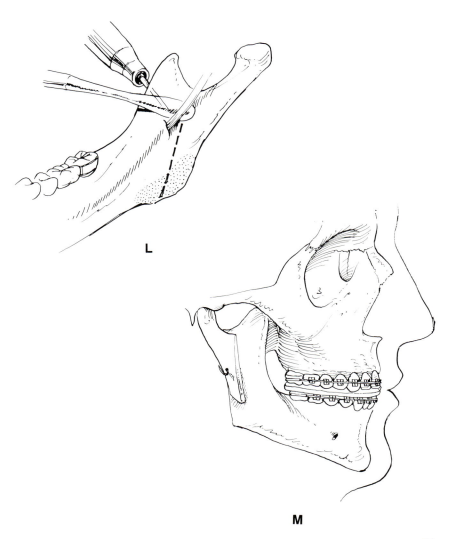

L

M

Modified sagittal ramus osteotomy

In general the following indications exist for the modified sagittal ramus osteotomy:

1. Symmetric and asymmetric mandibular advancement
2. Symmetric mandibular setback
3. Minor asymmetric mandibular setback
4. Vertical lengthening of ascending mandibular ramus

The sagittal split ramus osteotomy of the mandible has been used with increasing frequency for the correction of various dentofacial deformities. Despite the popularity of this operative approach, there is appropriate concern about the potential untoward sequelae associated with the procedure: significant swelling, excessive bleeding, serious injury to the inferior alveolar nerve, avascular necrosis or infection of the proximal segment, and skeletal relapse. These problems are directly related to several technical and biologic aspects of the sagittal osteotomy technique. In large part these are avoidable with some modifications in the procedure.

Excessive swelling. The swelling increases in proportion to the amount of soft-tissue dissection. When the lateral soft tissues (periosteum and masseter) are not reflected from the mandible, much of the excessive postoperative swelling is avoided. Further, the stripping of the masseteric-pterygoid sling from the inferoposterior border of the mandible is unnecessary. There is no reason to remove these muscles, because the proximal segment of the mandible will not be altered spacially and therefore muscle and bone relationships in this area will remain anatomically and functionally unchanged.

Excessive bleeding. Bleeding during the sagittal osteotomy comes from three areas: the posterior ramus area, medial ramus area, and intramedullary area. The various arteries and veins in each of these areas can be inadvertently cut during the blind stripping phases of the classic sagittal osteotomy. With the modified technique to be described here no blind posterior dissection or periosteal stripping of the masseteric-pterygoid sling is done. The medial dissection is done subperiosteally with good visibility and stopped just superior and posterior to the lingula. No retractor is inserted to the posterior border or the medial aspect of the mandible, and therefore there is little chance of tearing the inferior alveolar neurovascular bundle or encountering bleeding from the region posterior to it. Intramedullary bleeding is seldom, if ever, a problem and can be controlled by direct packing or bone wax after the segments are separated.

Inferior alveolar nerve injury. The inferior alveolar nerve can be injured in two locations: medial to the mandible before it enters the bone at the lingula and within the medullary component of the mandible where the split is accomplished. By direct visualization of the neurovascular bundle in the medial dissection and by not forcing a retractor posterosuperior to it, injury to the nerve

66

in this area is virtually eliminated. If the split is accomplished so the medial and lateral portions of the mandible are first torqued apart, the neurovascular bundle can be visualized before attempting to complete the split, and thus direct injury to the nerve within the marrow cavity generally can be avoided.

Avascular necrosis or infection of proximal segment. With the removal of most of the lateral and medial soft-tissue attachments to the ascending ramus of the mandible, the blood supply to the proximal segment is diminished. This reduced vascularity can account in part for some of the reported complications of infection and loss of this segment. If the masseter and medial pterygoid muscles as well as the major portion of the temporalis muscle are left attached, they afford an excellent vascular pedicle to the proximal segment of the ascending mandibular ramus.

Relapse. Two aspects of relapse are germane to this discussion: proper condylar positioning at surgery and allowing the muscles of mastication to remain in their original spacial relations with the mandible. By properly wiring the segments, as will be described, the condyle can be correctly repositioned in the glenoid fossa at surgery. Similarly this technique allows for the proximal segment of the mandible, with all the muscles of mastication attached to it, to remain in a normal, preoperative, anatomic, and functional spacial position.

The basic technique described and illustrated is for advancement of the mandible because this is the primary operative procedure we utilize for this purpose.

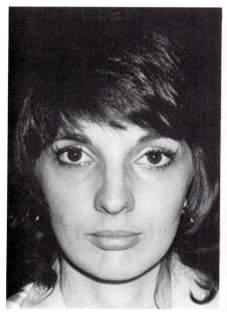 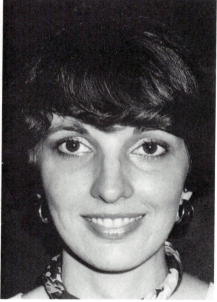

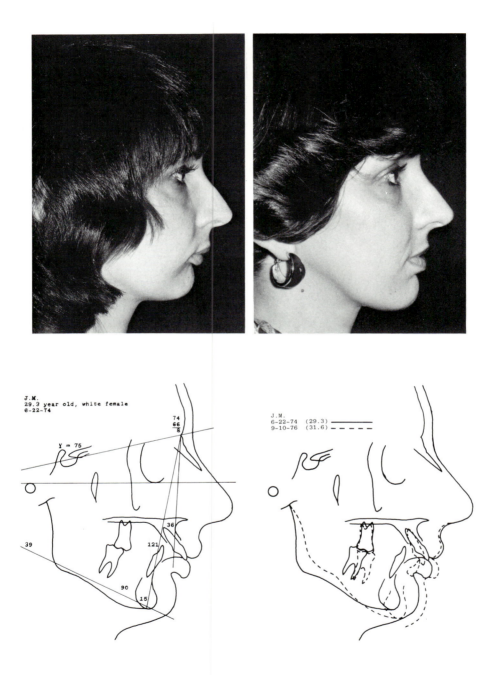

J.M.
29.3 year old, white female
6-22-74

Y = 75

74
66
8

36
121
39
90
15

J.M.
6-22-74 (29.3) ——————
9-10-76 (31.6) ------

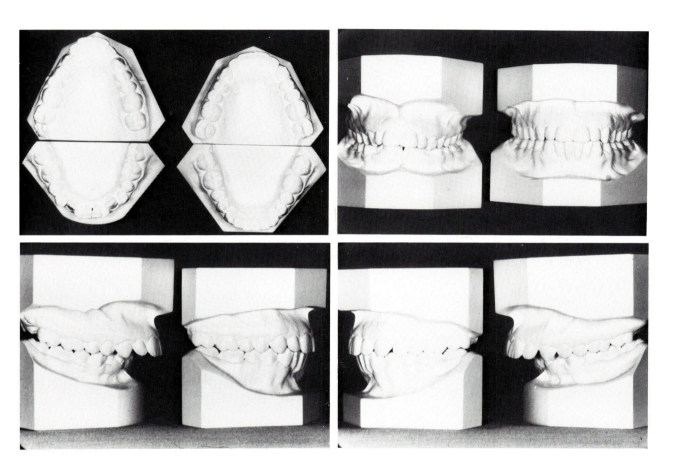

MODIFIED SAGITTAL RAMUS OSTEOTOMY

Plate 2-3

A. The illustrated case demonstrates a 10-mm class II occlusion and mandibular deficiency. With increasing magnitudes of mandibular advancement and when the sagittal osteotomy is utilized to correct mandibular prognathism, special modifications in the basic procedure to be described must be considered. These are discussed following a description of the basic sagittal osteotomy technique.

B. The anatomy of the masticator muscular attachments and ligamentous attachments to the mandible as well as the neurovascular foramina are illustrated. The basic principle of the modified sagittal osteotomy is to maintain the proximal portion of the ascending ramus in a normal anatomic position with virtually all of the associated soft tissues remaining attached, yet permitting unrestricted anterior, posterior, and vertical movement of the distal segment. Significant transverse movements (horizontal rotations) are not recommended with this technique because they cause asymmetric flaring of the proximal fragments, clinically manifested for many months postoperatively as unilateral facial fullness.

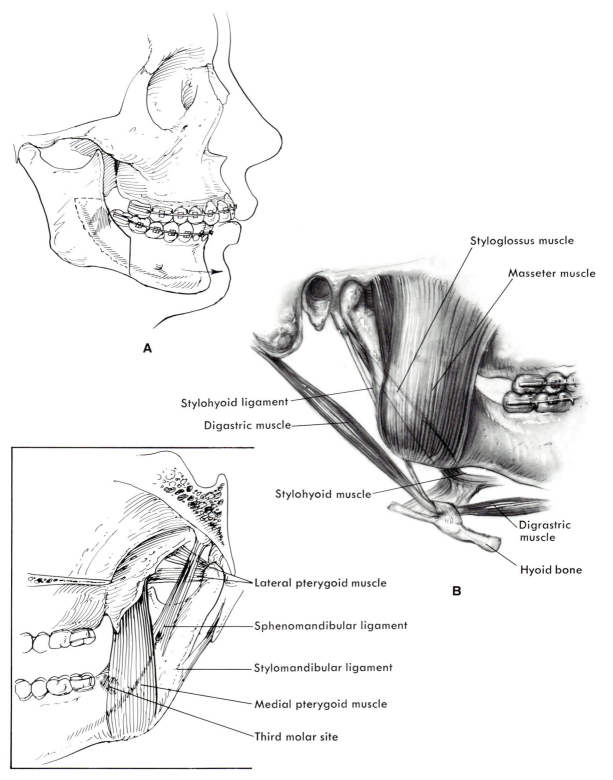

A

Styloglossus muscle

Masseter muscle

Stylohyoid ligament

Digastric muscle

Stylohyoid muscle

Digrastric muscle

Hyoid bone

B

Lateral pterygoid muscle

Sphenomandibular ligament

Stylomandibular ligament

Medial pterygoid muscle

Third molar site

MODIFIED SAGITTAL RAMUS OSTEOTOMY
Plate 2-3

C. A bite block is inserted between the teeth on the side opposite that to be operated on first. This projects the mandibular ramus anteriorly and makes access to it easier. An incision is made with a diathermy knife down to bone on the lateral aspect of the anterior border of the ramus approximately overlying the external oblique ridge from midway up the ascending ramus downward into the depth of the vestibule to about the mandibular first molar area. Making the incision lateral facilitates soft-tissue closure, which is always done with this technique after the teeth are wired into intermaxillary fixation. By not extending the incision more than halfway up the anterior border of the ramus the buccal fat pad is avoided.

The soft-tissue dissection is begun subperiosteally along the anterior border of the ramus upward toward the coronoid process. This is facilitated by firm retraction with a coronoid notch retractor concomitant with the soft-tissue dissection. *No lateral dissection is done of the ascending mandibular ramus.* The sigmoid notch is identified superiorly, and a bone clamp is placed high on the coronoid process to retract the soft tissues. Medially the soft tissues are generously reflected subperiosteally until the lingula and inferior alveolar neurovascular bundle as it enters the mandibular foramen are identified. The medial soft-tissue dissection is stopped slightly posterior and superior to the lingula. The sphenomandibular ligament can be stripped from the lingula with careful dissection for major advancements. While the medial soft tissues are being retracted the medial bone cut is made through only the lingual cortex and extends just posterior and superior to the lingula (a distance of approximately 15 to 20 mm from the anterior border of the ascending ramus and about 2 mm above the inferior alveolar neurovascular bundle where it enters the mandible). Care must be taken to ensure that the lingual cortex is cut through the entire length of the horizontal osteotomy or there will be an increased risk of a poor split.

D. Following completion of the horizontal medial osteotomy the bone cut is carried down the lateralmost aspect of the anterior border of the ascending ramus to the region of the second molar. This osteotomy is made parallel and directly adjacent to the lateral cortex. This is important so that when the actual split is done it will in effect separate the lateral cortex of the proximal segment from the medullary bone and medial cortex of the distal segment. When this occurs the inferior alveolar neurovascular bundle will almost always remain within the distal segment and is therefore seldom injured.

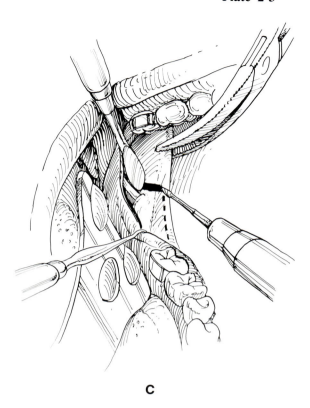

C

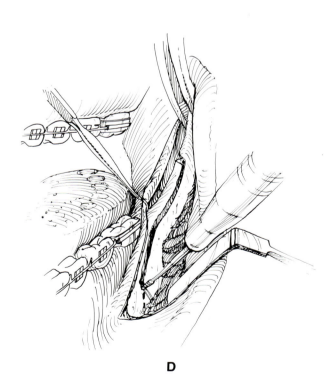

D

MODIFIED SAGITTAL RAMUS OSTEOTOMY

Plate 2-3

E. The coronoid clamp retractor and the bite block are removed to provide maximum relaxation and retraction of the soft tissues for the lateral soft-tissue dissection and osteotomy. The periosteum is elevated from the lateral aspect of the mandible in the molar area and off the inferior border of the mandible in the gonial notch area. A channel retractor is inserted beneath the inferior border of the mandible. The vertical osteotomy is generally done lateral to the second molar; however, in major advancements the vertical cut can be brought forward to the region of the premolar. The lateral osteotomy is carefully completed through the lateral cortex so as to avoid inadvertently severing the inferior alveolar neurovascular bundle, which can occur if this cut is carried too deep into the medullary bone. *The cut extends through both cortical plates of the inferior border of the mandible (insert).* Failure to do so will cause difficulties in splitting. The vertical thickness of the inferior border cortical bone varies and can be determined from the cephalometric or panographic radiographs.

F. With osteotomes all bone cuts are checked for their completeness through the cortex, especially at the inferior border of the mandible. Two osteotomes are then inserted and used as levers to separate the segments. One osteotome is inserted at the inferior border and levered off the distolateral cortex. The inferior border osteotome is placed low so that the inferior alveolar neurovascular bundle is not inadvertently traumatized. The second osteotome may be moved along the remainder of the osteotomy cut to any position between the segments where separation is not occurring. Both osteotomes are levered simultaneously, and the entire osteotomy site is observed to note whether the segments are beginning *to separate along their entirety.* This observation avoids pathologic fracturing of the lateral cortex of the proximal segment. If this method does not mobilize the entire length of the osteotomy, the osteotomies are again checked for completeness and the levering procedure repeated.

G. In adults as the osteotomes are used to pry the segments apart, the segments will often snap open. However, sometimes the split will greenstick on the posterior medial ramus area and the inferior medial area. These areas are where the fracturing occurs to complete the split between the segments. This occurs most often in younger patients and usually requires more prying and mobilization of the segments. In either instance when it is opened sufficiently so that the medullary area can be inspected, the area is irrigated and an attempt is made to visualize the inferior alveolar neurovascular bundle within the split. Generally it will be embedded within the medullary bone of the distal segment. If so, the split is completed with further levering.

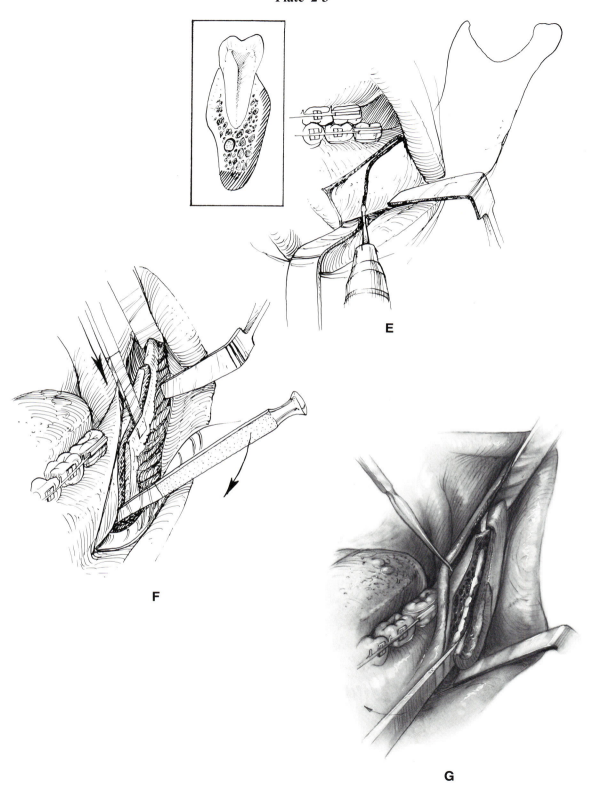

E

F

G

MODIFIED SAGITTAL RAMUS OSTEOTOMY

Plate 2-3

H. When the inferior alveolar neurovascular bundle is attached to or embedded in the proximal segment, the segment is rotated laterally and the neurovascular bundle freed from it. This is done by judicious removal of the overlying trabecular bone and teasing the bundle out of its bony canal with a curet.

I. With this technique the lingual cortex normally fractures as illustrated. This, however, will be dependent on (1) the posterior extent of the horizontal medial ramus, cut, (2) the completeness of the inferior border cut, and (3) the anatomy of the mandible.

J. When the horizontal medial ramus bone cut is made to the distal border of the mandible, the split may occur with the medial pterygoid muscle partially attached to the distal segment. If this occurs it is recommended that following mobilization of the segments a J periosteal elevator be inserted through the completed split so as to strip as much of the pterygoid muscle as possible from the distal segment.

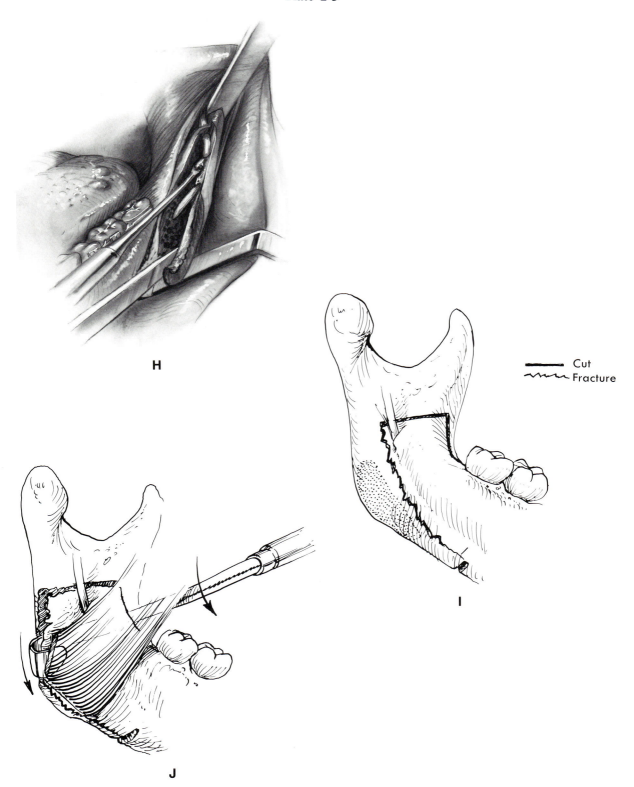

H

I

J

Cut
Fracture

MODIFIED SAGITTAL RAMUS OSTEOTOMY

Plate 2-3

K. With the distal segment grasped in one hand and the proximal segment stabilized with a bone clamp, the segments can be moved apart in an anteroposterior direction to relieve areas of soft-tissue attachment that may restrict good mobilization. At this time the J periosteal elevator can also be utilized, if necessary, by inserting it through the split to help relieve periosteal and other soft-tissue attachments on the distal segment.

   A moist sponge is placed between the fragments while the opposite side is being operated on to prevent the movement of the segments from damaging the nerve between them.

L. Interosseous holes are placed superiorly in the distal segment and inferiorly in the proximal segment, so that when a wire is passed and tightened, after securing the intermaxillary fixation, it seats the condyle in the glenoid fossa.

   When deciding exactly where to place the wire holes it is best to temporarily hold the teeth in their new occlusion and the proximal segment in the fossa so as to determine the best location for the wire holes. Wires, as illustrated, are passed but not tightened at this time. If the holes are placed excessively far apart when the wire is tightened it tends to rotate the proximal segment superoanteriorly. If they are not placed far enough superoinferiorly apart, tightening the wire can actually retract the condyle from the fossa.

M. The occlusal splint is inserted, intermaxillary fixation applied, and the wires tightened. The incisions are closed with running absorbable sutures. No drains are placed. The fixation is maintained for about 6 weeks, followed by appropriate jaw physiotherapy as discussed in Plate 2-1, *N*.

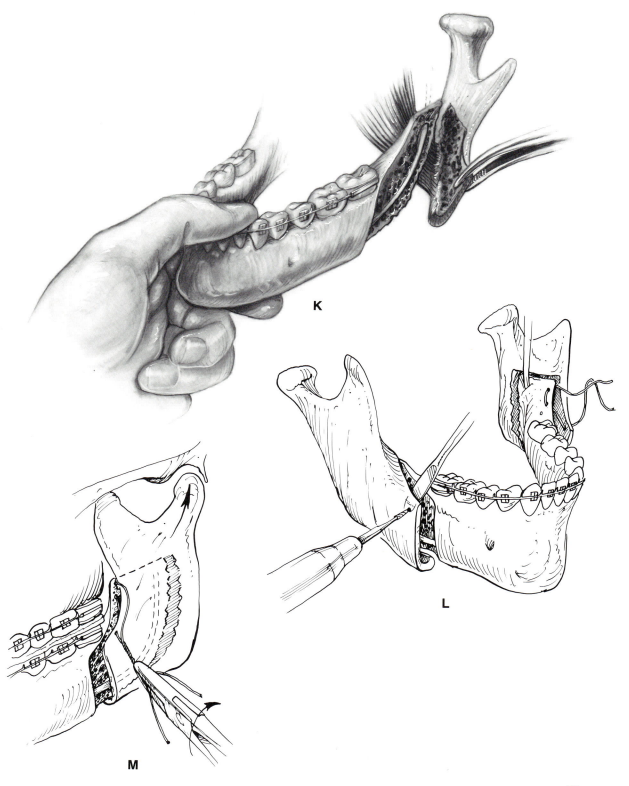

K

L

M

MODIFIED SAGITTAL RAMUS OSTEOTOMY

Major mandibular advancement (Plate 2-4)

Under certain circumstances variations in the sagittal osteotomy technique described must be considered. With major advancements (greater than 12 mm) the lateral vertical bone cut is brought forward to the first molar–second premolar area to increase the bone surface interface. In such instances there may also be a forward projection of the superior aspect of the distal segment when the proximal segment is properly distalized. It is best to reduce this with a mastoid bur so the interosseous hole can be positioned more posteriorly to prevent the wire from distracting the proximal segment superiorly and anteriorly.

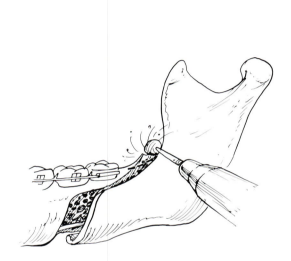

MODIFIED SAGITTAL RAMUS OSTEOTOMY

Mandibular prognathism (Plate 2-5)

A. When the modified sagittal ramus osteotomy technique is used to correct mandibular prognathism, distalization of the proximal segment is to be avoided to prevent skeletal relapse. This is accomplished after the split is completed by reflecting the medial pterygoid muscle from the medial aspect of the proximal segment, through the split, so when the distal segment is retracted it does not distalize the proximal segment.

B. Distalization of the proximal segment can be prevented by measuring the lateral cortex osteotomy accurately (as determined by cephalometric prediction tracings) and making certain at surgery that the anteroposterior relationship in this area is proper. The wire is then placed so that it exerts a light superior force vector to seat the condyle in the fossa but little posterior force vector.

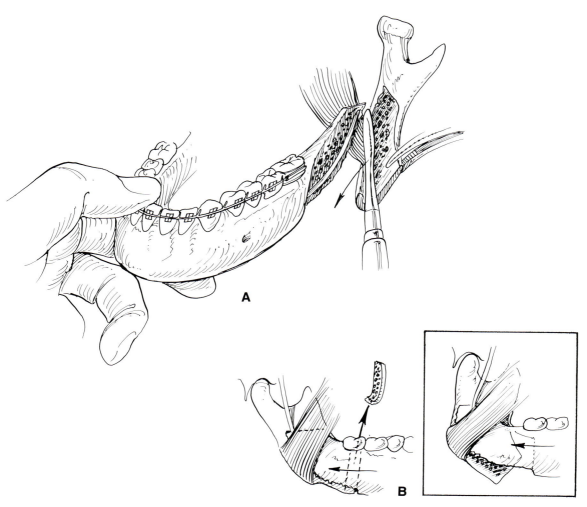

A

B

MODIFIED SAGITTAL RAMUS OSTEOTOMY

Impacted third molars (Plate 2-6)

A. Impacted mandibular third molars are generally removed at the same time as the sagittal osteotomy is performed. However, there are several special considerations. When a bony impaction with incomplete root formation is present, there is essentially no change in the procedure just described. At the time of splitting, the osteotomes are placed at the inferior border of the mandible and midway up the ramus, because prying directly over the area of the impacted tooth can result in pathologic fracture of the lateral cortex overlying the impacted tooth. When the split is completed, the tooth is simply removed through the split.

B. When the molar is fully formed and partially erupted, the incision and closure are modified. The incision is made as illustrated directly over the exposed portion of the crown to allow the soft tissues in the area of the partially erupted tooth to be closed primarily.

C. The bone cuts are similar and the split done as previously described. Following separation of the proximal and distal segments the tooth is removed through the split. If the roots are fully formed, the tooth may need to be sectioned to facilitate its removal.

D. Prior to placement of the intermaxillary fixation several interrupted sutures are passed through the medial soft tissue; however, the needles are left on them and they are retained with hemostats until after intermaxillary fixation is secured. At this time the needle is passed through the lateral aspect of the incision and the suture tied.

E. With fully formed deep vertical or horizontal impactions the mandible is structurally weakened in the area of the tooth, and considerable care must be exercised so as not to cause a pathologic fracture when the split is being made.

F. This will occur as illustrated and in effect creates a tangential mandibular angle fracture. If surgical experience with this technique is lacking, it is wise to remove these teeth 3 to 4 months before performing the sagittal osteotomy.

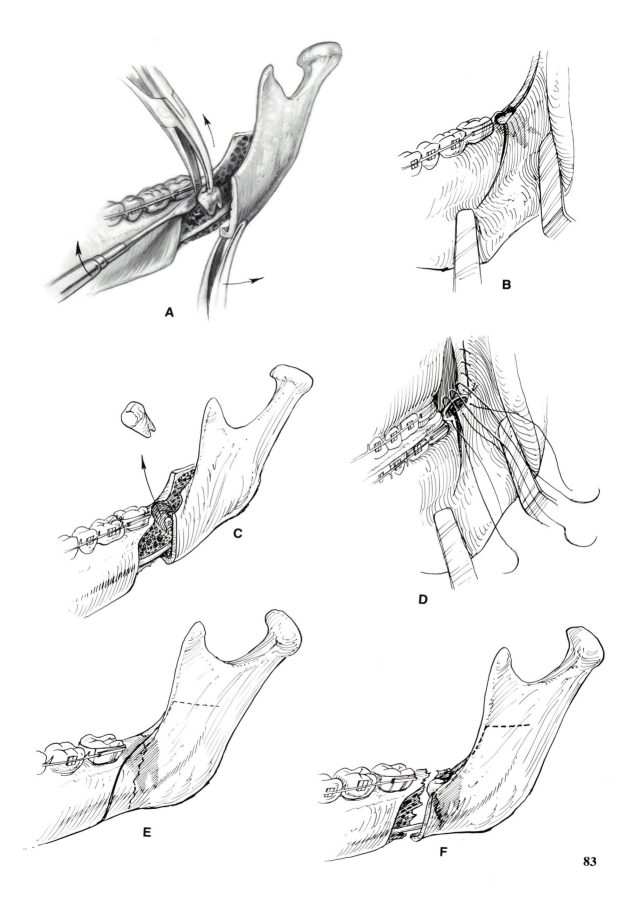

MODIFIED SAGITTAL RAMUS OSTEOTOMY

Suprahyoid myotomies (Plate 2-7)

A. In instances when the cephalometric prediction tracing reveals that the suprahyoid musculature will be lengthened ("stretched") over about 15% of its resting length, it is advisable to do suprahyoid myotomies simultaneous with the mandibular advancement. The magnitude of suprahyoid muscle stretch is determined by measuring from the midportion of the hyoid to the inferior midsymphysis area in the presurgical cephalometric tracing and repeating this in the prediction cephalometric tracing. The degree to which the suprahyoid muscles will be lengthened by the proposed surgery is determined by the difference of the two measurements. This difference is then divided by the resting length of the suprahyoid muscle initial measurement ($12 \div 35 = 34\%$) to give the percentage of lengthening. If the percentage of potential muscle lengthening is greater than 15% of the muscle resting length, then the suprahyoid myotomy is indicated. Excessive stretching of these muscles generally occurs in cases of major advancement and in those instances where there is counterclockwise rotational movement at the symphysis.

B. The suprahyoid myotomy consists of complete removal of the anterior digastric and geniohyoid muscles where they attach to the symphyseal area of the mandible. This is generally done transorally, although it can be done extraorally. Through an anterior vestibular incision the mandibular symphysis is degloved and the anterior digastric and geniohyoid muscles are removed. The digastrics are readily removed by inserting a periosteal elevator distal to their most distal area of insertion and pulling it forward while keeping it tightly on the bone.

C. The geniohyoid muscles are removed by cutting them with a diathermy knife close to where they attach to the mandible.

D. A two-layered closure of the vestibular incision is done with absorbable sutures, and a pressure dressing is applied for 5 days. This dressing is placed so as to maintain the lower lip superiorly and prevent it from being retracted inferiorly with healing *(insert)*.

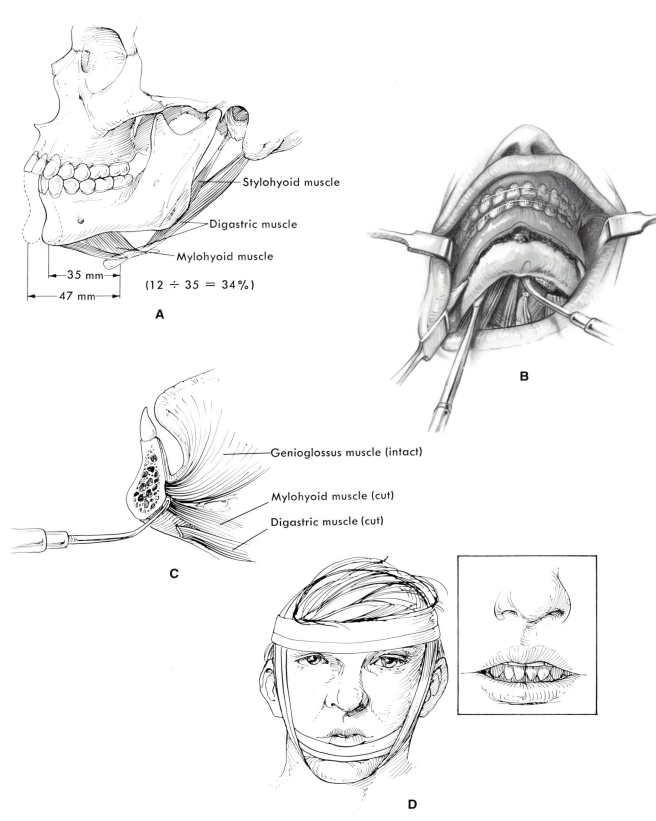

Stylohyoid muscle

Digastric muscle

Mylohyoid muscle

(12 ÷ 35 = 34%)

35 mm

47 mm

A

B

Genioglossus muscle (intact)

Mylohyoid muscle (cut)

Digastric muscle (cut)

C

D

85

Arcing ramus osteotomy

This surgical technique is useful for advancement of the mandible in certain instances. Although we prefer to utilize the modified sagittal osteotomy for advancement of the mandible in most cases, the arcing osteotomy is useful in:

1. Major mandibular advancements (greater than 10 mm) in high mandibular plane angle cases
2. Mandibular advancement in patients who have had previous surgery in the ascending ramus
3. Mandibular advancement with radiographically abnormal ascending ramus anatomy

The arcing ramus osteotomy is best done extraorally for reasons that will become apparent as the technique is described, although it has been suggested that it be done transorally. The principle of the procedure is to perform the osteotomy in a geometrically predetermined manner that permits the distal mandible to be advanced while leaving the condyle, coronoid process, and mandibular angle anatomically and spacially unchanged. Accordingly the major muscles of mastication will not change their spacial relationships with the mandible and therefore have no adverse effects on relapse. Similarly their function will be minimally altered. Further, the condyle is predictably properly repositioned in the glenoid fossa.

This technique is often referred to as the L or C ramus osteotomy; however, the arcing ramus osteotomy differs from these in its geometric precision, which has important implications with regard to relapse, bone healing, and masticatory function. Each of these is briefly commented on, followed by a detailed description of the planning and execution of the arcing ramus osteotomy.

Relapse. Although many factors are involved in relapse, those identified and germane to surgical techniques utilized for advancement of the mandible are adverse alteration (stretching, lengthening) of the muscles of mastication, distraction of the condyle from the glenoid fossa, and the rate of bone healing. With any procedure to reposition the mandible it is optimum if the spacial relationship between the major muscles of mastication and associated bone remain unchanged. The arcing ramus osteotomy achieves these objectives, as will be illustrated. When inadvertent distraction of the mandibular condyle from the glenoid fossa occurs with surgical repositioning of the mandible, relapse occurs. The arcing osteotomy is designed to prevent this, whereas the less precise but similar ramus procedure can cause, by the very nature of the lines of osteotomy, condylar distraction.

Bone healing. When two adjacent bone surfaces that have been fractured or osteotomized are viable (i.e., have a good blood supply), they heal and regain their physical characteristics in a predictable time. This permits function to be resumed at a prescribed time after surgery without adverse sequelae at the site of healing. However, if there is a significant compromise in the blood supply to either the distal or proximal bony segment of a healing osteotomy site, this time–physical properties–resumption of function sequencing must be varied. Simply put, it takes longer for dead bone to heal and thereby regain its physical properties than it does live bone. Accordingly, if early loads are placed on a site of delayed healing, movement (relapse) will occur.

Because in many of the ramus osteotomies virtually all soft tissues are removed from the proximal segment, thereby causing avascular necrosis and delayed healing, the stage is set for relapse. The arcing ramus osteotomy preserves the blood supply to the proximal segment and thereby avoids these specific problems. Moreover, when one segment is deprived of its blood supply it is more prone to infection or avascular dissolution.

Masticatory function. If certain rotational or tipping movements of the ascending mandibular ramus occur with surgery, as when the proximal portion of the ramus is rotated forward, they can have significant adverse effects on the biomechanics involved in mastication. This occurs because the muscles of mastication function best with specific spacial relationships to the mandible, and unfavorable alterations in these decrease the efficiency of muscle function. Such alterations are avoided with the arcing ramus osteotomy.

ARCING RAMUS OSTEOTOMY

Plate 2-8

A. The arcing ramus osteotomy is best suited technically for mandibular advancement in patients with the high mandibular plane angle type of skeletal morphology. Such a case is illustrated in which a severe class II malocclusion, slight open bite, and mandibular retrognathism are present.

    Because this procedure is predicated on precise preoperative planning to determine the exact location of the ramus osteotomy, the planning advocated by Hawkinson is described.

B. The exact line of the bone cut in the arcing osteotomy is determined from a carefully drawn composite cephalometric tracing (i.e., superimposed pretreatment and prediction tracing drawings). This tracing must include the coronoid process. Therefore it may be necessary to obtain an additional pretreatment cephalometric radiograph with the mouth open wide so that the entire mandible, including the coronoid process and condyle, can be accurately traced. This tracing of the mandible can then be superimposed in its entirety on the normal presurgical cephalometric radiograph to ensure an accurate tracing of the coronoid process of the mandible.

    A composite cephalometric tracing is then done of the presurgical and desired repositioning of the mandible, as illustrated. Two tangents are drawn from the tip of the presurgical coronoid and menton to their altered position, which occurs with the planned forward movement of the mandible. These two tangents are then perpendicularly bisected and the perpendicular bisections carried to the point where they intersect. This point of intersection is the *geometric center of rotation of the mandible as it moves from its presurgical position to the desired postsurgical position*. From the geometric center of rotation, arcs are traced with a compass across the presurgical mandibular ramus, and the one that anatomically appears most favorable (i.e., does not cut across the inferior alveolar neurovascular bundle) is selected to be made at surgery.

C. From this arc a line is drawn that passes to the anterior border of the ramus superior to the lingula, and an inferior cut is similarly planned in about the region of the molars. A template is made from any material that can be autoclaved, which allows for exact reproduction of the planned cut at surgery.

ARCING RAMUS OSTEOTOMY
Plate 2-8

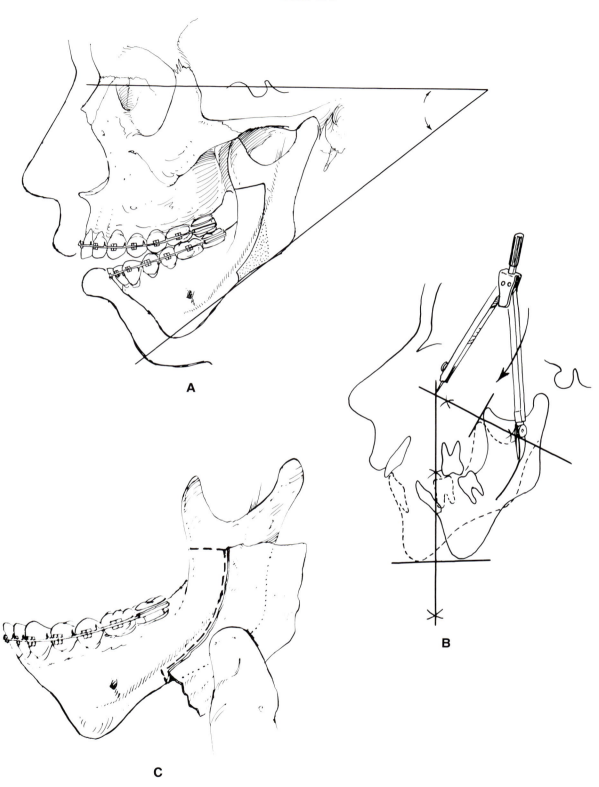

A

B

C

ARCING RAMUS OSTEOTOMY

Plate 2-8

D. If virtually all arcs scribed on the mandibular ramus from the center of rotation cross the inferior alveolar neurovascular canal, it is recommended that the arc that crosses it closest to the point where it enters the mandible be selected. When this is done, at surgery the area of the mandible overlying the entry of the inferior alveolar neurovascular bundle is decorticated laterally, and the neurovascular bundle identified within the marrow cavity of the mandible. It can then be retracted so that the medial cortical cut can be completed.

Before actually beginning the extraoral surgery it is often helpful to secure the occlusal splint to the lower teeth and place several class II intermaxillary elastics. These elastics will hold the mandible relatively stable and close to the desired final occlusion. This makes execution of the osteotomies easier because the distal mandible is partially stabilized. Moreover, placement of the definite intermaxillary fixation is easier on completion of the osteotomies bilaterally.

E. The soft-tissue incision, layered dissection, and exposure of the lateral aspect of the mandibular ramus are identical to that described in detail in Plate 2-1 with a few modifications. The incision for the arcing osteotomy is generally extended more anteriorly and the facial vessels ligated and cut to facilitate the required anterior exposure. Further, the lateral dissection *does not* include removal of the temporalis muscle from the coronoid. The medial dissection is also limited, with the *medial pterygoid being left attached*. Because the proximal segment will not be spacially altered with regard to its preoperative anatomic position, removal of these muscles is unnecessary and only reduces the vascularity to the proximal segment.

The template is used at the time of surgery to mark the location of the predetermined bone cuts on the lateral cortex. After marking the proposed cuts, a lateral cortical window is made, if indicated, so as to expose the inferior alveolar nerve where the arc crosses it. The superior horizontal cut and arcing cut, about halfway down the arc, are completed through both lateral and medial cortices. It is helpful to check these cuts for completeness on the medial aspect with a small curved osteotome.

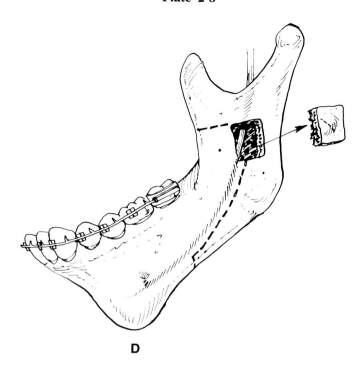

D

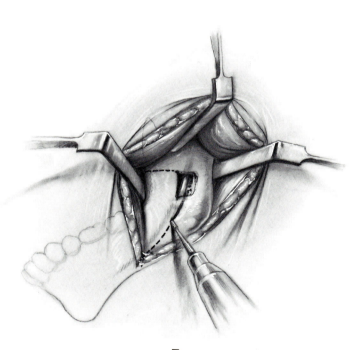

E

ARCING RAMUS OSTEOTOMY

Plate 2-8

F. To complete the medial cut in the region of the inferior alveolar neurovascular bundle, the nerve is retracted with a nerve hook.

Sagittally splitting the inferior aspect of the mandible will provide improved bony contact. Therefore the remainder of the arcing portion of the cut and inferior connecting cut in the molar area are then completed only through the lateral cortex and into the medullary bone. The inferior border is sagittally cut through with a fine fissure bur. A vertical cut is made through the medial cortex anterior to the angle to complete the sagittal aspect of the osteotomy. All osteotomy sites are checked with small osteotomes for completeness. The segments are then mobilized by insertion of osteotomes into the inferior border cut and in the arcing cut in the midramus area.

G. With advancement utilizing the arcing osteotomy the distal segment slides forward along the arcing portion of the cut, leaving the proximal segment including condyle, coronoid process, and mandibular angle anatomically unaltered in space. The separation of the lateral and medial cortices along the inferior portion of the cut avoids the large bone defect in this area, which is often visible and unesthetic clinically. On completion of both sides the patient is placed in stable intermaxillary fixation *before* the segments are wired. The segments are then wired so as to seat the condyle in the glenoid fossa. This is done by placement of holes and a wire so that as it is tightened it creates a superoposterior force vector on the proximal segment, which forces the condyle into the glenoid fossa.

H. It is not necessary to graft the bone defects to achieve normal healing with this osteotomy technique; however, the inferior defect will persist to some degree and can be esthetically objectionable, especially if it is large. Therefore bank bone can be added here. If autogenous bone is used, fresh cancellous strips are employed and actually accelerate the rate of bony union. In most major advancements it is advantageous to graft both defects, even with bank bone, to avoid not only the inferior border cosmetic defect but also the structural weakening of the mandible as a result of the superior defect.

An augmentation genioplasty is generally done simultaneously in patients with the high mandibular plane angle type of mandibular retrognathism, as in the illustrated case. The technique for doing this is discussed and illustrated in Chapter 4.

Plate 2-8

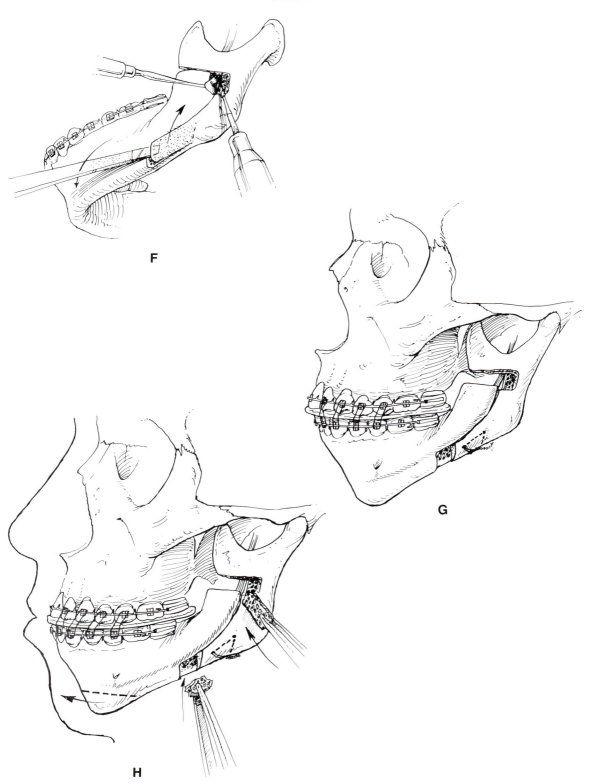

F

G

H

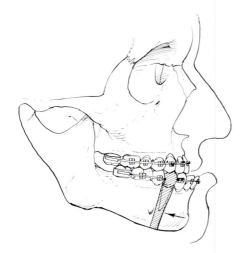

**ANTERIOR BODY
OSTECTOMY**

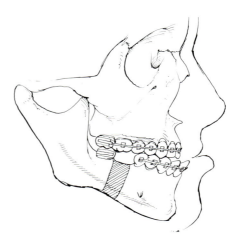

**POSTERIOR BODY
OSTECTOMY**

CHAPTER 3

Mandibular body surgery

The mandibular body ostectomy is an extremely versatile and stable procedure. It can be performed between adjacent teeth or through existing edentulous spaces or extraction sites. The mandibular body ostectomy is indicated for the correction of select cases of:

1. Mandibular prognathism
2. Class III open-bite deformity
3. Anterior crossbite in the adult

The mandibular body can be anatomically subdivided, relative to the location that the mental neurovascular bundle exits from the mandible, into the anterior body, that portion anterior to the foramen, and the posterior body. The reason for this anatomic distinction is predicated primarily on the technical consideration of the surgery required to perform the mandibular body ostectomy.

The anterior body ostectomy can be done without involvement of the inferior alveolar neurovascular bundle, whereas the posterior body ostectomy requires a more sophisticated surgical technique with intrabony identification, dissection out, and preservation of the inferior alveolar neurovascular bundle.

A one-stage intraoral technique is described and illustrated here for both the anterior and posterior mandibular body ostectomy. In addition it is often indicated to simultaneously widen or narrow the anterior arch width via a midsymphysis osteotomy, to alter the anterior, vertical, or transverse position of the chin via a genioplasty, or to rotate the posterior molar segment. The techniques for doing each of these is described and illustrated.

Anterior body ostectomy

The anterior mandibular body ostectomy is not, by definition, to involve the inferior alveolar neurovascular bundle posterior to the mental foramen. However, since the actual anteroposterior location of the mental foramen is quite variable, anywhere from distal to the cuspid to mesial to the first molar, the exact location of the mental foramen in each case must be accurately identified radiographically. When the planned mandibular body ostectomy is to be performed anterior to the mental foramen the technique is technically easy.

The anterior mandibular body ostectomy is indicated primarily in selected cases of mandibular prognathism, class III malocclusion when the posterior teeth are not in crossbite or the crossbite is dental (as opposed to skeletal) in nature and can readily be resolved with conventional orthodontics. In these instances the Class III molar occlusion is maintained and the Class III cuspid malocclusion and anterior crossbite are corrected to a normal relationship by the removal of either the first or second premolars and retraction of the anterior portion of the mandible.

As with the correction of other dentofacial deformities, carefully done model surgery and a cephalometric prediction tracing are imperative in planning the anterior body ostectomy. These are necessary to determine the actual size and shape of the vertical wedge of bone to be removed, the anterior and posterior mandibular arch width changes that will result from the proposed surgery, the possible need for simultaneous adjunctive procedures such as midline osteotomy or genioplasty, and to predict the soft-tissue changes.

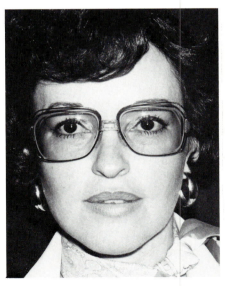 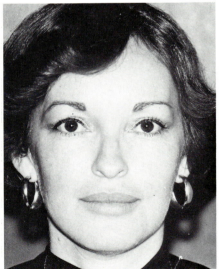

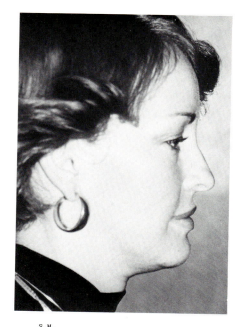

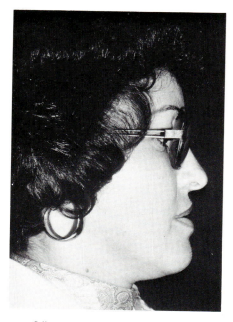

S.M.
12-8-75

Y = 64

78
82
-4

34

128

35

85

23

S.M.
12- 8-75 ——————
12-20-76 — — — —

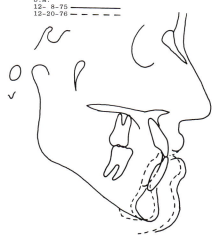

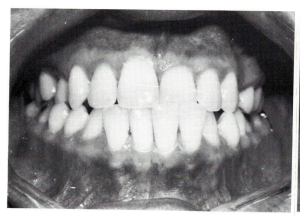

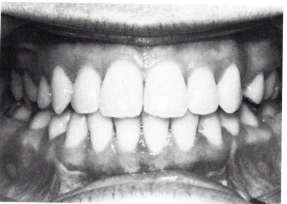

97

ANTERIOR BODY OSTECTOMY

Plate 3-1

A. In the case illustrated a moderate mandibular prognathism, class III cuspid and molar occlusion, and no posterior crossbite exist. This occlusal relationship is often present in such cases, or the posterior crossbite is minimal and can be corrected orthodontically. In this instance the first premolars will be removed, and following treatment the patient will have a class III molar and a class I cuspid occlusion.

   In some instances when a posterior crossbite does exist it can be corrected to a major extent with the surgery by narrowing the intermolar width. This is achieved via medial movement of both proximal segments. However, if this is to be done it must be remembered that the proximal segments will rotate around the condyle, and thus significant narrowing of the second molar area is impossible without associated ramus osteotomies. Carefully done model surgery, on an anatomic articulator, is important in such cases.

B. The gingival tissue is incised around the necks of the teeth, beginning one or two teeth distal to the proposed ostectomy site and carried anterior to the extraction site. Here it becomes vertical and tapers into the vestibule. Because the location of the mental nerve has been determined in this case to be distal to the extraction site, this incision is carried directly down to bone without concern about injury to the mental nerve.

C. The mucoperiosteal flap is then reflected posteriorly and inferiorly by subperiosteal dissection. As this dissection is being done the mental neurovascular bundle is readily identified and dissected out sufficiently to achieve good exposure of the proposed ostectomy site without undue stretching of the nerve. The soft-tissue dissection is continued to the inferior border of the mandible in the extraction area and the predetermined width of the body ostectomy outlined.

D. The mental foramen is often in or very near the actual line of the proposed ostectomy, especially when the ostectomy is to be done through the second promolar space. In such instances an anterior step osteotomy can be done to avoid dissecting out the inferior alveolar neurovascular bundle. The horizontal component is brought 2 to 3 mm in front of the mental foramen; then the inferior aspect of the ostectomy is completed.

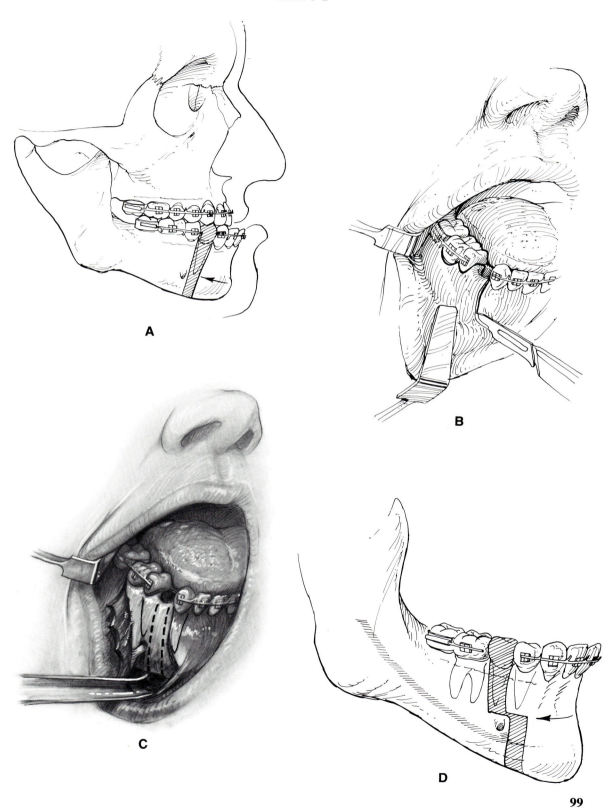

A

B

C

D

ANTERIOR BODY OSTECTOMY
Plate 3-1

E. A periosteal elevator is inserted lingually through the extraction site, sub-periosteally to protect the lingual soft tissues in the floor of the mouth. To do this it is generally necessary to minimally release the crestal gingivae of the adjacent teeth with a blade. The vertical ostectomy is completed through both cortices and the bone removed.

F. Care is exercised not to remove excessive crestal bone and thus avoid a serious and permanent periodontal defect. In this regard the ostectomy is done so that it is parallel or even somewhat convergent from buccal to lingual. If the ostectomy site is divergent from buccal to lingual a bone defect will result on the lingual, with creation of a periodontal defect *(insert)*.

G. Interosseous holes are placed through both buccal and lingual cortices at the inferior border of the mandible and a mattress wire placed and partially tightened. A bridle wire is placed around the necks of the teeth adjacent to the ostectomy and lightly secured. The ostectomy is then completed in an identical manner on the opposite side.

H. At this time the occlusal splint is tried. Generally there will be some small areas of bony interference in the ostectomy sites that prevent the splint from being completely and accurately seated in place. However, they can be readily visualized and removed. Following accurate seating of the splint, it is secured to the mandibular teeth by wiring the splint to the orthodontic lugs. The bridle wires and inferior border wires are then tightened.

Intermaxillary fixation is generally not necessary in these cases. However, it is important that the occlusal splint be constructed so that the mandibular teeth seat into it as far as possible, providing maximum stabilization.

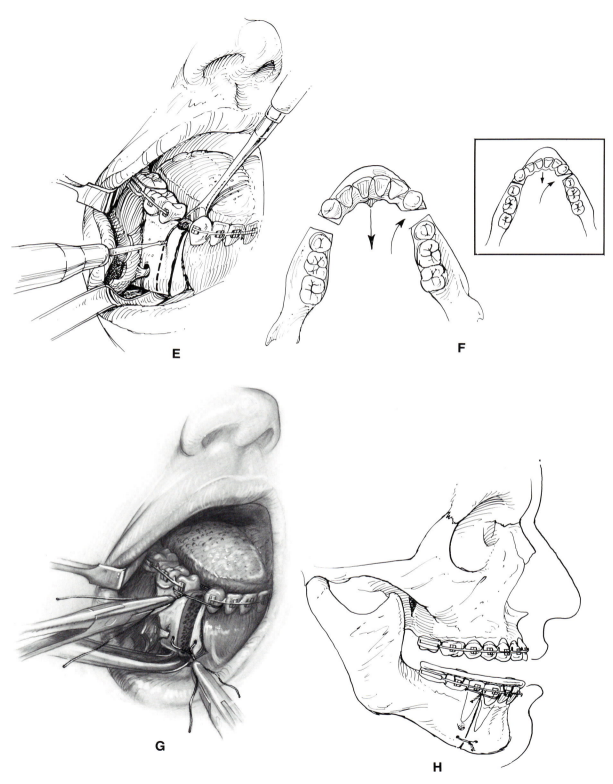

E

F

G

H

Posterior body ostectomy

The mandibular body ostectomy, which is to be performed distal to the mental foramen as ascertained radiographically, of necessity involves the intrabony identification, dissection out, and preservation of the inferior alveolar neurovascular bundle. Perhaps because of this the posterior mandibular body ostectomy is often not considered. Regardless, in instances where there are missing posterior teeth, in selected cases with class III open-bite deformity, and when simultaneous maxillary and mandibular procedures are to be done, this procedure must be considered. In the latter instance when the mandibular body ostectomy, as opposed to ramus osteotomies, is done the mandibular surgery can be done first and there will be an "intact" mandible to advance the maxilla to. This results in a much more stable overall treatment result.

The feasibility of performing this procedure depends on carefully done definitive model surgery in which not only correction of the anteroposterior discrepancy but the transverse changes and rotational effects on the mandibular condyles are judged. Generally with the posterior mandibular body ostectomy the proximal segments must be rotated somewhat medially or the midline of the symphysis must be osteotomized to widen the interarch distance so that properly oriented distal and proximal segments result. Although it is sometimes possible to perform only the posterior body ostectomies of the mandible, it is more often necessary to simultaneously perform adjunctive mandibular osteotomies to achieve the desired esthetic, functional, and occlusal results. Those simultaneous mandibular procedures most often indicated are:

1. Simultaneous midsymphysis osteotomy
2. Simultaneous horizontal osteotomy
3. Simultaneous sagittal ramus osteotomy

The midsymphysis osteotomy is indicated to widen or narrow the anterior arch width to make it compatible with the posterior mandibular arch and maxilla. On occasion it may be indicated to perform an ostectomy through an incisor space to accommodate a maxillary-mandibular anterior tooth mass discrepancy. The simultaneous horizontal symphysis osteotomy or genioplasty is often indicated to reduce excessive anterior face height, straighten a deviated chin, or even augment the chin. The simultaneous sagittal ramus osteotomy can be utilized to upright unusually tipped posterior teeth and close posterior spacing.

Each of these adjunctive procedures is described and illustrated following the description and illustration of the posterior mandibular body ostectomy.

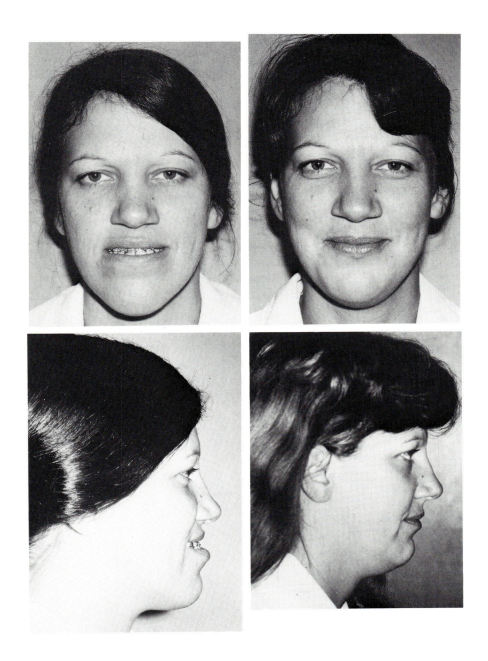

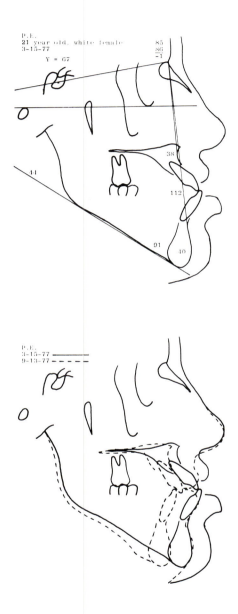

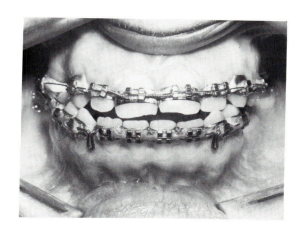

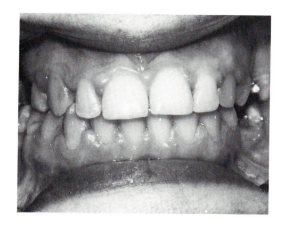

POSTERIOR BODY OSTECTOMY

Plate 3-2

A. The illustrated case demonstrates mandibular prognathism, Class III malocclusion, slight posterior crossbite, and the mandibular first molars missing. Bilateral posterior mandibular body ostectomies will be performed.

B. An incision is made around the cervical margins of the teeth, beginning one tooth distal to the proposed ostectomy site and carried at least one tooth anterior to the site and extended vertically into the vestibule. This incision can be extended posteriorly up the external oblique ridge for more relaxation. However, it is more important that adequate anterior relaxation be achieved. For this reason, in part, it is preferable to extend the incision anteriorly to the first premolar. In addition, when it is extended anteriorly like this it can be made into the sulcus by cutting directly down to bone without possible injury to the mental nerve.

C. The attached gingiva and mucoperiosteum are reflected inferiorly by subperiosteal dissection exposing the mental nerve as it exits from its foramen. The mental nerve is released from the surrounding periosteum and the soft tissues reflected from the entire lateral and inferior border of the mandible in the region of the proposed ostectomy. A channel retractor is inserted beneath the inferior border of the mandible in the area of the planned ostectomy.

D. Calipers are used to mark the lateral cortical bone where the vertical ostectomy cuts are to be made, as predetermined by the model surgery and the cephalometric prediction tracing. In addition, at the level of the inferior alveolar neurovascular bundle, as determined by the radiographs, an additional "window" is marked for removal to aid with identification and mobilization of the inferior alveolar neurovascular bundle. With a bur the lateral cortex is carefully cut along the proposed lines as marked. The cortex is then cut through superiorly and inferiorly, joining one vertical cut with the other.

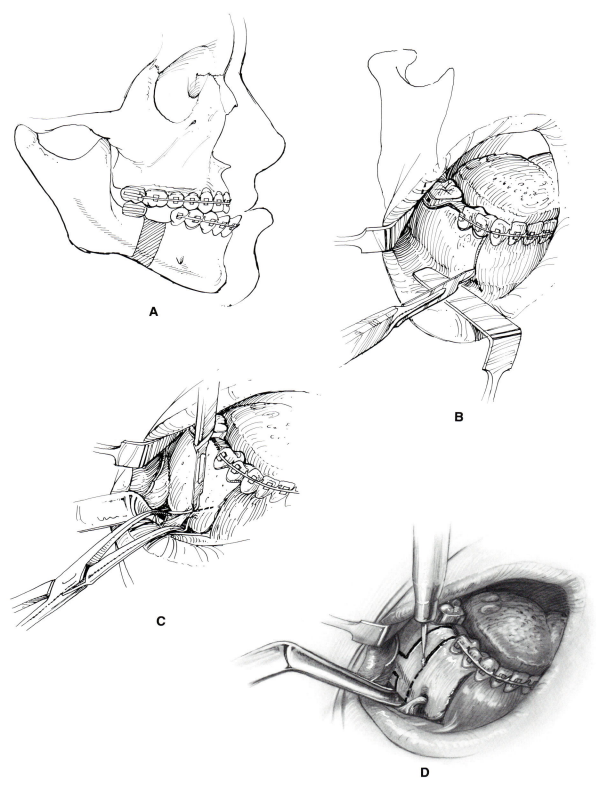

A

B

C

D

POSTERIOR BODY OSTECTOMY

Plate 3-2

E. The lateral cortex is then fractured off with an osteotome, exposing the medullary bone. In the region of the inferior alveolar neurovascular bundle the medullary bone is carefully removed with a curret to identify and expose the inferior alveolar neurovascular bundle. Generally there is a rather rigid but thin cortical bony canal surrounding the bundle.

F. After the inferior alveolar neurovascular bundle is well exposed and mobilized, the lingual ostectomy is done. In doing this a periosteal elevator is inserted from the superior incision to elevate the lingual mucoperiosteum adjacent to the ostectomy site and protect the lingual soft tissues while these bone cuts are being made.

G. With the bundle retracted laterally and inferiorly the vertical osteotomies are completed as well as the horizontal osteotomy, which is made low behind the neurovascular bundle. A horizontal strut of lingual cortex is maintained below the bundle.

H. The portion of the inferior cortex that maintains continuity to the mandible remains. It is important to maintain this cortical strut and the continuity of the mandible so that when the opposite side is being ostectomized the manipulations of the mandible do not crush and stretch this nerve, as they would if the ostectomy were completed. A through-and-through hole is drilled in the proximal and distal segments of the mandible below the level of the nerve. A 24-gauge mattress wire is passed but not tightened. The ostectomy is then *totally completed on the opposite side* and the inferior border wire and a bridle wire around the teeth adjacent to the ostectomy site tightened.

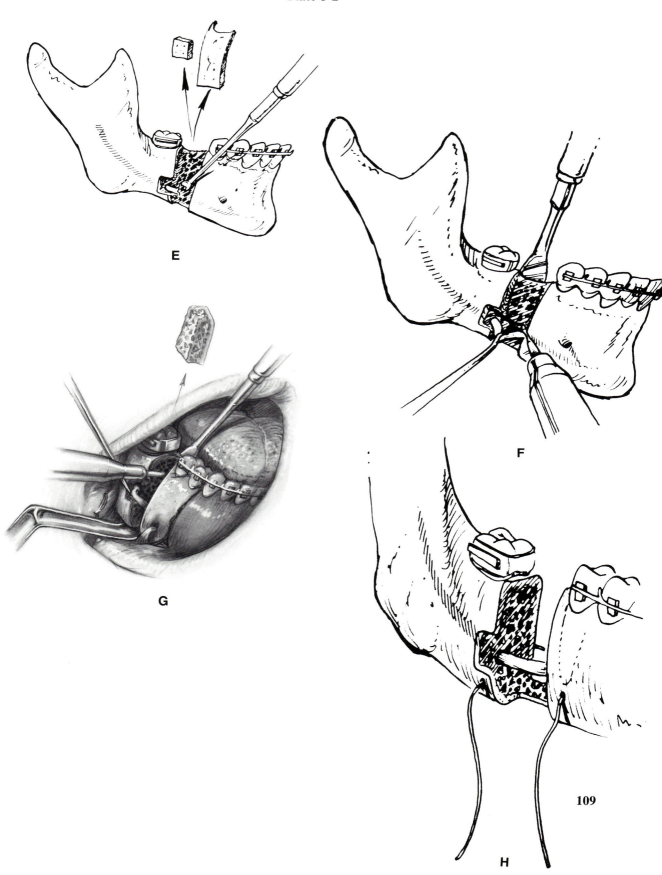

E

F

G

H

109

POSTERIOR BODY OSTECTOMY
Plate 3-2

I. Following completion of the opposite ostectomy and passive wiring, the original side is completed. The remaining strut of inferior cortex is removed, and the neurovascular bundle is gently retracted superiorly for access. A bridle wire is placed around the adjacent teeth, and the occlusal splint is tried in place.

J. Often the splint will not passively seat as there will be small areas of bone preventing the ostectomy site from being completely closed. These areas are most often on the lingual.

K. These areas of interference can be readily visualized and removed. In general it is better to have to remove some additional bone at this time than to originally remove an excessive amount. When an excessive amount is removed and poor bone contact results in the interdental area, a serious periodontal problem can occur.

L. When the teeth seat well into the occlusal splint, the splint is wired directly to the orthodontic brackets on the mandibular teeth, the inferior border and bridle wires are tightened, and the incisions closed before the jaws are placed in intermaxillary fixation. Again it is important that the splint be constructed so that the mandibular teeth seat deeply into it to prevent the various segments from being inadvertently tipped or rotated from their desired position.

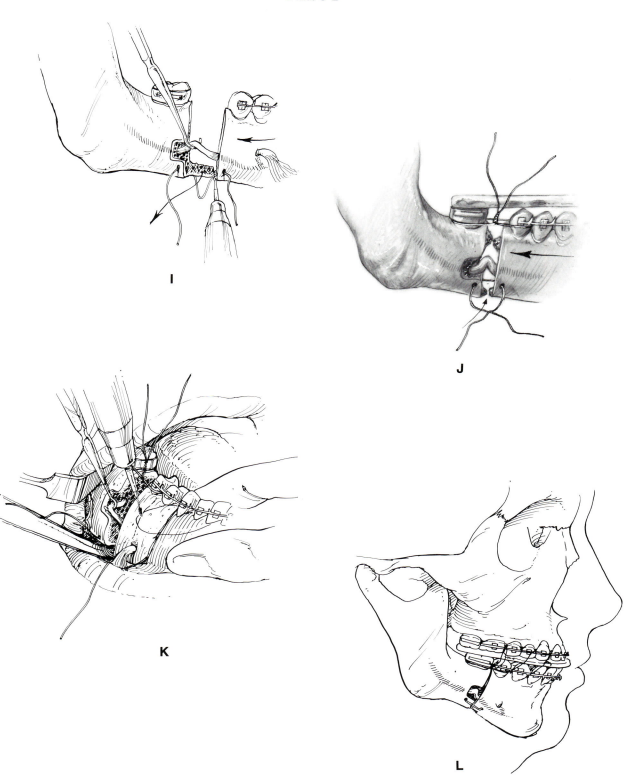

I

J

K

L

POSTERIOR BODY OSTECTOMY

Simultaneous midsymphysis osteotomy (Plate 3-3)

A. When the mandibular body ostectomy is performed with a simultaneous midsymphysis osteotomy, the lateral circumdental incisions are extended anteriorly and joined in the midline. From the depth of the vestibular incision a midline incision is made up to but not through the attached gingiva between the incisor teeth. Minimal reflection is done of this mucoperiosteal flap. The labial cortical bone is cut through from the inferior border of the mandible between the teeth to about 3 mm below the height of the crestal bone. At the *subapical level* the vertical osteotomy can be completed through both the labial and lingual cortices down to and through the inferior border of the mandible. In general, attempts to complete the lingual cortical cut in the area *between* the teeth will result in injury to the tooth roots unless they are unusually far apart (i.e., a diastema is present).

B. A thin, sharp osteotome is then used to complete the superior portion of the osteotomy between the teeth. A finger is placed lingually to detect the osteotome as it perforates the lingual cortical bone. The osteotome is directed from a superior or inferior angle so as to cut the lingual cortex with the corner of the osteotome. In this manner there is less chance of creating an adverse fracture of the lingual plate.

C. When the transverse mandibular molar width is to be *significantly narrowed,* it may be necessary to remove a small portion of the inferior lingual cortical bone so that the incisor teeth will not be separated as the segments rotate medially. This can be done by gently separating the segments with a periosteal elevator and using a bur to remove a portion of the lingual cortex directly. A heavy-gauge interosseous mattress wire is placed through both cortices in the inferior portion of the symphysis to stabilize the segments. However, this is not tightened until the splint is fitted and secured to the mandibular teeth.

D. Conversely, if the transverse mandibular molar width is *significantly increased,* a small amount of the inferior labial cortical bone may have to be removed.

POSTERIOR BODY OSTECTOMY

Simultaneous midsymphysis osteotomy (Plate 3-3)

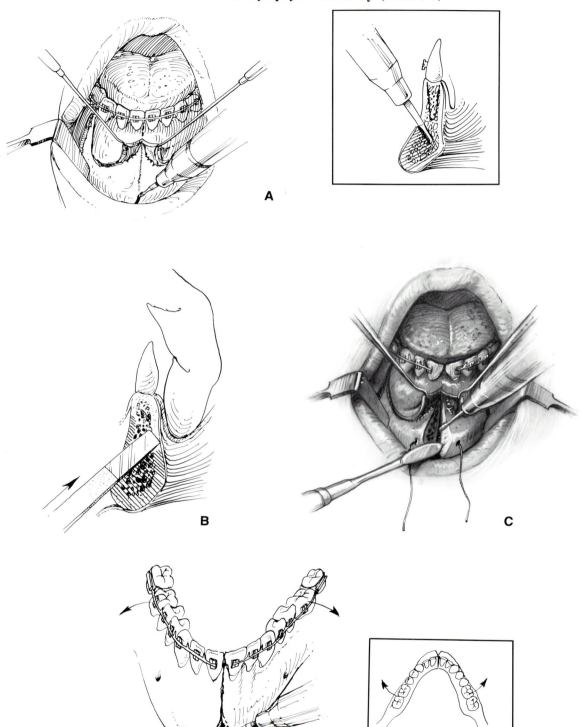

A

B

C

D

113

POSTERIOR BODY OSTECTOMY

Simultaneous horizontal osteotomy and vertical osteotomy (Plate 3-4)

A. A simultaneous horizontal osteotomy may be indicated to reduce an excessive vertical anterior facial height, straighten a deviated chin, or increase the projection of pogonion. In the case illustrated there is need to achieve all three of these objectives. In addition a maxillary-mandibular tooth mass discrepancy exists such that a central incisor will be removed and a midline ostectomy done. Vertical reference lines are made on the chin to accurately determine horizontal shifts. The proposed ostectomies are outlined. The horizontal ostectomy is completed as described in detail in Chapter 4, Genioplasties.

B. After the bony cuts are made and bone removed, an interosseous symphysis mattress wire and occlusal splint will provide stability to the superior segment. The genioplasty segment is repositioned superoanteriorly and stabilized to the mandible with two interosseous wires that pass in a figure-of-eight fashion through the labial cortex of the superior segment and lingual cortex of the inferior segment.

POSTERIOR BODY OSTECTOMY

Simultaneous horizontal osteotomy and vertical osteotomy (Plate 3-4)

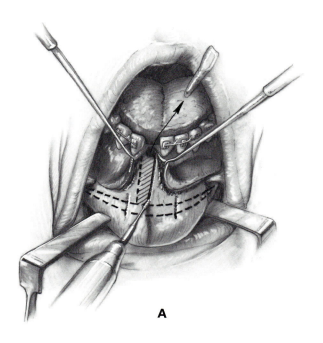

A

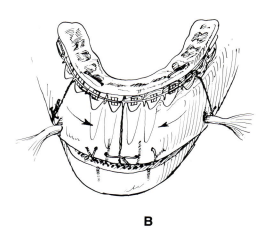

B

POSTERIOR BODY OSTECTOMY

Simultaneous sagittal ramus osteotomy (Plate 3-5)

A. The combination of a mandibular sagittal ramus osteotomy and a mandibular body ostectomy on the same side will permit uprighting of posterior teeth (labially, buccally, or medially) and closure of an edentulous space.

B. The soft-tissue incision is like that for the sagittal osteotomy except that the incision is extended farther anteriorly to about the premolar area in the depth of the mandibular vestibule to provide access for the mandibular body procedure. The mandibular sagittal ramus osteotomy is completed first as described in Chapter 2, the interosseous wire placed passively, and moist sponges inserted between the split segments to minimize trauma to the inferior alveolar neurovascular bundle during the body ostectomy procedure.

C. The body ostectomy is completed as previously described. If the posterior teeth are to be uprighted, as in this illustrated case, a large wedge-shaped section of bone is indicated for removal with the widest portion at the inferior border of the mandible.

D. Following completion of the body osteotomy the segment containing the mandibular molars is rotated forward and upward. An occlusal splint and bridle wire provide stability at the occlusal level. An interosseous wire is placed at the inferior border. Intermaxillary fixation is maintained for 6 weeks.

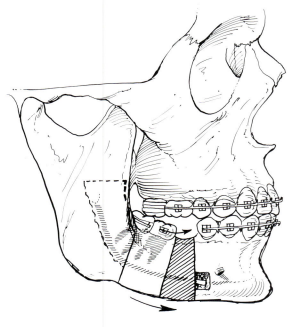

A

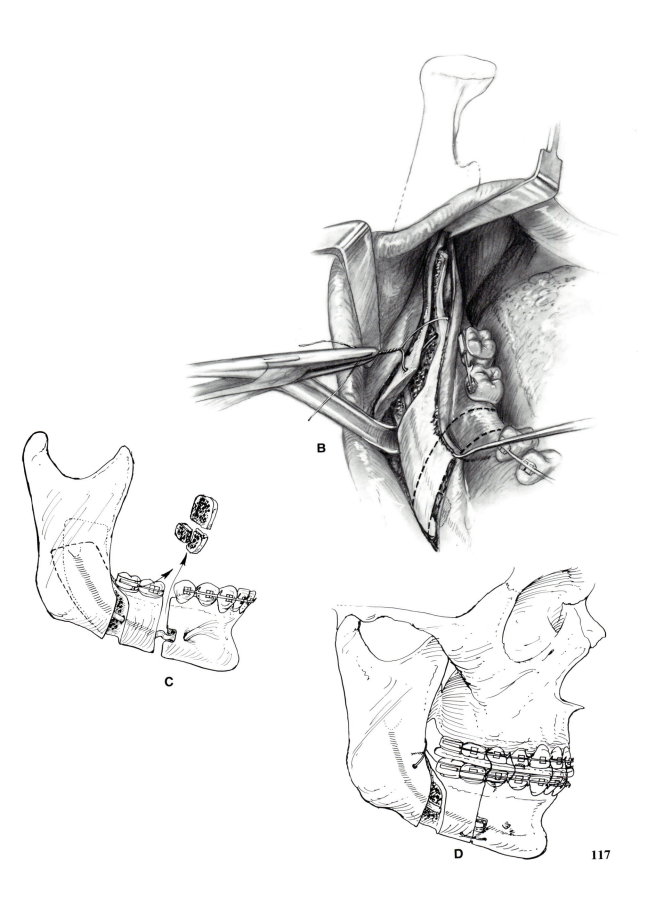

B

C

D

117

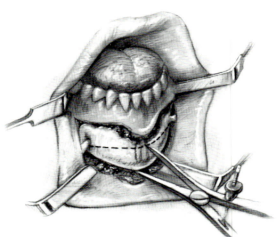

**AUGMENTATION
GENIOPLASTY**

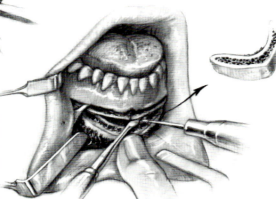

**REDUCTION
GENIOPLASTY**

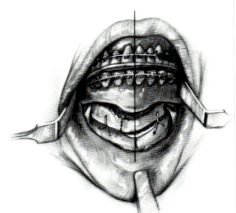

**STRAIGHTENING
GENIOPLASTY**

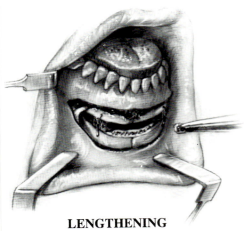

**LENGTHENING
GENIOPLASTY**

CHAPTER 4

Genioplasties

The morphology of the mandibular symphysis is highly variable in all three planes of space: posteroanterior, vertical, and transverse. Each of the various skeletal types (e.g., class II deep bite, class II open bite) tend to have "typical" morphology. The morphology of the mandibular symphysis, however, is highly variable in different individuals, even with the same basic types of dentofacial deformities. Accordingly the chin must be independently considered in the overall surgical treatment planning in order to achieve optimal esthetic and functional results.

Basically, genioplasties can augment, reduce, straighten, or lengthen the external chin. They are most often incorporated as adjunctive procedures and are done simultaneously.

In this chapter the techniques for performing the various types of genioplasties are illustrated and described in detail.

Augmentation genioplasty

The indications for augmentation genioplasty are predicated more on full-face than profile esthetics. In individuals with normocephalic or brachyocephalic faces, good esthetic results are usually achieved with a horizontal osteotomy and advancement of the inferior border of the mandible. Individuals with dolichocephalic faces (i.e., tapered or narrow chin) usually benefit esthetically more from lateral as well as posteroanterior augmentation with an appropriately shaped alloplastic implant or lateral chin alloplastic augmentation accompanyir the horizontal osteotomy.

The augmentation genioplasty is commonly employed as an adjunctive procedure in concert with various orthognathic techniques, such as mandibular advancement surgery, superior repositioning of the maxilla, anterior maxillary surgery, or mandibular subapical procedures, and occasionally as an isolated procedure in individuals who have an acceptable occlusion but a contour-deficient chin.

In treatment planning for a genioplasty, frontal as well as profile soft-tissue and skeletal morphology must be considered in order to assess the overall objectives to be achieved by the procedure. Basically, the surgeon must determine what alterations in the transverse, anteroposterior, and vertical dimensions are indicated and design an appropriate procedure to achieve these objectives. There is no standard operation for all patients. People most often see themselves from the frontal facial view. In this regard the frontal facial change is more important than the profile changes. Therefore the optimal esthetic change must be achieved in the frontal facial view. The amount of anteroposterior and vertical change for optimal facial balance can be determined primarily from the cephalometric evaluation. The transverse change, however, can only be determined by careful clinical evaluation of the patient.

There are two basic types of augmentation genioplasties: the sliding horizontal osteotomy of the mandibular symphysis and alloplastic augmentation of the mandibular symphysis. The indications for each of these are:

1. Horizontal osteotomy
    a. Increase chin projection when the facial morphology is normocephalic or brachycephalic
    b. Alter lower third vertical facial height and increase chin projection
2. Alloplastic augmentation
    a. When an anterior mandibular subapical osteotomy is done in conjunction with a genioplasty so as to avoid a second operation
    b. Increase chin projection and lateral bulk when the face, especially the chin, is dolichocephalic

These two basic augmentation genioplasty procedures are discussed and illustrated on the following pages.

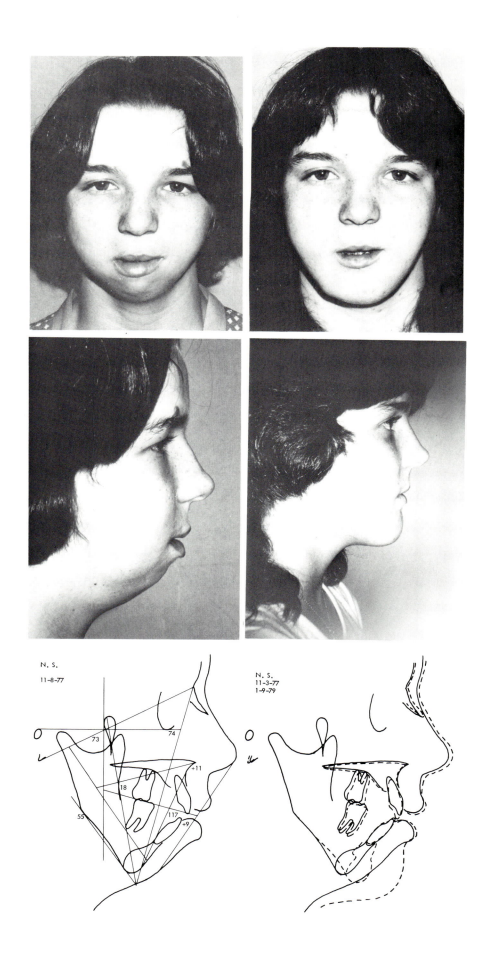

N. S.
11-8-77

73   74   +11   18   55   117   +9

N. S.
11-3-77
1-9-79

HORIZONTAL OSTEOTOMY

Plate 4-1

A. Most all genioplasties can be performed through the same basic intraoral approach. The incision we use is made in the lower lip with a diathermy knife approximately 15 to 20 mm from the depth of the vestibule in the midline when the lip is extended. The lip is pulled out with one hand so that it is kept tight, and this hand is used to help orient the incision so that it is not carried too deep toward the cutaneous surface. The incision is carried down into the obicularis oris muscle and then directed tangentially toward the mandible so that some muscle as well as mucosa remains in the flap adjacent and attached to the dentoalveolus. This will permit a two-layer soft-tissue closure. The incision extends laterally toward the depth of the vestibule in the cuspid area. The posterior extent of the incision is to the area adjacent to the cuspid–first bicuspid area but superior to the level of the mental foramen. This incision and the two-layer closure when appropriately sutured provide good superior support to the lip and prevent dehiscence of the incision.

B. Once the incision is carried to the bone the entire inferior border of the symphysis is degloved by subperiosteal dissection. The mental nerves are exposed by dissecting posteriorly along the inferior border of the mandible in the bicuspid area and elevating the mucoperiosteum. The mental neurovascular bundle can be safely and easily identified with this method.

The subperiosteal dissection is then extended above the mental neurovascular bundle and the initial incision extended posteriorly above the bundle if better exposure is necessary. The periosteum around the bundle is incised for relaxation to minimize retraction tension.

The digastric muscles are moved from the mandible to reduce the muscle tension they otherwise would exert on the advanced bone. The geniohyoid muscles remain attached and provide a major portion of the vascular supply to the osteotomized segment.

The periosteum that has been reflected off the inferior border of the mandible is incised transversely to permit soft-tissue relaxation to provide adequate coverage when the chin is advanced so lower lip height can be maintained. Generally the anteroposterior dimension of the symphysis is about 8 to 12 mm, so advancements of this magnitude can be done in a straightforward manner.

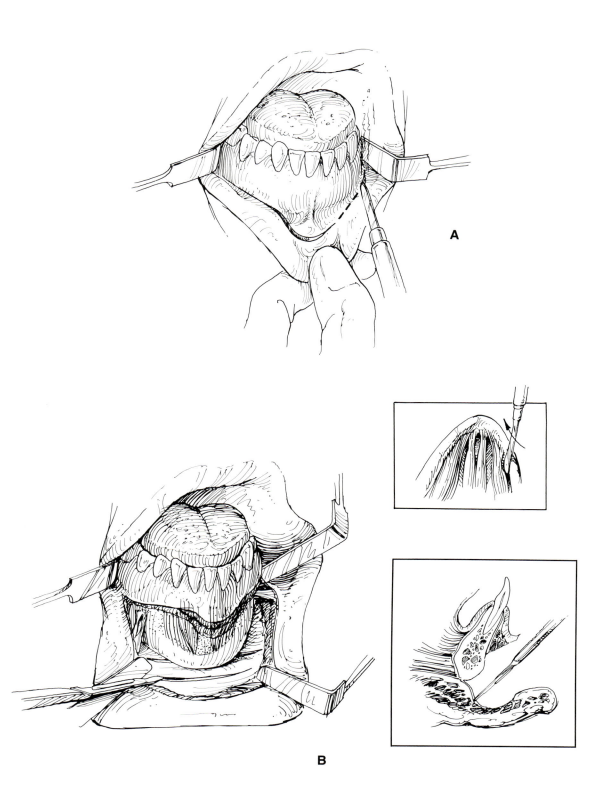

A

B

HORIZONTAL OSTEOTOMY

Plate 4-1

C. The bone cut is made so that the maximum amount of bone is advanced without injuring the cuspid apices or mental nerves. The horizontal osteotomy is made at least 4 to 5 mm below the apices of the cuspids and 3 to 4 mm below the level of the mental foramen so as not to jeopardize these structures. The angle at which the anteroposterior horizontal aspect of the osteotomy is made can predictably alter facial height simultaneously with advancement. The exact angle of the cut is planned from the cephalometric prediction tracing. Varying the angle of the cut can maintain, reduce, or even lengthen the lower third face height. The posterior extent of the horizontal osteotomy and its vertical relationship in the bicuspid area can be accurately transposed from the prediction tracing to the patient at surgery by relating these aspects to the anatomic position relative to the mental foramen.

D. The bone cut is completed through both the labial and lingual cortices. Care is given to be certain that the osteotomy is completed through the lingual cortex at the posterior extent of the bone cuts so that aberrant pathologic fracture of the lingual cortex will not occur in this area.

E. Following completion of the cut bilaterally the lingual aspect of the cut is checked for completeness with an osteotome, and the segment is then mobilized inferiorly. The mobilized segment is pedicled to the geniohyoid muscle and some lingual periosteum. Once the segment is mobilized any lingual cortical irregularities, which may prevent an even sliding forward of the inferior segment, are removed under direct visualization.

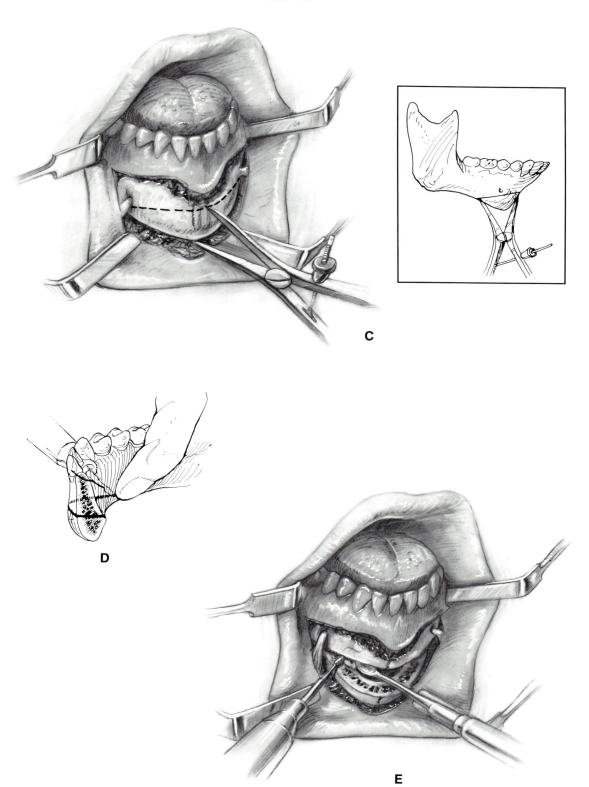

C

D

E

HORIZONTAL OSTEOTOMY
Plate 4-1

F. There are numerous methods to stabilize the inferior segment. The methods described here are those that we most often employ. Holes are placed through the lingual cortex of the mobilized inferior segment and buccal cortex of the stable superior segment in the midline and on each side. *The lateral holes in the inferior segment are placed distal to the superior holes* so the wire, as it is tightened, pulls the mobilized portion of the chin forward to the desired degree. To facilitate placement of the lateral holes the mobilized segment can be slightly overadvanced the desired degree and the lateral holes drilled in alignment with the lateral holes in the stable segment. Figure-of-eight wires or mattress wires are placed through these three holes and tightened. Proper placement of the wires prevents posterior displacement of the segment and allows gradual tightening to achieve the desired degree of advancement. The predetermined degree of advancement is achieved by direct measurements.

G. An alternative wiring technique is to place holes through both cortices of the lateral aspect of the superior segment. Wires are passed through these holes and then circumferentially around the inferior segment. Notching the inferior border at the appropriate area for the desired degree of advancement will keep the wire and segment from slipping out of place. This technique is useful for more major advancements or when the two segments will overlap some.

H. The incision is closed in two or three layers with absorbable sutures. The first suture of each layer is placed in the midline to properly align the soft tissues. The deep sutures are placed so as to maximally elevate the lip. By suturing the periosteum from the lip flap to the periosteum of the gingival flap, good support will be provided to the lip. Note that the periosteum has been incised along the inferior border of the symphysis to permit adequate soft-tissue relaxation.

I. With major advancements the periosteal relaxing incision should be made and relaxation obtained by pulling the lip and chin tissue up and out. If this is not done the lower lip may be retracted with the subsequent scarring and heal inferiorly, resulting in unsightly excessive exposure of the lower teeth and difficulty for the patient in closing the lips. A supportive chin dressing is applied to support the soft tissues holding the lip up, also eliminating dead space so better definition of the labiomental fold will be achieved.

126

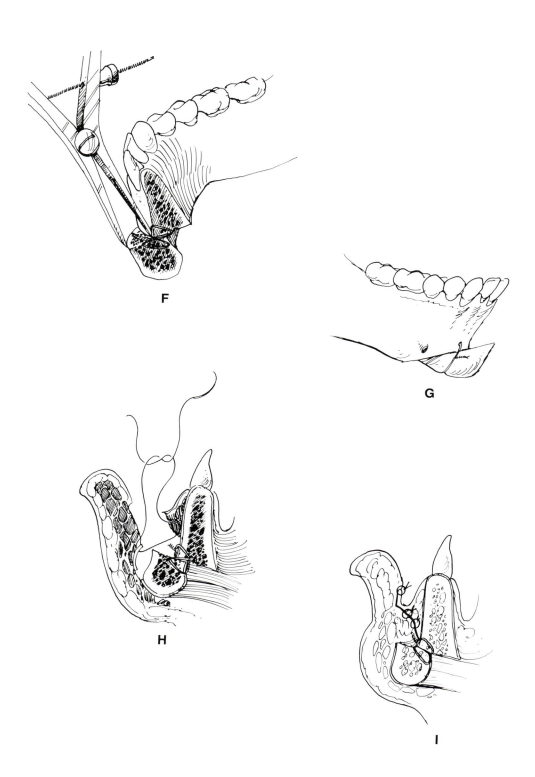

F

G

H

I

HORIZONTAL OSTEOTOMY

Plate 4-1

J. The variation in angulation of the horizontal osteotomy can shorten or lengthen the lower third facial height. The greater the acute angle of the osteotomy relative to the mandibular plane, the greater the tendency to shorten the facial height. In cases of severe microgenia two levels of oste-otomies can be done to telescope the advancement forward to achieve twice the amount of advancement, yet maintaining good bony contact between all segments.

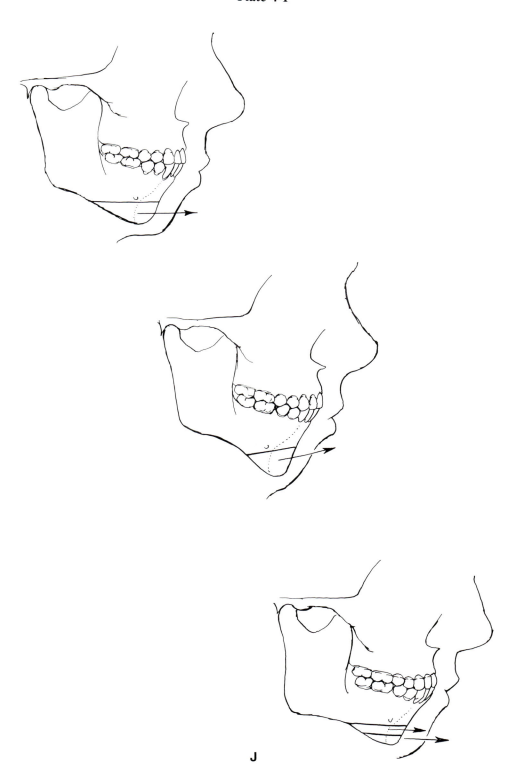

J

ALLOPLASTIC AUGMENTATION
Plate 4-2

A. Alloplasts have been used in genioplasties for many years. Technically the procedure is easier than the horizontal osteotomy. The use of an alloplast for chin augmentation is of significant advantage when a mandibular subapical procedure is done simultaneously; thus a second operation is avoided. Because alloplasts can be readily shaped at the time of operation, they are more versatile when lateral augmentation of the symphysis is desired as well as for additional chin projection in persons with tapered chins. The case illustrated involves a dolichocephalic facial type with a tapered chin. Horizontal osteotomy often tends to make this type of patient appear to have a *more tapered chin when viewed frontally.* By proper shaping of the alloplast, as illustrated, bulk can be added laterally to eliminate the pointedness of the chin.

ALLOPLASTIC AUGMENTATION
Plate 4-2

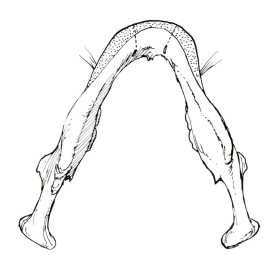

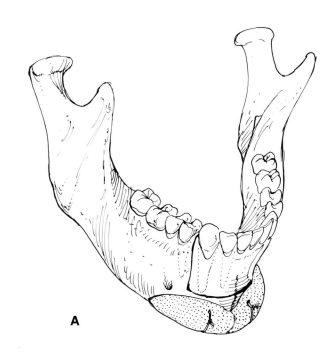

A

131

ALLOPLASTIC AUGMENTATION

Plate 4-2

B. The incision and dissection is performed exactly as described for the horizontal osteotomy genioplasty (Plate 4-1). The periosteum reflected from the inferior border of the symphysis is incised and generously separated to achieve relaxation so that the presurgical lip height can be maintained. In some individuals, particularly in cases of high angle where a large alloplastic implant is being placed, extensive soft-tissue undermining well into the neck through this periosteal incision may be required to obtain sufficient soft-tissue relaxation. On completion of the soft-tissue dissection the implant is shaped and placed temporarily in place for visual inspection of the external appearance and to test for adequate soft-tissue relaxation. The degree of anteroposterior augmentation can be accurately ascertained from the cephalometric evaluation. The lateral augmentation, however, must be determined from a thorough clinical evaluation. Two holes are then placed on each side of the mandibular symphysis at its inferior border and wire inserted to stabilize the implant. The wires will be passed through the body of the implant at the desired superoinferior position.

C. The alloplastic implant, which has been appropriately shaped at the time of surgery, is wired in place with care so that it is well centered. Centering the implant is done by marking the midline of the implant and aligning this with the facial, dental, or skeletal midline, whichever is appropriate. Lower third facial height can be slightly altered by the positioning of the implant in a vertical reference to the inferior aspect of the symphysis. Placing the implant slightly above the inferior aspect of the symphysis will give the illusion of shortening the face. Placing the implant as low as possible relative to the inferior border will give the impression that the face has been lengthened. The more inferior the placement of the implant and the broader its base contact on the bone, the less underlying bone resorption occurs. The incision is closed in layers and the supportive chin dressing applied as described for the horizontal osteotomy (Plate 4-1, *H* and *I*).

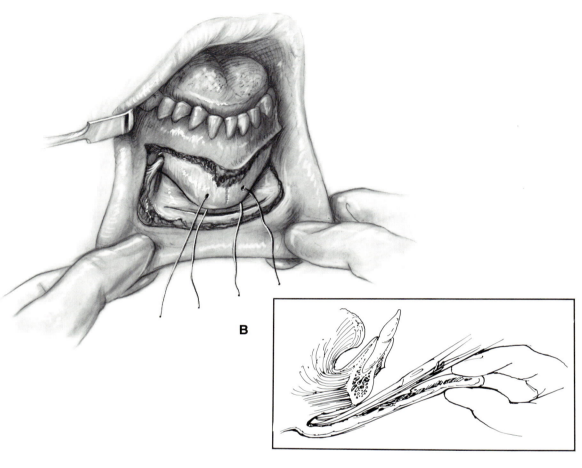

B

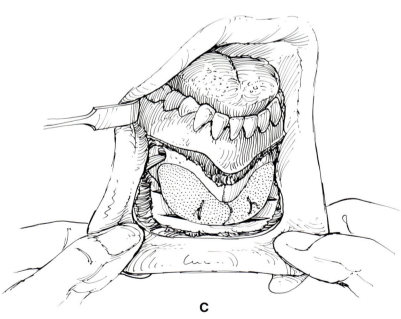

C

Reduction genioplasty

Two basic aspects of treatment planning for macrogenia are important: (1) an exact delineation of the anatomic-morphologic type of macrogenia that exists and (2) utilization of a surgical approach that will give predictable results. Each of these is briefly discussed.

First the frontal and profile esthetic features of the patient with macrogenia must be evaluated clinically and radiographically. This is important because some individuals with "cephalometric macrogenia" do not appear to have large chins clinically, and vice versa. Variations in soft-tissue thickness must also be assessed because that aspect definitely affects the esthetics. When soft-tissue thickness in the chin area is significantly less or greater than normal, the amount of alteration of the osseous support could be greater or lesser for the desired esthetic result than would be required if soft-tissue thickness is normal. Next, correlation of the clinical and radiographic examination is done, and it is determined whether clinical and radiographic macrogenia exists. It is helpful to divide osseous macrogenia into three subgroups, depending on the vectors of growth involved. The first subgroup involves overgrowth primarily in the anterior direction. The second subgroup shows primarily an increase in growth vertically. The third subgroup demonstrates increased growth in both a downward and an anterior direction and is manifested by an increased lower facial height and an increased anterior projection of the chin. Obviously there is a continuum from one type to the next, but in most circumstances one type predominates. These different entities must be approached surgically in different ways if the specific deformity is to be optimally corrected.

In the past macrogenia has generally been ignored or treated most often by simply degloving the symphysis and cutting off a given amount of the inferior aspect. This technique provides extremely poor and unpredictable results. Although the osseous height is decreased, the soft tissues *do not* demonstrate predictably the same change and in fact may increase in thickness in the submental area to where no appreciable change is noted. To achieve predictable esthetic results the symphysis *must not* be degloved with this operation, and therefore the actual removal of bone must be done between the apices of the teeth and the inferior portion of the symphysis. The technique is illustrated as follows.

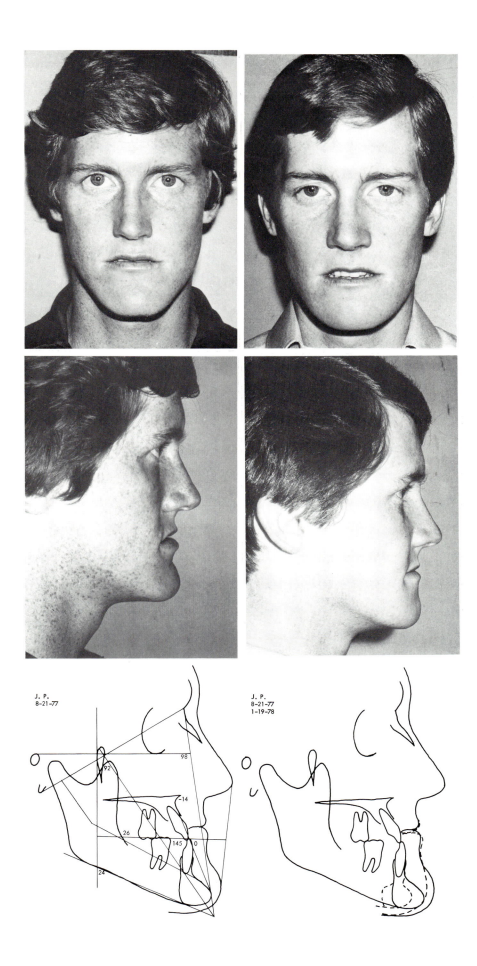

J. P.
8-21-77
1-19-78

REDUCTION GENIOPLASTY

Plate 4-3

A. A reduction genioplasty can be achieved to decrease the size of the chin vertically, anteroposteriorly, or in both directions as determined by esthetic and cephalometric criteria. Like augmentation genioplasties, this surgical procedure is most often done in conjunction with other orthognathic surgical procedures to obtain optimum treatment results. However, the surgical technique varies significantly from that described for augmentation genioplasty. The three subgroups are illustrated here. In the case illustrated (morphology similar to that of subgroup three) both vertical and anteroposterior reduction is to be accomplished.

B. The initial soft-tissue incision is made in the labial vestibule exactly as described for the augmentation genioplasty; however, the anteroinferior aspects of the symphysis *is not* degloved. The anterior and inferior periosteum and overlying soft tissues remain attached to the inferior aspect of the symphysis, yet exposing an adequate amount of bone beneath the tooth root apices to complete the indicated surgery. However, directly below the mental foramen the soft tissues and periosteum are reflected off the inferior border to facilitate completion of the ostectomy through the inferior border. This minimal dissection will not jeopardize the final soft-tissue result. The midline of the symphysis is marked to maintain symmetry. In addition, if the combined anteroposterior and vertical reduction is to be done, it is most helpful to make vertical referent lines laterally in the bicuspid area to facilitate accurate repositioning of the mobilized inferior segment. This will better correlate the repositioning of the segment relative to the desired result on the prediction tracing. The predetermined amount of vertical bone to be removed is measured and removed as high as possible (4 to 5 mm below the tooth apices) to maintain a maximum amount of periosteum and soft-tissue attachment to the inferior symphysis segment. The indicated ostectomy generally tapers to the width of the bur as it goes posteriorly beneath the mental foramen, but the posterior width is individually determined from the prediction tracing to obtain the optimum desired esthetic results.

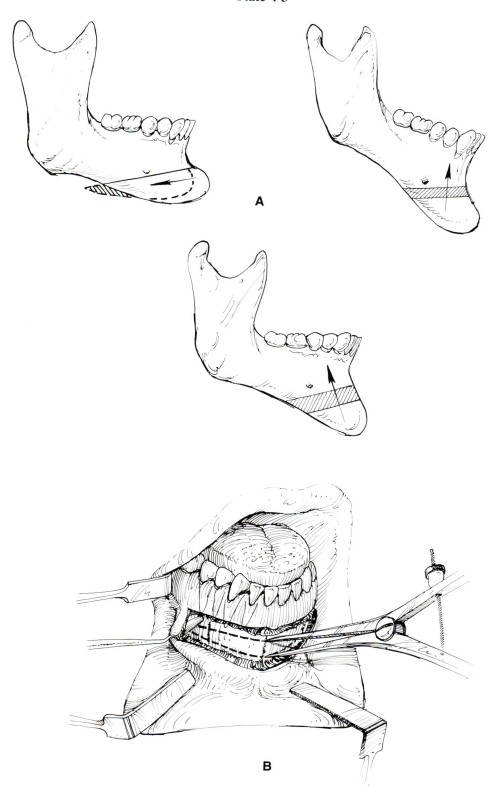

A

B

REDUCTION GENIOPLASTY
Plate 4-3

C. The two horizontal osteotomies are completed with a saw or bur, the lower cut being completed first. The superior osteotomy is then done and the bony wedge removed. It is easiest to mobilize the inferior segment following the inferior horizontal osteotomy and then complete the superior osteotomy to mobilize the wedge to be removed. The geniohyoid or genioglossus muscles, or both, will need to be detached from the segment. This is best done with a diathermy knife. The inferior portion of the symphysis with its attached soft tissues is mobilized inferiorly and with good direct visualization the superior and inferior lingual cortical margins checked for bony interferences.

D. Interosseous holes are placed through the superior buccal cortex on each side just distal to the area of the canine apices, and a properly located hole is made in the inferior segment. The location of the hole in the inferior segment is determined by manipulation of the mobilized segment into the predetermined position, as determined by the lateral referent line, and placing the interosseous hole directly below the superior hole.

After the wires are tightened the posterior corners are inspected and reduced if they protrude excessively. This is usually not much of a problem, because as the inferior border moves posteriorly it will be within the horizontal confines of the stable posteroinferior border of the mandible, which is wider than the anterior intrabody width. The surgical area is thoroughly irrigated, soft tissues closed in layers, and a supportive chin dressing applied. With this basic technique a predictable 80% to 100% soft tissue to osseous change can be anticipated, depending on the degree of change in the anteroposterior and vertical directions.

138

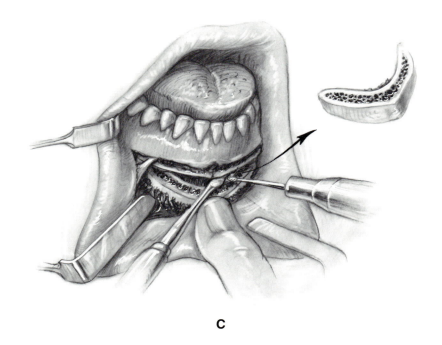

C

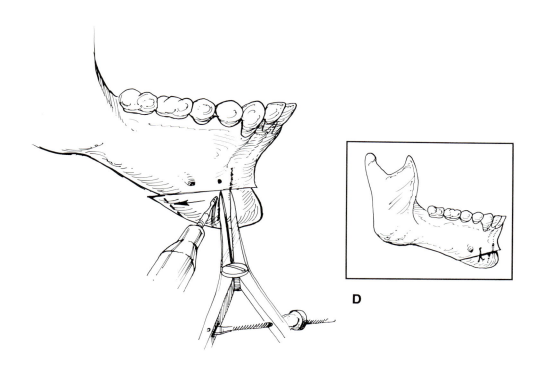

D

Straightening genioplasty

Straightening genioplasty is indicated in many patients with facial asymmetries in which the chin asymmetry is not completely corrected by appropriate repositioning of the jaws and occlusion. Some of the conditions necessitating this procedure for optimal treatment results are laterognathism, hemifacial microsomia, condylar hyperplasia, temporomandibular joint ankylosis, and simple chin asymmetry. This procedure, like other genioplasty procedures, is usually combined with other orthognathic surgical procedures.

The predictability of this procedure is predicated not only by careful planning but, like the reduction genioplasty, by maintenance of the optimum possible amount of soft tissues attached to the inferior segment. With significant asymmetry of the osseous chin component there is also a component of soft-tissue asymmetry. If the soft tissues are totally reflected from the inferior border, they *will not* rotate equally to the osseous change. Therefore the soft tissues must remain normally attached to the mobilized segment so that a soft tissue to bone change can be achieved.

Although a horizontal osteotomy is recommended to achieve straightening, because this technique will produce the most predictable result, alloplasts can be used similarly. However, when alloplasts are utilized the soft-tissue chin (external contour and muscles) does not move predictably, and thus the underlying supporting structures may be precisely straightened, yet the soft-tissue drape both at rest and during animation remains asymmetrical. This can be minimized by reflecting substantial periosteum and soft tissues off the symphysis and body of the mandible and then independently rotating and securing the soft tissues to the stabilized alloplast.

The use of the horizontal osteotomy to straighten the chin is illustrated.

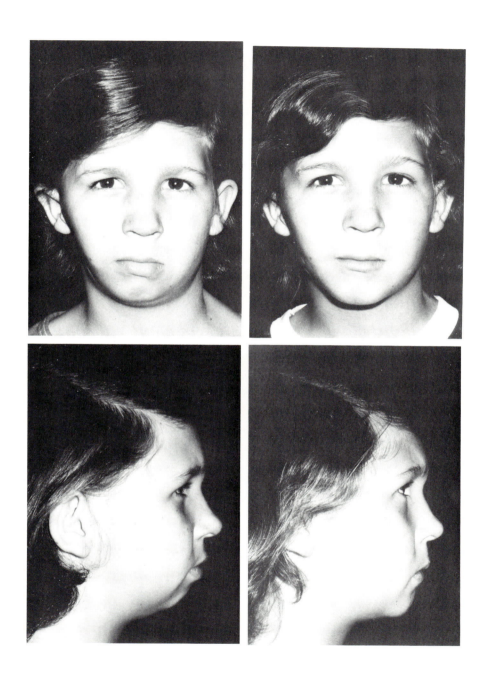

141

STRAIGHTENING GENIOPLASTY

Plate 4-4

A. In many instances the indicated orthognathic surgical procedure that corrects the major musculoskeletal disharmony and places the teeth into proper occlusion does not optimally straighten the chin, either transversely or vertically. In these instances a straightening genioplasty is simultaneously planned. Frequently this is done in conjunction with anteroposterior, vertical, or transverse augmentation or reduction of the chin. In these cases the degree of anteroposterior, vertical, or transverse alteration is determined primarily from the clinical evaluation because the amount of change will differ from the left to right sides. The surgical approach is the same as described for genioplasties.

B. The principles of this surgical procedure are essentially identical to those described for reduction genioplasty. The incision is the same, and the mandibular symphysis *is not degloved*. The midline of the symphysis is marked, and the appropriate bone cut is made. The segment is repositioned and stabilized with interosseous wires to match the facial midline. A layered closure is made and supportive chin dressing applied.

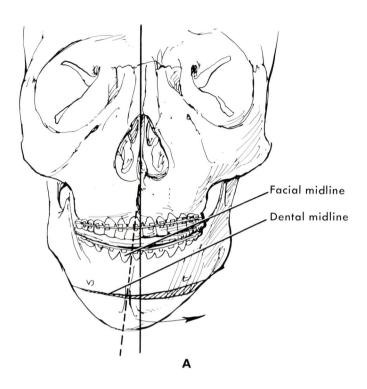

Facial midline

Dental midline

A

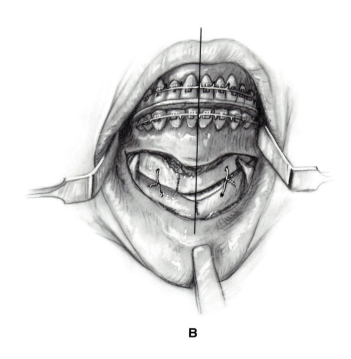

B

Lengthening genioplasty

Many patients with short vertical lower third faces, especially those with class I or class II deep bites, have as the primary deformity a decreased anterior mandibular vertical dimension. This condition is exactly the converse of macrogenia. To improve facial esthetics in those who will not benefit from mandibular advancement with clockwise rotation or a total subapical mandibular osteotomy with lengthening, a lengthening genioplasty should be considered.

The esthetic and cephalometric workup should be utilized to determine the magnitude of lengthening as well as any possible indication for simultaneous anterior or posterior repositioning of pogonion. With this procedure optimum osseous stability is achieved when the grafting is done utilizing a combination of three small cortical blocks for vertical stability and packing the remaining portion of the defect with fresh autogenous cancellous bone.

The technique is discussed and illustrated.

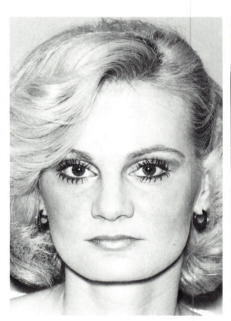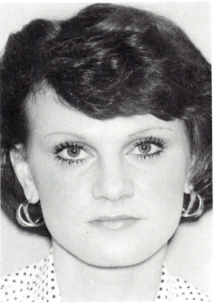

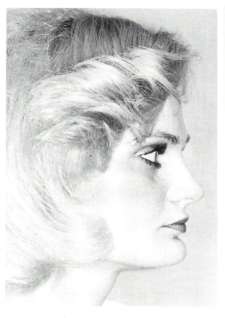

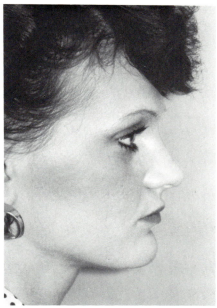

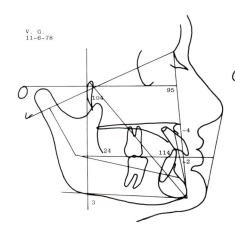

V. G.
11-6-78

95

104

24

114

-4

-2

3

V. G.
11-6-78 ― ― ―
12-8-78 ―――――

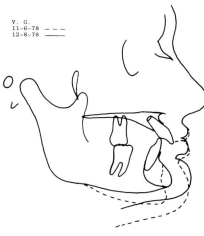

LENGTHENING GENIOPLASTY

Plate 4-5

A. This procedure is illustrated in a typical patient with a very short lower third face, satisfactory upper tooth–to–lip relationship, prominent labiomental fold, and a class I occlusion (which was obtained by conventional orthodontics). Utilizing the lengthening genioplasty procedure, the chin can simultaneously be advanced or retruded, as determined from the clinical evaluation and cephalometric prediction tracing to obtain balance with the middle third face.

B. The surgical approach is the same as for other genioplasties. However, there is variation relative to the periosteal attachment to the inferior aspect of the symphysis, depending on the clinical assessment of the patient. The patient must be evaluated clinically while standing with the mouth open to the point where the lips are relaxed and are just slightly apart. If the lower teeth are well below the level of the lower lip, equal to or in excess of the amount of vertical augmentation, then the periosteum and soft tissues *should not* be reflected from the inferior border of the symphysis (as in the reduction genioplasty and straightening genioplasty). However, if the lower lip is relatively short and the teeth are even with or above the level of the lower lip, then the periosteum and soft tissues must be reflected from the inferior border and the periosteum striated so the lip can be lengthened relative to the downward movement of the inferior aspect of the symphysis.

   In instances where this procedure is indicated there is generally less than a normal amount (vertical distance) of bone between the mandibular anterior teeth apices and the inferior border of the mandible. This makes the soft-tissue dissection and bone cut technically difficult when it is indicated to keep the periosteum and soft tissues attached to the inferior border, as discussed in the criteria above.

C. In doing the osteotomy, an attempt should be made to carry it as far posteriorly as possible, even to the anterior aspect of the gonial notch. On completion of the osteotomy interosseous holes and mattress wires are placed laterally through both labial and lingual cortices but are not tightened until after the bone grafts are inserted. Two or three blocks of cortical bone are shaped to provide the correct amount of inferior repositioning and stabilization. One block is placed anteriorly and one laterally on each side.

D. The desired vertical lengthening is checked with calipers, and the anteroposterior change is verified by the lateral vertical reference lines. The major bony defect is then packed with fresh autogenous cancellous bone so that rapid osseous union will occur. The wound is closed in layers and a supportive chin dressing applied.

146

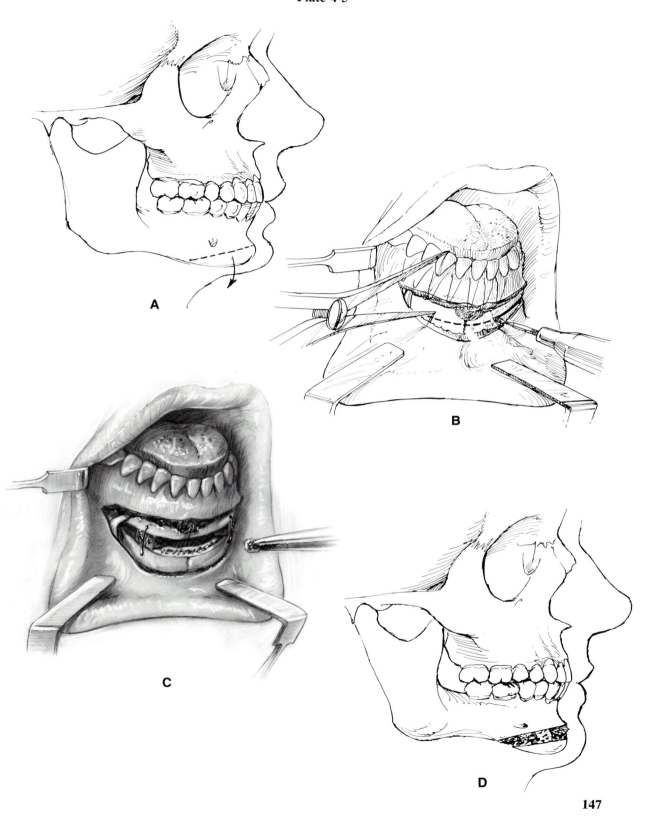

A

B

C

D

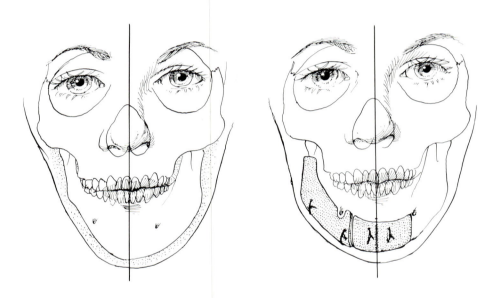

**ALLOPLASTIC AUGMENTATION
OF MANDIBLE**

CHAPTER 5

Alloplastic augmentation of mandible

When vertical and transverse mandibular body and ascending ramus deformities exist secondary to congenital, developmental, or acquired causes and good jaw function is present, alloplastic mandibular augmentation is a realistic alternative to bone grafting or dermal-fat grafts. In many such instances treatment results with alloplasts are better than with bone (as the amount of bone augmented decreases unpredictably with time following surgery) and with dermal-fat grafts (which also decrease in size). Moreover, many alloplasts can be readily carved or contoured and therefore can be more ideally shaped at the time of surgery.

Alloplastic augmentation of mandible

Full-face moulages have been advocated for this type of surgery to allow for precise presurgical construction of the implants. Despite their obvious usefulness, we have by and large abandoned these and rely on *direct preoperative* measurements from the patient's face and lateral and posteroanterior cephalometric radiographs with soft-tissue markers incorporated. A simple manner in which soft-tissue markers can be employed in the cephalometric radiographs is to paint fine lines with barium on the patient's face bilaterally. These are best placed in a vertical manner overlying the ascending mandibular ramus and more anteriorly in the premolar area. When the lateral and posteroanterior cephalometric radiographs are taken these lines are visible soft-tissue markers and provide a means of measuring the actual magnitude of both skeletal and soft-tissue asymmetries. From these clinical and radiographic measurements the alloplast can be shaped very close to the ideal before surgery, and finishing adjustments can be made at the time of the operation.

The surgical approach to augment the mandibular body or ramus or both can be either intraoral or extraoral. Each approach has its advantages and disadvantages. To date we have placed the majority of mandibular alloplastic implants via the intraoral route and have had few problems with postoperative infection that necessitated the removal of the implant. These results, however, are predicated on careful technique.

Illustrated and described is the basic intraoral approach for placement of a large alloplastic implant to reconstruct a vertically and transversely deficient mandible.

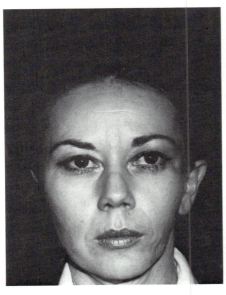 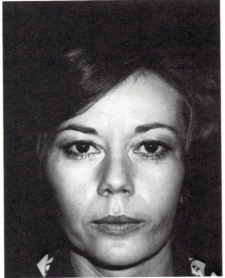

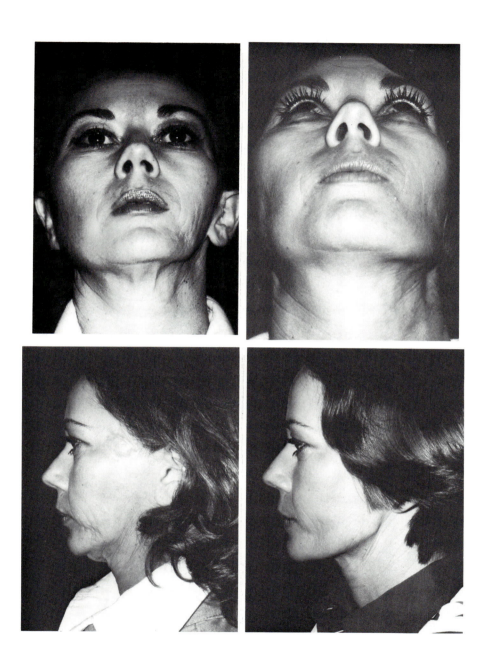

151

ALLOPLASTIC AUGMENTATION OF MANDIBLE
Plate 5-1

A. This case demonstrates both a vertical and transverse osseous deficiency on the right mandibular body and ramus. The alloplastic implants were prepared presurgically by the method described to a size slightly larger than desired so that precise contouring can be achieved at the time of surgery.

B. The patient has good jaw function, and the existing mandible is not considered structurally compromised to the degree that autogenous bone grafting is preferred. The incision is made down to bone, starting about halfway up the lateral aspect of the ascending ramus and carried to the distolateral aspect of the second molar. From here it is made around the necks of the teeth to the distal aspect of the first premolar on the same side and then extends tangentially into the vestibular sulcus. With this anterior extension the incision can be made down to bone in the labial sulcus with impunity because it is anterior to the exiting mental nerve. The anterior portion of the incision is identical to that described for alloplastic augmentation genioplasty (see Plate 4-1, *B*). This entire incision placement and subsequent closure is extremely important in that a watertight closure with primary healing must occur with alloplastic augmentation of the mandible to avoid infection.

C. Through this incision the entire lateral aspect of the ascending ramus, body, and entire symphysis are exposed via a subperiosteal dissection. To achieve sufficient soft-tissue relaxation for placement of the large implant the periosteum around the mental nerve, at the posterior border of the ramus, and along the entire inferior border of the mandible is reflected and multiple relaxing incisions are made through the periosteum. These relaxing incisions permit finger pressure to be used to develop a large ''pocket'' for the implants without excessive overlying soft-tissue tension. It is imperative that the soft tissues be well relaxed overlying the implant to prevent it from being secondarily forced into the bone. Releasing incisions in the periosteum can be placed in additional areas but are best kept in the inferior and posterior portions of the dissection.

152

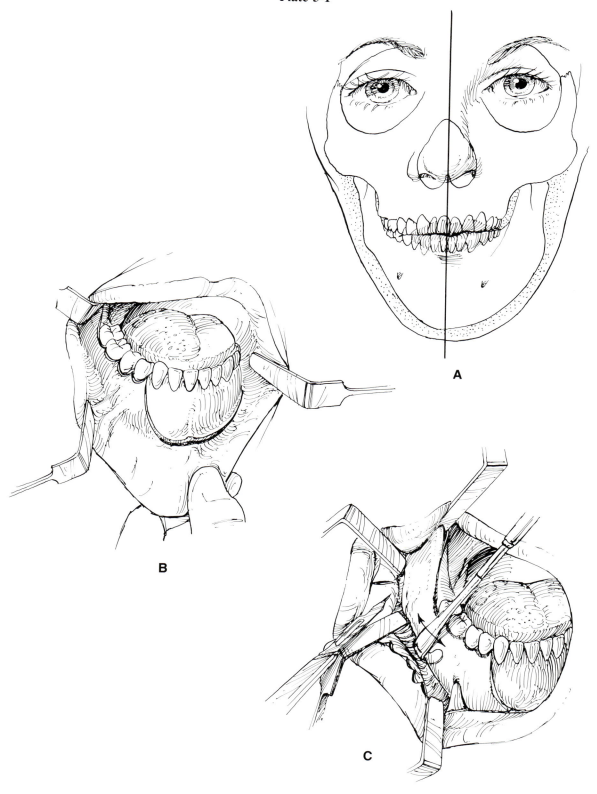

A

B

C

ALLOPLASTIC AUGMENTATION OF MANDIBLE
Plate 5-1

D. When excellent soft-tissue relaxation has been achieved by a combination of adequate periosteal relaxing incisions and manual stretching, the entire area and oral cavity are irrigated with copious amounts of sterile saline and the preformed mandibular alloplastic implants placed into the site for a test fit. When the implants are in place there should be no excessive soft-tissue pressure and it must adapt properly to the mandible. If excessive soft-tissue pressure exists, further releasing incisions are made to eliminate this. Adjustments to modify and reshape the implants are usually necessary (i.e., around the mental nerve and at its edges) so that they have a fine taper where they meet with the mandible.

   After the implants are judged to be properly contoured and well fitting and the soft tissues properly released, the implants are removed and the entire surgical site is again irrigated with copious amounts of sterile saline and the implants rinsed with saline. Hemostasis in the surgical site is important to avoid hematoma formation.

E. The lateral mandibular ramus and body implant of the type illustrated "locks" beneath the inferior and posterior border of the mandible and is therefore generally self-stabilizing. It may not require wire stabilization to the mandible. The need for wiring is determined by whether the implant *rests passively in the proper position without any tendency to displace*. Symphyseal or chin implants always require wiring to the inferior border of the mandible to ensure that they do not become displaced.

   If Proplast is the implant material used it is injected with about 5 million units of aqueous penicillin in 10 ml sterile saline. This is done to flush the implant out and will act much like a subcutaneous injection of the antibiotic.

   The incision line is then tightly closed with interrupted sutures. The posterior incision is closed with circumdental sutures, and anteriorly the incision is closed in layers. An external pressure dressing is applied to further aid in stabilizing the implants, reduce the possibility of hematoma formation, and minimize edema.

F. The corrected skeletal and soft-tissue facial deformity is illustrated.

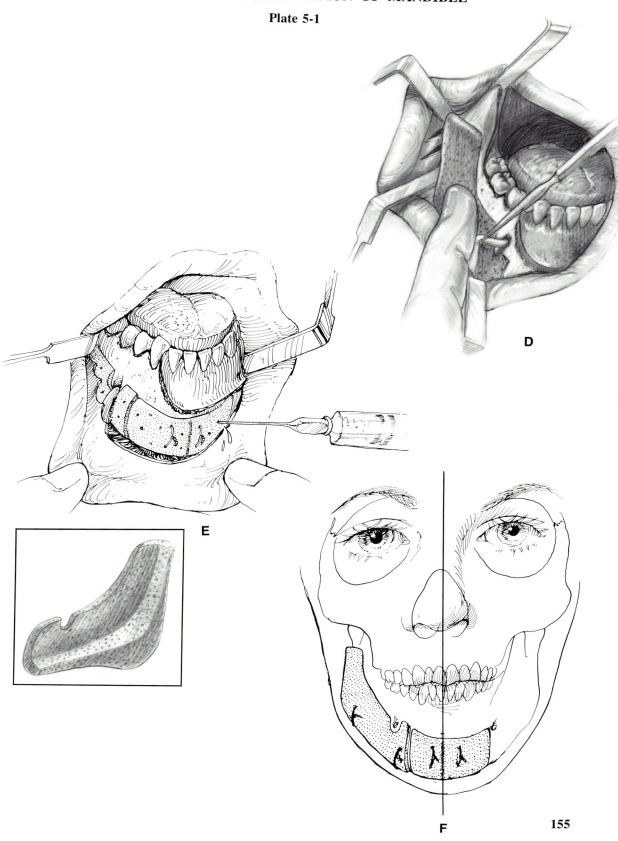

D

E

F

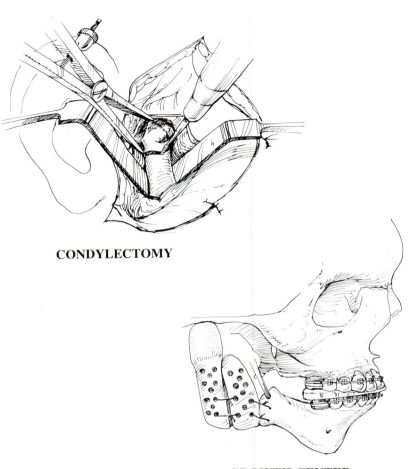

CONDYLECTOMY

**GROWTH CENTER
TRANSPLANTATION**

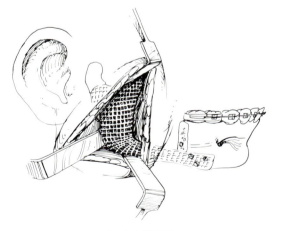

**ALLOPLASTIC
REPLACEMENT OF
MANDIBULAR CONDYLE**

CHAPTER 6

Temporomandibular joint surgery

In this chapter discussion of surgery of the temporomandibular joint is limited to those conditions involving the temporomandibular joint that are causative of or directly related to dentofacial deformities. In these instances condyle surgery must be considered in the overall treatment. Condylectomy, growth-center transplantation, and alloplastic replacement of the condyle are the surgical techniques most often indicated. These three procedures as they relate to dentofacial deformities are sequentially discussed in this chapter.

Condylectomy

The most common pathologic conditions requiring condylectomy in orthognathic surgery are condylar hyperplasia and osteochondroma. The abnormal growth in either condition, causing excessive increase in length and size of the condylar head and neck, will create various degrees of facial asymmetry. The severity of the resultant deformity is dependent on the age of onset, rate of abnormal growth, duration of abnormal growth, and actual type of abnormal growth.

Condylar hyperplasia most often occurs between the ages of 15 and 19 years but can occur at any age. Development of this condition in childhood or adolescence will result in increased vertical dimension of the condylar head and neck. In addition there is generally unilateral vertical elongation of the mandibular body with bowing of the inferior border, posterior open-bite deformity on the involved side, and chin shift toward the normal side. Moreover, in children significant skeletal and dental compensations occur with this condition and may include excessive vertical growth of the ipsilateral maxillary dentoalveolus, resulting in a canted maxillary occlusal plane; a crossbite on the normal side; shifting of the mandibular teeth toward the affected side; and shifting of the maxillary teeth toward the normal side. In effect these latter conditions tend to mask the developing deformity because they help to keep the teeth together in some semblance of occlusion.

When condylar hyperplasia develops in the adult the condition is not usually associated with the extensive compensatory growth factors or the severe dental compensations that are observed in adolescents. Inasmuch as these compensations do not tend to occur, the diagnosis is often made earlier because the individual notices his or her occlusion changing.

The specific form of surgical treatment for condylar hyperplasia depends on whether active growth is occurring or the pathologic growth process has been arrested. When the process is active, as ascertained by serial records taken 3 to 6 months apart, condylectomy is indicated to eliminate further abnormal growth and the associated skeletal and dental compensations. In addition condylectomy must also be considered when the condyle is excessively or unusually enlarged in order to establish definitive histopathologic diagnosis, when its enlargement (usually of a bulbous type) interferes with function, or when the patient has temporomandibular joint pain *specifically related to the abnormal condyle*. These conditions most often occur with osteochondromas of the mandibular condyle.

When condylar hyperplasia is of long standing with an arrested pathologic growth process and no pathologic temporomandibular function as documented by history, clinical examination, and appropriate records, condylectomy need not be incorporated in the surgical treatment. In these instances the deformity is corrected by any combination of procedures indicated to optimally improve facial esthetics and masticatory function. Procedures that may be indicated to produce the optimum esthetic and functional results in these instances are:

1. Contralateral ramus osteotomy
2. Ipsilateral ramus osteotomy
3. Ipsilateral reduction of the inferior border of the mandibular body
4. Straightening genioplasty
5. Maxillary leveling procedures

Clinical and histopathologic differentiation between condylar hyperplasia and osteochondroma of the mandibular condyle is not always clearcut. Generally osteochondroma of the mandibular condyle is differentiated from condylar hyperplasia by radiographic appearance. In condylar hyperplasia the involved condyle per se is not grossly abnormal anatomically; however, the condylar neck is excessively elongated. In osteochondroma of the mandibular condyle the condylar head is usually significantly enlarged and appears bulbous. Osteochondroma of the condyle usually occurs after the age of 25 years. Signs and symptoms may include developing open bite on the involved side, shift of chin to normal side, temporomandibular joint dysfunction, temporomandibular joint pain, and preauricular enlargement. Condylectomy is the surgical treatment of choice to eliminate the temporomandibular joint dysfunction or pain. When this is the indicated treatment, a bone graft or an alloplastic replacement is usually indicated in the adult patient to provide a functional joint. In the growing patient a growth-center transplant is usually indicated. If the condition has been of long duration, then dental and skeletal compensations may also occur, which may require adjunctive maxillary and mandibular procedures to optimally correct the existing deformity.

A description of the basic surgical technique for condylectomy in these two conditions is presented, followed by a description of vertical shortening of the mandibular body as is often indicated in concert with condylectomy in condylar hyperplasia. The various other adjunctive procedures that may be indicated for optimal functional and esthetic results include ramus osteotomies and genioplasties. These procedures are described in Chapters 2 and 4. Leveling of the maxilla is described in Chapter 8.

CONDYLECTOMY

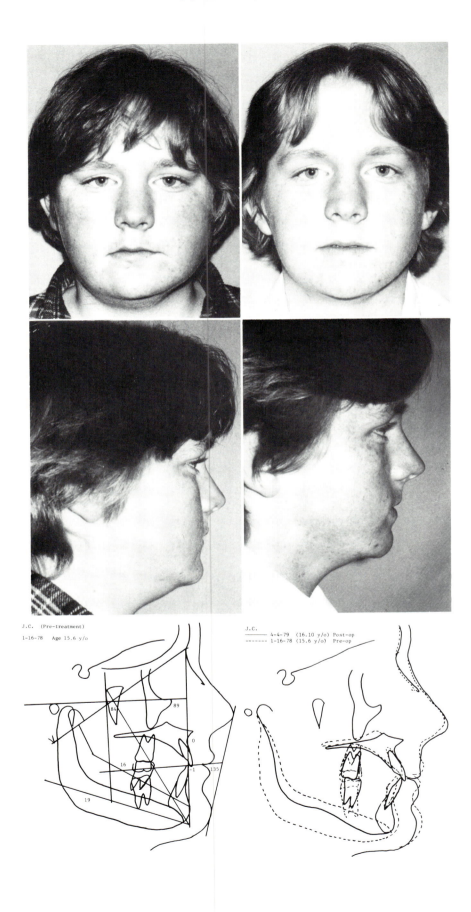

J.C. (Pre-treatment)

1-16-78   Age 15.6 y/o

J.C.

——— 4-4-79 (16.10 y/o) Post-op

------- 1-16-78 (15.6 y/o) Pre-op

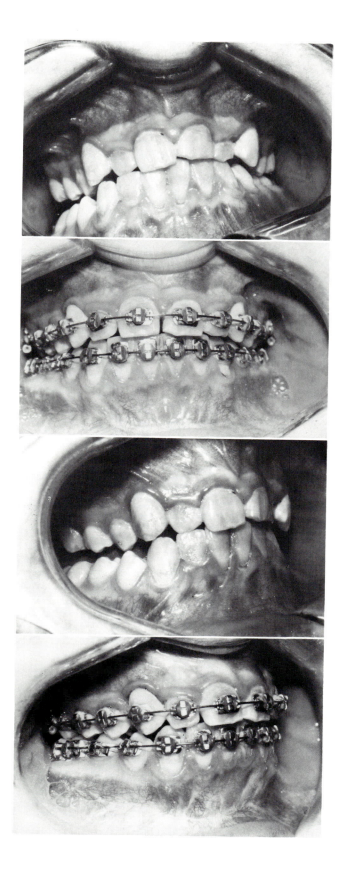

CONDYLECTOMY

Plate 6-1

A. The illustrated case demonstrates right condylar hyperplasia that has been actively growing for several years. The patient has an elongated condylar head and neck, increased ipsilateral mandibular body height, slight posterior open bite, a crossbite on the normal side, and a shift of the chin toward the normal side. Presurgical orthodontic treatment was done to eliminate the dental compensations, which always make the occlusion worse, yet permit optimum surgical correction of the overall dentofacial deformity. Primary emphasis in this section is on the condylar surgery.

B. The superficial temporal artery and vein are medial to the posterior aspect of the ramus at the level of the earlobe, then pass posterior and lateral to the ramus at the level of the condylar neck. They then course superiorly just anterior to the tragus of the ear. Adjacent to the superior helix the zygomatic-orbital artery branches off in an anterosuperior direction accompanied by its associated vein. The auriculotemporal nerve courses superiorly adjacent but posterior to the superficial temporal artery. The temporal branches of the facial nerve and the transverse facial vessels are also in close proximity to the condyle. In condylar hyperplasia the venous vascularity in the area of the temporomandibular joint is often increased.

   The preauricular approach to the temporomandibular joint is utilized to perform the condylectomy. The hair in the area is shaved and drapes positioned to expose the anterior aspect of the ear, lateral canthus of the eye, corner of the mouth, and angle of the jaw. Moist cotton is placed in the external auditory canal to prevent debris from collecting there during surgery.

CONDYLECTOMY

Plate 6-1

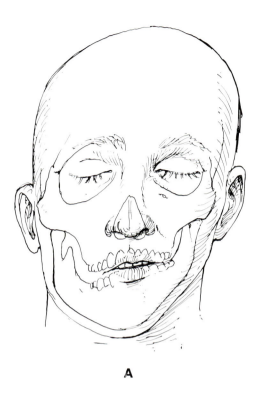

A

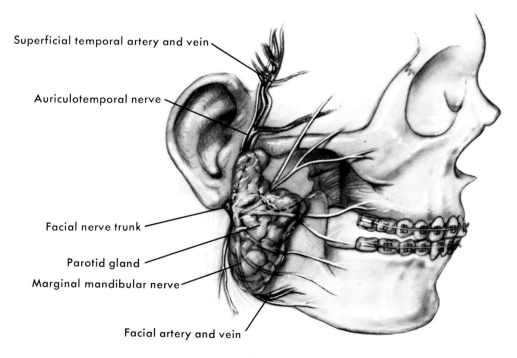

Superficial temporal artery and vein

Auriculotemporal nerve

Facial nerve trunk

Parotid gland

Marginal mandibular nerve

Facial artery and vein

B

CONDYLECTOMY

Plate 6-1

C. The incision is made in the skin creases just anterior to the ear and extends from the base of the lobe to the base of the superior helix. The incision is then directed at an angle of approximately 120° in an anterosuperior direction for approximately 2 cm. This incision is contained within the hairline. This will permit excellent exposure of the condyle. The initial incision is made through the skin and into the subcutaneous tissues. The skin is then undermined for several millimeters to pass superficially and anteriorly to the temporal vessels and auriculotemporal nerve. Once anterior to the superficial temporal vessels and auriculotemporal nerve, the superior limb of the incision is carried to the depth of the temporal fascia, which is readily identified superiorly above the zygomatic arch. By dissecting this tissue plane the temporal branch of the facial nerve will be in the superficial flap. Dissecting inferiorly in this plane downward will expose the fascia covering the zygomatic arch directly over the temporomandibular joint capsule. The dissection is carried forward, exposing the articular eminence and inferiorly exposing the temporomandibular joint capsule. The soft-tissue flap created can now be sutured down anteriorly for retraction.

D. A T incision is made through the fascia overlying the zygomatic portion of the temporal bone and lateral aspect of the temporomandibular joint capsule. The vertical limb of this incision extends down onto the neck of the condyle. The temporomandibular joint capsule and overlying fascia are reflected off the condylar head and neck.

E. Retractors are placed anteriorly and posteriorly to the condylar neck to afford good exposure. Calipers are used to accurately remove the excess condyle and neck as predetermined by the case workup. Generally the degree of ostectomy is determined by the degree of vertical change desired as well as the need to remove an adequate amount of condylar growth center in the case of active growth. For example, if a 5 mm posterior open bite is to be closed, at least this amount of condyle will have to be removed to close the open bite. Similarly this amount is usually adequate to remove the active growth center. In instances when the ipsilateral maxilla is severely elongated and will be simultaneously shortened, a considerably greater amount of condyle head and neck may be indicated for removal. If no open bite exists and no maxillary surgery is to be done, about 5 mm of the condylar head is excised to eliminate the active pathologic growth process. The ostectomy is completed with a fissure bur. Because the internal maxillary artery is in close approximation to the medial aspect of the condylar neck, care must be exercised as the bur cut approaches the medial soft tissues.

CONDYLECTOMY

Plate 6-1

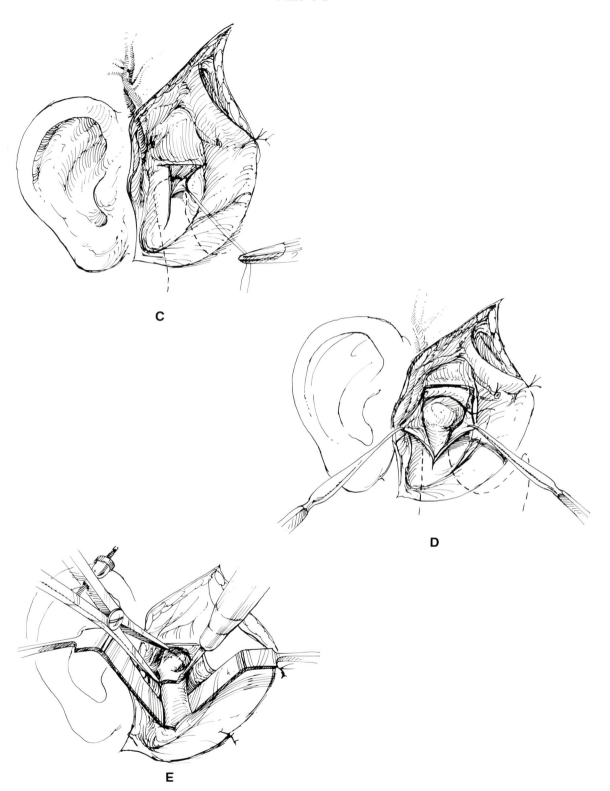

C

D

E

CONDYLECTOMY

Plate 6-1

F. To remove the mobilized condylar head, it is distracted in a lateroinferior direction, and the lateral pterygoid muscle is removed from the condylar head and neck with a diathermy knife.

G. The sharp edges of the condylar neck are smoothed. The surgical site is inspected and irrigated. The meniscus will generally be unaffected and is left intact.

H. As the condylar stump assumes its new position in the glenoid fossa, the mandible will rotate in a superoposterior direction. The capsule, as well as the subcutaneous tissues and skin, is closed in layers. The ear is carefully irrigated to prevent blood clots from forming against the tympanic membrane. A pressure dressing is applied over the surgical site for 2 days to eliminate hematoma formation under the flaps and to minimize facial edema. If no simultaneous ramus osteotomies are done, intermaxillary elastics are applied postoperatively to control the occlusion. These are used for progressively decreasing periods over 3 to 4 weeks. If simultaneous ramus procedures are done the patient is treated as any patient undergoing ramus osteotomies would be (see Chapter 2).

CONDYLECTOMY

Plate 6-1

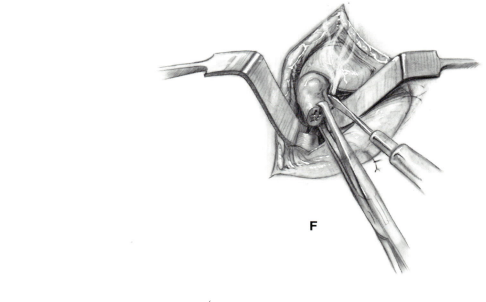

F

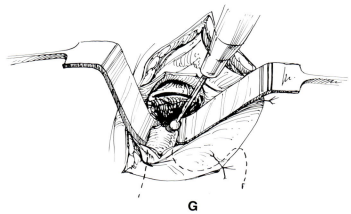

G

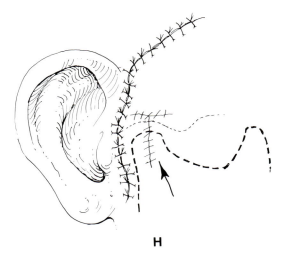

H

167

SPECIAL CONSIDERATION
CONDYLECTOMY

Condylectomy for large osteochondromas of mandibular condyle (Plate 6-2)

A. Large osteochondromas of the mandibular condyle can cause pain and masticatory dysfunction as well as some of the compensatory skeletal and dental changes usually associated with condylar hyperplasia. However, because these patients are generally older when the tumor develops there are usually less compensatory changes in the dento-osseous structures.

    When the osteochondroma is relatively small and involves primarily the condylar head, the surgery can be done through a preauricular approach as described and illustrated for condylectomy. In other instances, as in this case, the lesion may be very large and difficult to treat properly via only the preauricular approach. In these circumstances it is often beneficial to utilize a combined preauricular-submandibular approach to facilitate removal of the lesion and simultaneously reconstruct the temporomandibular joint.

B. The preauricular approach permits direct access to the tumor to facilitate its removal. After exposure of the tumor as completely as possible, its removal is facilitated by sectioning it and removing it piecemeal. Osteotomes are often helpful to complete the medial sectioning. In sequencing the removal of the tumor it is best to remove the medial aspect last, after the lateral aspect has been removed, so that if severe bleeding is encountered better direct access to it will be possible. The lateral pterygoid muscle will be attached to the most anterior portion of the tumor and must be removed.

C. Through the submandibular approach a subcondylar ostectomy can be done for removal of the inferiormost portion of the lesion or to provide excellent access for immediate reconstruction.

D. The temporomandibular joint is reconstructed with a costochondral graft or alloplastic substitute as illustrated. In the growing child it is always preferable to utilize an autogenous costocondral graft.

    Intermaxillary fixation is applied prior to the insertion of the new condyle so that the proper anteroposterior and vertical relationships can be maintained. Postoperatively when a prosthesis is used a course of intermittent, intermaxillary elastics is started, with progressive use of the jaw over 4 to 6 weeks. For the postoperative course when a costochondral bone graft is used, see Plate 6-4, *J*.

Condylectomy for large osteochondromas of mandibular condyle (Plate 6-2)

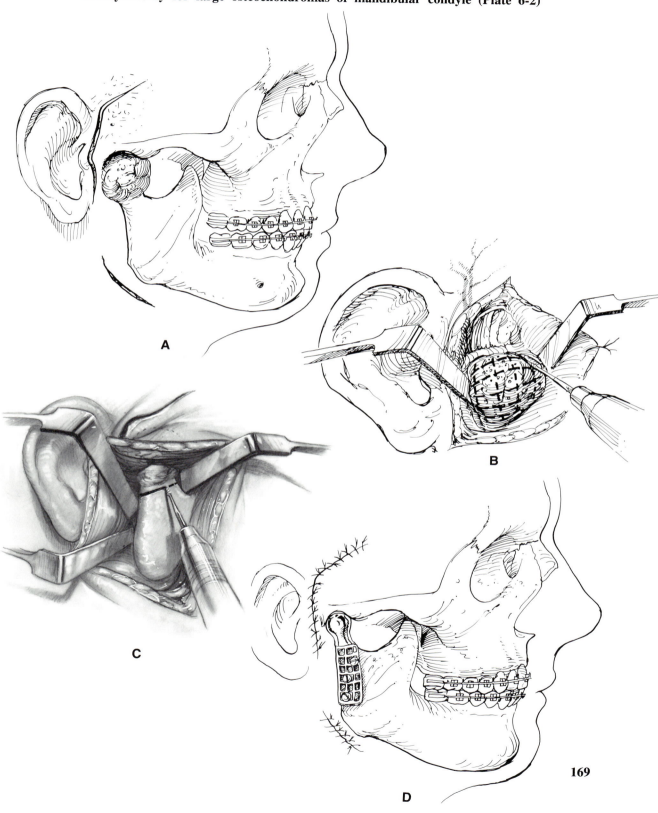

A

B

C

D

169

CONDYLECTOMY

Vertical reduction of ipsilateral mandibular body (Plate 6-3)

A. When condylar hyperplasia occurs during active growth there may be *excessive* vertical height of the mandibular body on the affected side that warrants correction to optimize facial symmetry. A vertical height reduction of the inferior border of the mandible can be accomplished via an extraoral or intraoral approach. The inferior alveolar canal may be located above or below the level of the intended ostectomy, as determined by preoperative radiographs. If located above the level of the proposed osteotomy the horizontal cut is simply made without concern for injury to the neurovascular bundle. When the inferior alveolar neurovascular bundle is located in the region of the proposed ostectomy, the procedure must be done so as to identify it and dissect it out.

B. The intraoral approach is our preference in most instances in order to avoid a facial scar. An incision is made with a diathermy knife beginning about one third of the way up the ascending ramus, overlying the external oblique ridge, into the buccal sulcus, and extending anteriorly to about the midsymphysis area. A subperiosteal dissection is done beginning anterior to the mental nerve, exposing it and dissecting it out. Next the entire lateral aspect and inferior border of the mandible are exposed from the angle to the symphysis.

The predetermined amount of bone to be removed is measured and scored. The horizontal osteotomy is made just through the lateral cortical plate. Anterior to the mental foramen the cut can be made through both the lingual and buccal cortices. Vertical osteotomies through the lateral cortical bone are then made to facilitate its removal with an osteotome.

CONDYLECTOMY

Vertical reduction of ipsilateral mandibular body (Plate 6-3)

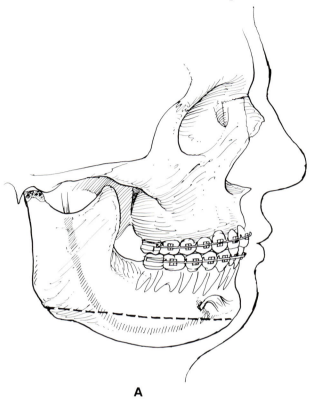

A

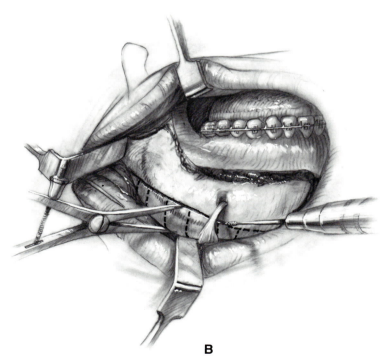

B

CONDYLECTOMY

Vertical reduction of ipsilateral mandibular body (Plate 6-3)

C. Small segments of the lateral cortex can then be removed carefully and the inferior alveolar neurovascular bundle identified within the medullary bone. Following removal of the lateral cortex the neurovascular bundle is carefully dissected out by removing the trabecular bone overlying it with a curret.

D. After it is dissected out in its entirety the neurovascular bundle is gently retracted to provide access to the lingual cortex. The ostectomy of the lingual cortex is then done and the inferior section of bone removed. The neurovascular bundle is left exposed under the new inferior border of the mandible.

   When the soft tissues are closed the periosteum is sutured so that it adheres tightly to the inferior border of the mandible. This may necessitate excision of some periosteum; however, if this is left lax and a hematoma forms between the periosteum and new inferior border, additional bone will form that will in part negate the desired result.

E. A postoperative pressure dressing is always applied to minimize facial edema, eliminate hematoma formation, and ensure close approximation of the soft tissue to the new mandibular structure so that an optimum soft-tissue change will occur. This dressing is to be left in place for 5 to 7 days postoperatively. Long-term radiographic follow-up usually will demonstrate a new cortical inferior border around the neurovascular bundle creating a new intrabony canal.

CONDYLECTOMY

Vertical reduction of ipsilateral mandibular body (Plate 6-3)

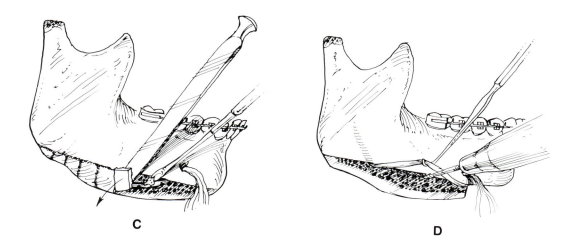

C

D

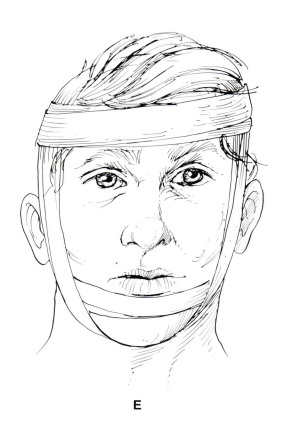

E

Growth center transplantation

Whenever the actively growing patient is missing a condyle (as in hemifacial microsomia), the condyle is destroyed (as in ankylosis), or the condyle must be removed because of neoplasia, consideration must be given to replacing it with an autogenous growth center. Available clinical and experimental studies suggest that the best growth center transplant for replacement of the mandibular condyle is an autogenous costochondral rib graft.

In instances where consideration is being given to a grafting procedure there must be *real* benefits to the proposed surgery. In many individuals with hemifacial microsomia in which there is only moderate alteration of the condylar structure, craniofacial growth and facial appearance do not significantly worsen with growth, and consequently costochondral growth center grafting is not indicated. In these mild cases various ramus osteotomies in concert with activator therapy produce predictably good results. However, when the entire condyle is missing and facial, skeletal, and dental asymmetry exist at an early age, costochondral growth center transplantation in concert with unilateral rotation and advancement of the affected side will produce improved growth and thereby minimize the adult deformity.

Similarly in children with temporomandibular joint ankylosis discovered prior to the development of significant secondary facial deformities, arthroplasty and resumption of good mandibular function often result in *good* subsequent facial growth.

However, when young patients are seen with ankylosis and significant secondary deformities already exist, growth center transplantation offers a means of immediate correction of much of the existing deformity as well as optimum potential for improved future growth. The technique for autogenous costochondral rib growth center transplantation is described and illustrated.

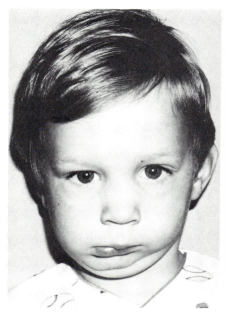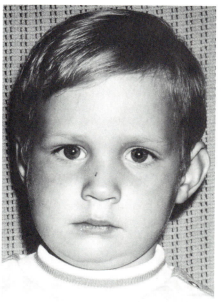

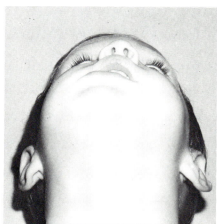

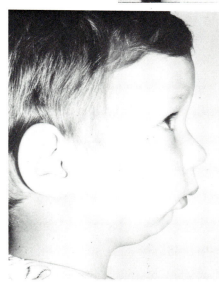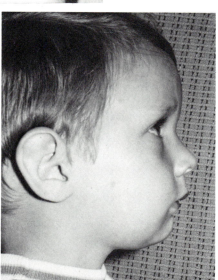

GROWTH CENTER TRANSPLANTATION

Plate 6-4

A. The illustrated case demonstrates hemifacial microsomia in a 10-year-old girl. There is significant facial asymmetry with an aplastic right condyle and ascending mandibular ramus. The maxilla is moderately canted such that the affected side is about 4 or 5 mm shorter than the unaffected side. The occlusion is class I on the left and class II on the right. Mild to moderate soft-tissue involvement is present.

B. The submandibular approach (see Chapter 2) provides good access to the residual mandibular ramus. However, special care must be exercised when reflecting the soft tissues from the ascending mandibular ramus, because the inferior alveolar neurovascular bundle may have an abnormally located foramen. It may, on occasion, even enter from the lateral aspect of the residual ascending mandibular ramus. A careful subperiosteal dissection is done to elevate the soft tissues from the lateral, posterior, and medial aspects of the ramus, yet preserving the inferior alveolar neurovascular bundle. All the soft tissues must be removed from the mandibular ramus because it will be moved a considerable distance both anteriorly and inferiorly. Usually in the young patient the submandibular approach permits good access to the temporal bone in the region of the deformed glenoid fossa because of the short distance between the glenoid fossa region and the angle of the mandible.

C. However, difficulty in identification of the fossa area may be encountered when attempting this dissection from the submandibular approach. The surgeon has three options in dealing with this problem: (1) carefully carry the dissection superiorly from the submandibular approach until the glenoid fossa area is adequately identified, (2) supplement the submandibular approach with a preauricular approach to facilitate the dissection and graft placement, (3) or place the growth center transplant into the soft tissues where the existing condylar remnant exists and accept a ''pseudoarthrosis'' in this area. The severity of the overall temporal bone, glenoid fossa, condylar, and soft-tissue deformity helps dictate the most judicious approach. In this case the former surgical approach is illustrated.

With finger palpation over the region of the glenoid fossa and while visualizing the operative site from below, a combination of sharp and blunt dissection is carried superiorly until the temporal bone is encountered. This dissection should be directed toward the lateralmost aspect of the temporal bone in the region of the glenoid fossa. To carry the dissection medially can produce troublesome bleeding.

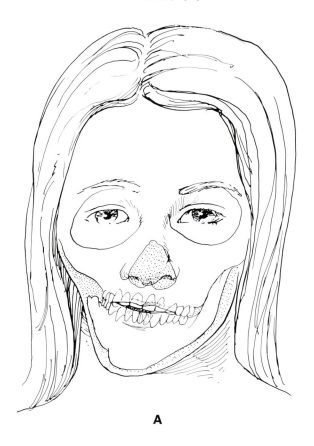

A

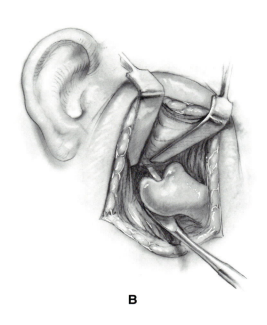

B

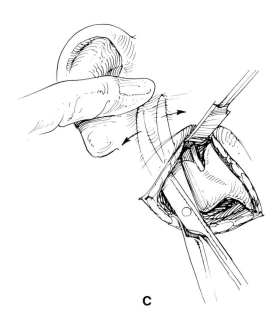

C

D. The costochondral graft is usually taken from the fifth or sixth rib. It must be remembered that in the very young child the cartilaginous portion of the ribs extends toward the midclavical line. Inasmuch as only 1 cm of cartilage is to be obtained with several centimeters of bone, the location of the chest incision may be slightly more lateral in the very young child.

E. The required amount of rib with about 1 cm of attached cartilage is removed.

F. This is done via a subperiosteal dissection of the major bony portion of the graft and a supraperiosteal dissection of the costochondral junction area to help maintain continuity between cartilaginous and bone interphase of the graft.

G. If a small tear in the pleura occurs, the patient's lungs can be manually expanded, because a nasotracheal tube is in place, and sutured. If a large tear occurs or the leak is not stopped with suturing, a chest tube is placed for a few days. The area is closed in layers with subcuticular skin sutures.

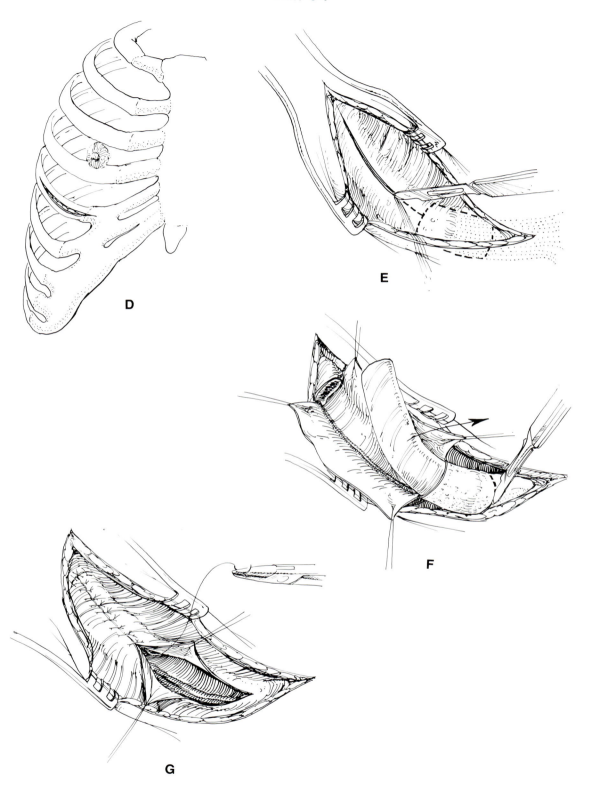

D

E

F

G

H. Before attempted placement of the graft the mandible must be repositioned anteriorly and inferiorly in the desired position. This is predetermined by model surgery and accomplished at surgery with an occlusal splint and intermaxillary fixation. When the maxillary occlusal plane is canted upward on the affected side, the bite can be opened with an occlusal splint to level the lower occlusal plane. To place the mandible in this position may necessitate a contralateral ramus osteotomy. In all cases it is desirable to "overcorrect" the existing facial, skeletal, and occlusal deformity with the splint. Frequently it may be necessary to do a suprahyoid myotomy for major movements. This can be accomplished through the submandibular approach. With a periosteal elevator the digastric muscles are reflected off the inferior border of the mandible and the geniohyoid muscles off the genial tubercles.

Holes are made through the cortices of the osseous portion of the rib to expedite its revascularization and healing. The graft is then placed in position and secured with several interosseous wires.

I. In severe cases of hemifacial microsomia when the major portion of the ascending mandibular ramus is absent or the degree of mandibular advancement is great, it may be necessary to utilize multiple rib sections, which can be obtained through the same chest incision. Only one need be obtained with cartilage attached.

J. The soft tissue is closed over the graft in multiple layers and a pressure dressing applied. Postoperatively a lengthened ramus and mandibular advancement have been achieved. Significant remodeling can be expected with resorption of the inferior aspect of the graft. The degree to which this occurs is variable and dependent on the existing soft-tissue deficiency. The mandible is stabilized anteroposteriorly and vertically with an occlusal splint and intermaxillary fixation for 3 to 6 weeks. The splint is generally wired to the mandible via circummandibular wires. Therefore progressive jaw function is resumed with the splint (which has opened the bite on the deformed side) being maintained for 6 to 12 months with selective grinding after the primary healing phase to allow for vertical growth of the maxillary alveolus with erruption of the maxillary posterior teeth. Subsequent growth is unpredictable.

Residual soft-tissue and osseous deficiencies can be further corrected by alloplastic and soft-tissue augmentation procedures at a later date. Generally these are best done after puberty.

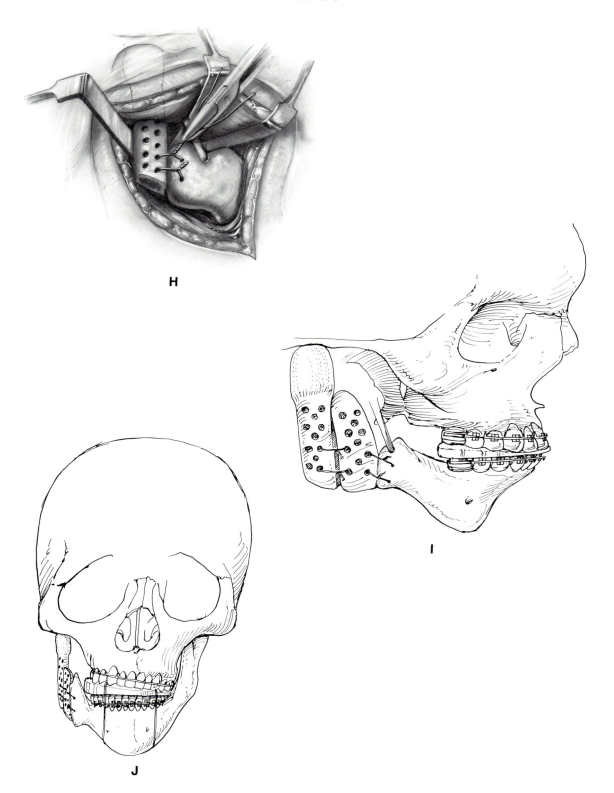

H

I

J

SPECIAL CONSIDERATION

GROWTH CENTER TRANSPLANTATION

Massive ankylosis in child with facial deformity (Plate 6-5)

A. This is an illustrative case of massive ankylosis of the right temporomandibular joint in a 3-year-old boy, which has been present, by history, since shortly after birth and has resulted in a severe facial, skeletal, occlusal, and functional deformity. The mandible is deviated toward the ankylosed side.

B. There is a class II malocclusion and crossbite on the affected side. Radiographically a large radiopaque mass is present, obliterating the joint space and continuous with the zygomatic arch.

C. The submandibular approach, as described in detail in Chapter 2, provides good access to the ankylosed mandibular condyle in a child of this size because the vertical distance from the angle of the mandible to the glenoid fossa is not great. A subperiosteal dissection is done of the lateral, posterior, and medial aspects of the mandible. The temporalis muscle is reflected off the coronoid process and the coronoid process removed because it is generally hypertrophied and will interfere with advancement of the mandible. A subcondylar osteotomy is done to free the mandibular ramus and mobilize it. The pathologic bone is removed in part and an attempt made to identify the residual meniscus so that the graft can be placed against it.

D. In more severe cases it is virtually impossible to dissect through the bone and preserve the miniscus. A new fossa can be constructed, however, by reshaping and slightly hollowing out the residual osseous mass of the ankylosed condylar head. The costochondral graft can then be inserted into this new fossa.

E. The occlusal splint is inserted and secured to the mandible with circummandibular wires. Intermaxillary fixation is applied as well as craniofacial suspension if needed (i.e., circumzygomatic suspension). The autogenous costochondral graft is placed so that the cartilaginous portion is abutted against the base of the ankylosed condyle or more optimally the meniscus. This will be the new joint mechanism. The graft is wired to the posterior aspect of the ramus. Intermaxillary fixation is maintained for 2 to 4 weeks, and then the occlusion is controlled with intermittent elastics for an additional 4 to 12 weeks. During this time every effort is made to keep heavy loads off the healing graft and to achieve full mandibular opening. This is done with a combination of jaw exercises and intermaxillary elastics.

182

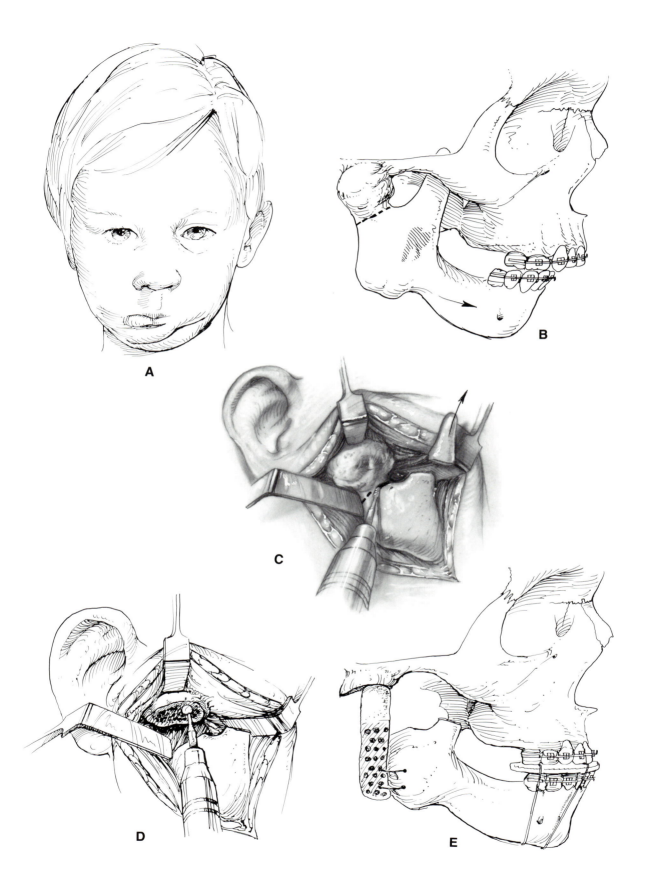

A

B

C

D

E

Alloplastic replacement of mandibular condyle

Generally there is little indication for alloplastic replacement of the mandibular condyle in the correction of dentofacial deformities. Although multiple applications of the alloplastic replacement of the mandibular condyle have been proposed, we restrict its use to adults in the case of some neoplastic processes that require resection, occasional congenital deformities without condyles (hemifacial microsomia), and in unusual cases of rheumatoid arthritis. In all circumstances it must be appreciated that any alloplast is subject to subsequent stress fracturing, poor interphase bonding to the bone, and possible infection. Regardless, in the unusual case where it is deemed advisable this approach can be utilized to either correct or prevent significant dentofacial deformities.

Each case will dictate the exact size and nature of the alloplastic condylar replacement. In some instances it will only be necessary to replace the condyle itself, whereas in others the condyle and various portions of the ascending mandibular ramus may require simultaneous reconstruction. Such a case is illustrated.

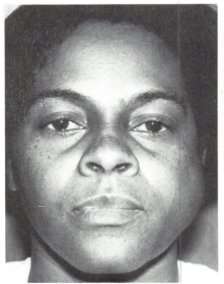 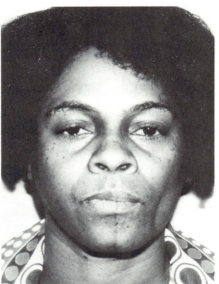

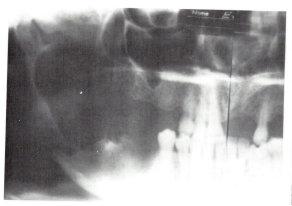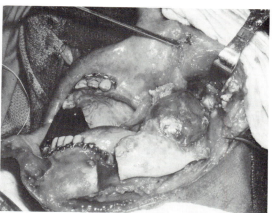

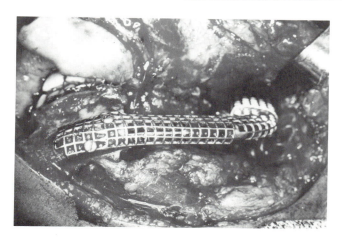

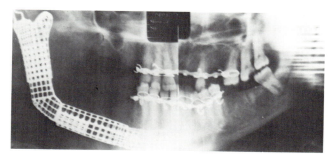

ALLOPLASTIC REPLACEMENT OF MANDIBULAR CONDYLE

Plate 6-6

A. A large biopsy-proved ameloblastoma of the entire right mandible including the condyle in a 39-year-old woman is illustrated. The laminograms of the area indicate that the tumor has perforated the buccal and lingual cortices in several areas. Therefore a primary supraperiosteal resection of the ascending ramus, including the condyle, and immediate reconstruction with an alloplastic replacement are planed. The alloplast is prefabricated to size from a cephalometric radiograph.

B. An extended submandibular incision is used to expose the entire lateral, posterior, and inferior aspect of the mandible. After this the bone cut is made through the planed area in the body, and with lateral retraction of the proximal segment the medial supraperiosteal dissection is carried superiorly. The entire proximal segment is then removed and the specimen inspected for possible areas of perforation.

C. If such areas are present, additional soft tissue is removed in these areas and submitted for frozen-section examination. When it is felt the entire area is free of tumor, the preformed alloplastic replacement is inserted with the teeth in intermaxillary fixation. It is secured to the distal mandibular segment with several screws. Generally intermaxillary fixation is maintained for 3 weeks. Thereafter intermittent jaw exercises and intermaxillary elastics are used for an additional 3 to 6 weeks.

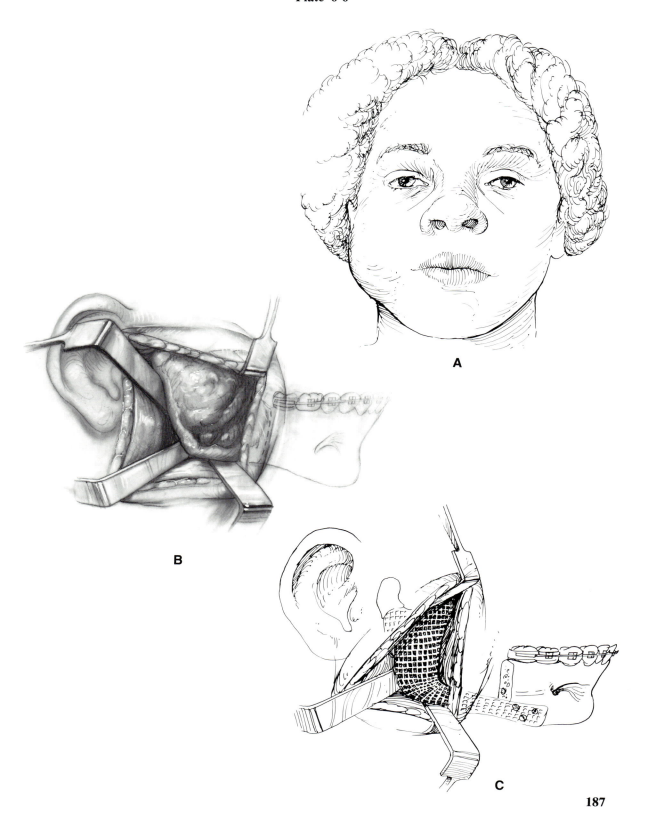

A

B

C

PART TWO

MAXILLARY SURGERY

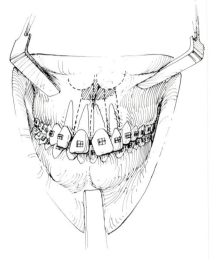

**SINGLE-TOOTH DENTO-OSSEOUS
OSTEOTOMIES**

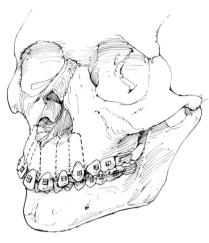

ANTERIOR MAXILLARY OSTECTOMY

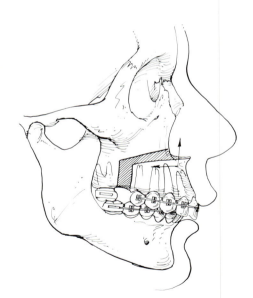

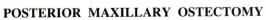

POSTERIOR MAXILLARY OSTECTOMY

CHAPTER 7

Segmental maxillary surgery

Segmental maxillary surgery is commonly indicated in the correction of dentofacial deformities where only a portion of the maxillary arch requires repositioning for functional and esthetic reasons. While a number of different specific operative approaches have been proposed for the various segmental maxillary procedures, the specific procedures described in this chapter are predicated on our clinical experience and laboratory studies by a number of individuals. In this regard they have been proved to be biologically and clinically successful and predicated on the following basic surgical principles:

1. Maintain an adequate amount of attached, viable soft tissue to the mobilized segments in order to provide sufficient vascularity to them
2. Provide maximal direct visualization of all areas to be osteotomized or ostectomized
3. Achieve good mobilization of the segments to allow for passive repositioning in the predetermined position
4. Maintain optimal periodontal health
5. Provide good bony contact between the stable and mobilized segments to effect rapid bone union

In this chapter the techniques for single-tooth dento-osseous osteotomies, the anterior maxillary ostectomy, and the posterior maxillary ostectomy are sequentially described and illustrated.

Single-tooth dento-osseous osteotomies

Any surgical approach to perform single-tooth dento-osseous osteotomies must be predicated on the basic surgical principles put forth in the introduction to this chapter. These principles are not theoretical but practical in that minor infractions of them when performing single-tooth dento-osseous osteotomies may result in complications. Meticulous treatment planning and surgical technique is of the utmost importance.

There are two basic operative approaches to performing single-tooth dento-osseous osteotomies: (1) the one-stage technique in which the segments are mobilized and repositioned during a single operation and (2) the two-stage technique in which osteotomies and ostectomies at the first operative setting are done through only one cortical plate (usually the palatal) and then 4 weeks later the osteotomies and ostectomies are completed through the opposite cortex and the segments mobilized and repositioned. Both of these surgical approaches are discussed.

One-stage single-tooth dento-osseous osteotomies. In order to consider a one-stage procedure there must be sufficient interdental space between adjacent tooth roots so that a fine osteotomy can be made completely between the tooth roots without injury to them, the dento-osseous segments can be mobilized and repositioned into the desired relationship, and adequate attached soft tissue to the mobilized segments can be maintained. This means that periapical radiographs and articulated dental models are essential in planning for such a procedure. The radiographs will help determine the periodontal health, bone-tooth relationships, and interdental spacing. The models are sectioned to ascertain the *feasibility* of making the necessary interdental cuts, to achieve the desired occlusal result, to accurately determine the amount and direction of movement for each segment, and to construct stabilizing appliances. The stabilizing appliance is generally an occlusal acrylic splint or orthodontic arch wire.

The one-stage surgical approach is most applicable when one to three single-tooth or small dento-osseous segments are to be repositioned and the type of movement to be accomplished is uncomplicated. With the one-stage procedure it is *difficult* to execute major rotational movements, significant posterior repositioning, and alignment of multiple anterior single-tooth dento-osseous segments where adjacent root apices are in very close approximation.

The one-stage technique is usually done from the labial aspect. There are two basic soft-tissue approaches: (1) *a horizontal vestibular incision,* which is generally preferred because it provides excellent surgical access yet maintains good soft-tissue predicles to the segments, and (2) *multiple vertical incisions,* which are sometimes more advantageous, especially in cases where large diastemas are present or a significant vertical change in the position of the dento-osseous segments is required.

Two-stage singe-tooth dento-osseous osteotomies. All small-segment dento-osseous osteotomies can be done in two surgical stages if desired. There are some conditions where the two-stage procedure is indicated or preferred. These conditions include simultaneous movement of multiple (three or more) single-tooth dento-osseous segments when tooth roots are very close together, the need for closure of multiple *large* diastemas, movement of multiple small segments considerable distances, necessity to remove palatal bone for posterior repositioning, and significant rotational movements of segments. The two-stage technique has advantages over the single-stage technique in these conditions because it is technically easier, safer, and more biologic.

Generally the first stage of the two-stage procedure is accomplished with the patient under local anesthesia. A full palatal flap is reflected, and the indicated palatal osteotomies or ostectomies are completed. Four weeks later, through a vestibular incision (generally horizontal), the buccal osteotomies and ostectomies are done and the segments mobilized, repositioned, and stabilized.

Both the one- and two-stage surgical approaches for the movement of small dento-osseous segments are illustrated and described. In addition the coordination of orthodontics with these surgical procedures is discussed.

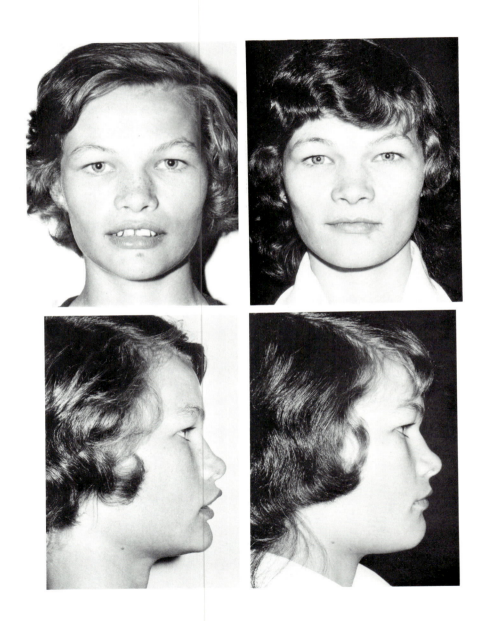

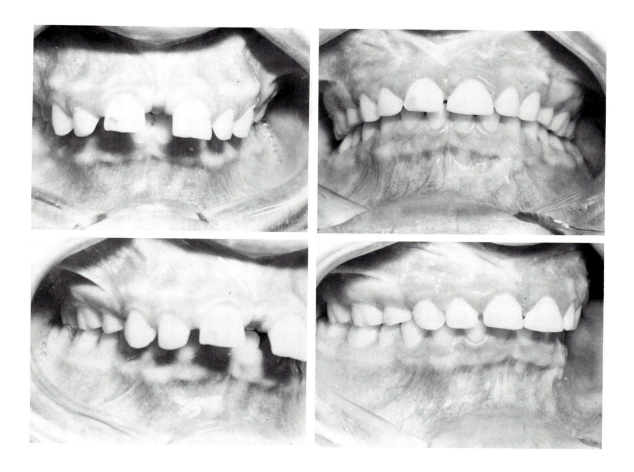

ONE-STAGE SINGLE-TOOTH DENTO-OSSEOUS OSTEOTOMIES: HORIZONTAL INCISION

Plate 7-1

A. The illustrated case demonstrates three procumbent and slightly extruded anterior teeth. These malaligned teeth will be surgically repositioned via a one-stage procedure followed by orthodontic tooth movement to refine their positions.

B. A high horizontal vestibular incision is made extending one tooth distal to those being mobilized. In this case the incision will extend from above the right lateral incisor to the left cuspid. The mucoperiosteal tissues are reflected superiorly, exposing the anterior nasal spine and piriform apertures of the nose. With a periosteal elevator the nasal mucoperiosteum is reflected from the anterior floor of the nose and piriform aperture area. The anterior aspect of the cartilaginous nasal septum is elevated from the vomerine groove in the nasal crest of the maxilla. This dissection is done carefully without tearing the nasal mucoperiosteum.

The oral mucoperiosteum is reflected inferiorly only to the level of the attached gingiva in order to maintain a good buccal pedicle to the mobilized segments. The interdental alveolar crestal bone is not exposed unless large diastemas (4 to 6 mm) are being closed. Vertical interdental osteotomies are made through the labial cortex with a fine-fissured bur. These osteotomies extend from the anterior aspect of the nasal floor inferiorly to about the level of the attached gingiva, which is about 4 mm above the alveolar crestal bone.

When minimal space exists between adjacent tooth roots or diastemas are not present, the labial vertical osteotomies are made only through the outer cortex and completed through the palatal cortex with fine osteotomes. A finger is placed on the palatal mucoperiosteum to detect the osteotome or bur as it perforates the palatal cortex.

When diastemas exist some interdental bone will have to be removed, and the entire interdental osteotomy or ostectomy can be made with a bur. However, care is taken to *initially remove less interdental bone* than predetermined, because there is a tendency to remove an excessive amount. When diastemas dictate removal of crestal bone it is imperative that some crestal bone around both adjacent teeth be preserved in order to avoid the secondary development of serious periodontal defects. After mobilization of the dento-osseous segments, when they are being positioned in the splint, additional interdental bone can always be removed. The osseous interferences are more easily identified at that time.

The alveolar crestal bone is thin and is readily sectioned with a fine osteotome directed inferiorly. This avoids excessive elevation of the buccal pedicle and excessive removal of alveolar crestal bone, as occurs when a bur is used.

196

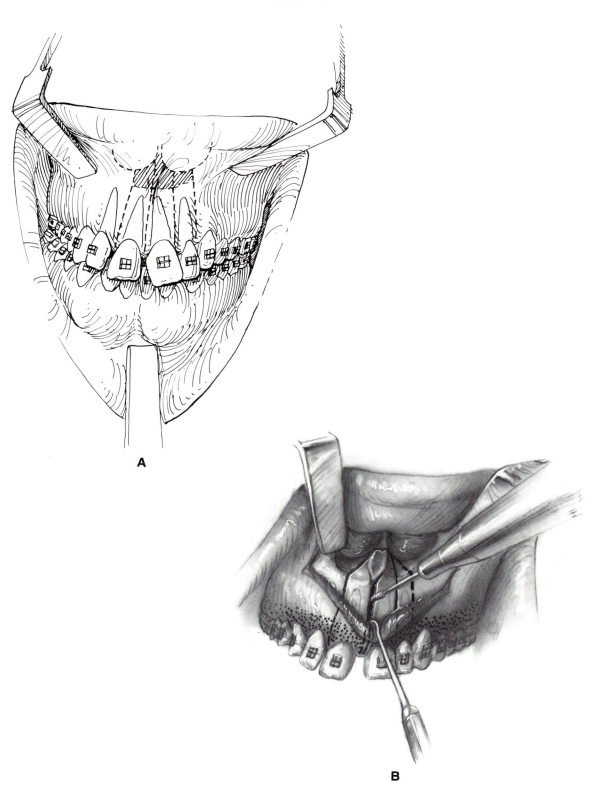

A

B

ONE-STAGE SINGLE-TOOTH DENTO-OSSEOUS OSTEOTOMIES: HORIZONTAL INCISION

Plate 7-1

C. Generally the vertical interdental osteotomies extend into the anterior floor of the nose. Because of the curvature of the maxillary arch, the interdental osteotomies are generally convergent as they are made posteriorly. Therefore a horizontal palatal cut is rarely necessary to connect the palatal portion of the interdental osteotomies. If, however, following completion of the vertical cuts the segments cannot be easily mobilized, or if the roots are aligned so that the vertical osteotomies are not convergent posteriorly, it may be necessary to use a curved osteotome transnasally to make a horizontal palatal osteotomy to facilitate mobilization of the segments.

D. On completion of the initial vertical interdental osteotomies or ostectomies, the alveolar osteotomies, and palatal cuts, the dento-osseous segments are mobilized by manipulation with an osteotome placed between the segments. When initiating mobilization of the segments it is best to place the osteotome so it will not injure the apices or crestal bone. Approximately midway between the teeth apices and crestal alveolar bone, so as not to damage either, is a good location, as some pressure on the cementum is inconsequential. The segments are carefully mobilized with slow, deliberate levering movements so as not to inadvertently detach the palatal or buccal soft-tissue pedicles, which can occur with fast shearing movements. Sufficient mobility must be achieved to passively reposition the individual segments in their predetermined position in the occlusal splint.

Plate 7-1

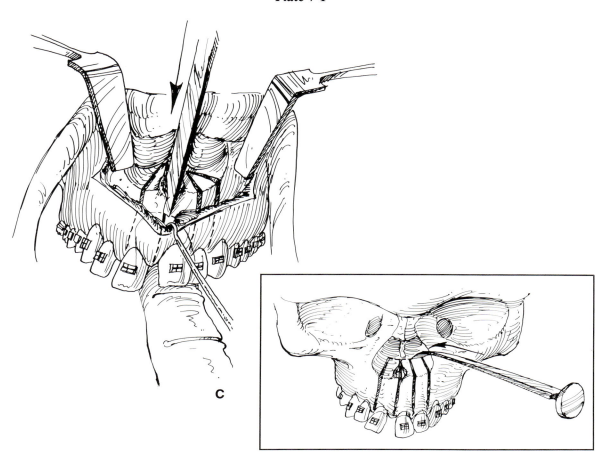

C

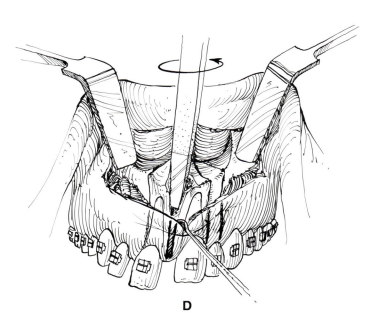

D

E. When the segments appear to be adequately mobilized an attempt is made to place the individual dento-osseous segments into the preformed occlusal acrylic splint. It is important that the splint (which is constructed from the surgery on the dental models) is made such that the maxillary teeth "key" well into it. The splint is secured to the stable portion of the maxillary dentition, and an attempt is made to position the individual mobilized teeth into it. While attempting to place the mobilized dento-osseous segments into the splint any areas of bone interference that prevent their proper placement can be detected by direct visual inspection and judiciously removed with a bur. After positioning the segments in the splint any subapical bone that protrudes into the nose can be removed so long as in doing so the root apices are not endangered.

F. The individual segments are stabilized in the splint with 26-guage wire, and generally no intermaxillary fixation is necessary. If no postsurgical orthodontic tooth movement is to be undertaken the splint is left in place for about 6 weeks until bony union normally occurs. It is then worn at night for an additional month as a retainer and tooth positioner.

When postsurgical orthodontic tooth movement is to be done the splint can be removed 7 to 10 days after surgery and an orthodontic arch wire immediately inserted to finalize the occlusion. *At this time rapid movement of the entire previously mobilized dento-osseous segments can be achieved with normal orthodontic forces.* If this sequence is followed, finishing orthodontics can often be completed within an additional 3 to 4 weeks, before bone healing is completed. However, when orthodontic forces are applied to the mobile dento-osseous segments this early postoperatively, the patient must be seen at least once a week so that careful control of the movement of the dento-osseous segments can be accomplished. When orthodontic forces are applied early and the patient is *not* appropriately followed up, the segments will move rapidly, possibly into undesirable positions where they will undergo bony union and result in a new malocclusion.

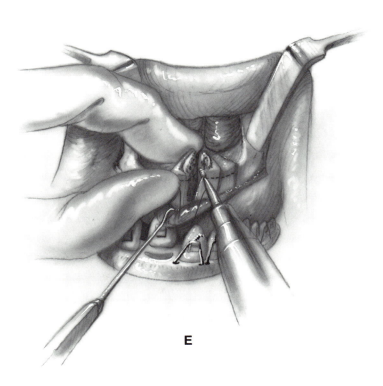

E

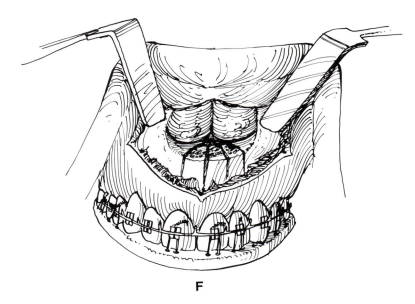

F

ONE-STAGE SINGLE-TOOTH DENTO-OSSEOUS OSTEOTOMIES: VERTICAL INCISIONS

Plate 7-2

A. When the one-stage technique is to be employed and multiple large (4 to 6 mm) diastemas are present or major vertical repositioning of a tooth or teeth is to be achieved, multiple vertical interdental soft-tissue incisions are preferred. The vertical incisions permit the labial mucoperiosteal pedicle to move more freely with and therefore remain attached better to the individual dento-osseous segments. However, additional care during the soft-tissue dissection must be exercised so that the labial mucoperiosteal pedicle is not inadvertently stripped from the dento-osseous segments.

In the case illustrated an ankylosed central incisor is present. Inadequate space is available for its proper placement in the arch, because the lateral incisor has drifted mesially. Model surgery confirmed the feasibility of moving the lateral incisor slightly distolaterally to open the space and simultaneously moving the central incisor into its proper position.

Because the central incisor, its associated bone, and its attached labial soft-tissue pedicle will require considerable vertical movement, multiple vertical incisions are to be used. The vertical incisions are made in a divergent direction as they are extended superiorly to provide a broad-based mucoperiosteal vascular pedicle. Inferiorly these incisions are carried through the interdental papillae on the segments moving significantly inferiorly. A viable attached labial pedicle is essential in this case because with the required amount of movement the palatal mucoperiosteum will likely be avulsed from the dento-osseous segments to some degree.

B. Minimal reflection on the soft-tissue flaps is done to expose the interdental bone in order to maintain the maximum attached soft-tissue pedicle to the mobilized segments. The flaps are carefully retracted and all of the interdental osteotomies completed with a fine-fissure bur through the labial cortex only, stopping about 3 to 4 mm above the alveolar crestal bone. *The vertical interdental osteotomies must be parallel to one another or slightly convergent at their superior aspect.* If they are divergent superiorly it will be impossible to move the dento-osseous segment inferiorly after it is mobilized.

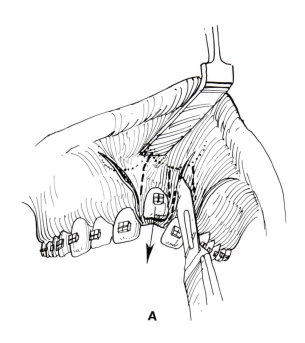

A

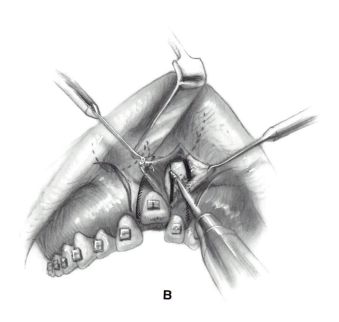

B

C. A thin osteotome is used to complete the vertical osteotomies between the teeth. A finger is maintained on the palate to detect the osteotome as it completes the cut through the palatal cortex. The curvature of the maxillary arch and the location of the maxillary tooth roots makes it feasible and desirable to angle the osteotomies in a converging direction from labial to palatal, as illustrated in the insert. When this is done the mobilization of the segments is easy.

An osteotome is used to lever between the segments to facilitate their mobilization. Levering against the apices or crestal bone must be avoided. If the segments do not mobilize, the cause is usually incomplete osteotomies of the palatal bone, and the osteotomies are checked for completeness.

D. If it is not possible to make the interdental osteotomies convergent posteriorly, a thin curved osteotome can be inserted transnasally and used to complete the osteotomies on the palatal bone.

E. Following mobilization of the segments the occlusal splint is inserted and ligated to the stable maxillary teeth, and an attempt is made to position the mobilized segments in the splint and to ligate them in place. It is best to first place the smaller dento-osseous segments in the splint. If any of the segments cannot be properly positioned in the splint, direct inspection of the interdental osteotomy sites while attempting to place it in the splint will disclose areas of bony interference, and these are judiciously removed.

The postoperative fixation, with or without orthodontics, is the same as discussed for horizontal incisions.

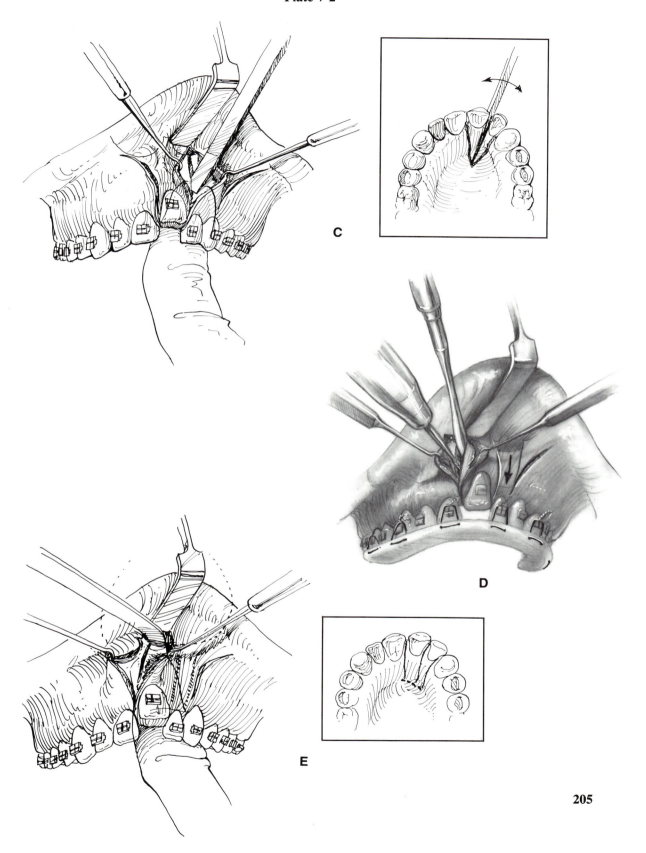

C

D

E

TWO-STAGE SINGLE-TOOTH DENTO-OSSEOUS OSTEOTOMIES
Plate 7-3

A. In the illustrated case an Angle's class II, division I malocclusion is present with multiple anterior maxillary diastemas. The patient has previously had upper first premolars removed and incomplete orthodontic treatment. Model surgery revealed the feasibility of surgically repositioning the anterior six teeth as individual dento-osseous segments and producing a class I cuspid occlusion with good overjet and overbite. Following surgery the occlusion will be refined with finishing orthodontics. Because of the large diastemas, the significant amount of repositioning indicated, and the necessity of removing palatal bone to accomplish the necessary dento-osseous movements, the two-stage technique was selected for this case.

B. In the two-stage procedure the first surgical stage is generally performed on the palate by elevating a full-thickness palatal mucoperiosteal flap. The incision for this flap is made about 3 mm from the necks of the teeth, extending just distal to the proposed location of the most posterior interdental osteotomy. This incision minimizes periodontal problems and facilitates suturing. As the palatal mucoperiosteum is reflected the nasopalatine vessels are severed and the entire anterior bony palate exposed.

   Depending on the indicated movement of the dento-osseous segments, as dictated by the occlusion and *predetermined from the model surgery,* either palatal osteotomies or ostectomies are required at this stage. If the dento-osseous segments are to be moved anteriorly, as in an anterior crossbite or straightening of crowded teeth, only palatal osteotomies are required. If diastemas are to be closed, as in the illustrated case, and the dento-osseous segments are to be moved posteriorly, *palatal ostectomies* are required. The exact size of the midpalatal ostectomy is predicated on the distance that the anterior dento-osseous segments will be moved posteriorly as predetermined from the model surgery. The midpalatal ostectomy is carried through the palatal bone to the nasal mucoperiosteum, while the interdental cuts are completed only through the palatal cortical bone. *The entire alveolar crestal bone is always left intact during the first surgical stage.*

C. The palatal mucoperiosteal flap is replaced and sutured. A moist sponge is used to apply pressure to the repositioned palatal flap and is held tightly against the anterior hard palate for 30 minutes after surgery by the patient. This will prevent hematoma formation beneath the flap and eliminate the need for a palatal stent or splint.

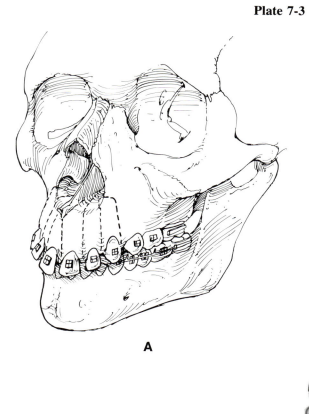

A

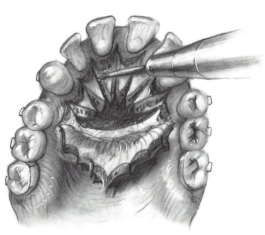

B

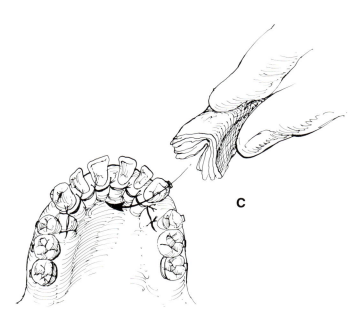

C

D. *Four weeks after the completion of the first stage* the second stage is done. This period permits adequate revascularization by the palatal flap of the bone-tooth segments that will be mobilized and yet is not so long as to permit complete bony repair from the first stage. The same general guidelines, as discussed previously for the single-stage technique, determine flap design. If possible a horizontal vestibular incision is utilized, because it provides a good buccal pedicle and affords excellent visibility of the bone, tooth roots, and anterior nasal floor. This incision can be used in almost all instances except when multiple large diastemas (greater than 5 mm) exist, in which case multiple vertical soft-tissue incisions are best.

In cases where a large midline maxillary diastema exists with an abnormal frenulum, a midline vertical excision of the frenulum can be combined with the horizontal vestibular incision without significant compromise of the labial pedicle vascular supply.

E. Following the soft-tissue dissection the anterior aspect of the nasal crest of the maxilla is removed. Next the planned interdental osteotomies and ostectomies are done. *When diastemas exist, as in this case, only about one half as much interdental bone is initially removed, as compared with the measured width of the diastemas.* Moreover, at the alveolar crestal bone area the ostectomy is carefully completed so that crestal bone remains around the cervical margin of both adjacent teeth. Generally when the diastemas are only 3 to 4 mm no crestal bone is removed at this time, as following sectioning of the crestal bone with an osteotome, because of its compressibility, and the diastemas can be manually closed.

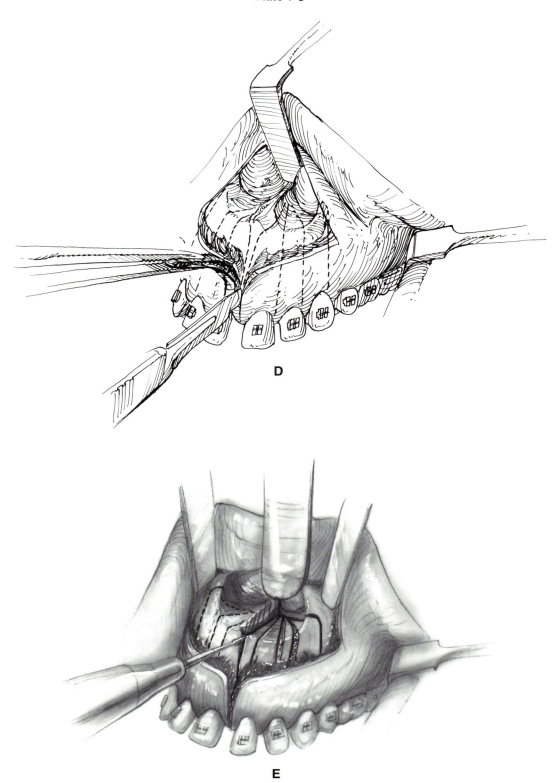

D

E

TWO-STAGE SINGLE-TOOTH DENTO-OSSEOUS OSTEOTOMIES
Plate 7-3

F. If diastemas are not present the alveolar crestal bone can be sectioned with a fine osteotome and the other bone cuts can be checked for completeness with an osteotome. The segments are then carefully mobilized with digital pressure or levering with an osteotome interdentally. Minimal pressure should be applied to the crestal bone and root apices. Following mobilization of the multiple segments they are checked for placement in the preformed acrylic occlusal splint. If bony interferences exist they can be removed with direct visualization.

G. When using the horizontal vestibular incision to close moderate diastemas (3 to 4 mm) it is helpful to make a horizontal soft-tissue incision along the crest of the alveolus to avoid entrapment and compression of the interdental soft tissues as the two adjacent teeth are moved together.

Once final adjustments are made and all segments fitted into the splint, it is secured to the stable teeth, and the individual mobilized dento-osseous segments are similarly stabilized. Incisions are closed with absorbable suture. When no postsurgical orthodontics are to be done the splint is left in place for about 6 to 8 weeks until bony union occurs. It is then worn at night for several months as a retainer. When postsurgical orthodontics are to be done it is advantageous to begin active postsurgical orthodontics about 10 days after surgery. When this is done the patient must be seen weekly because rapid movement of the unhealed dento-osseous segments will occur. Ideally with this regimen the finishing orthodontics will be completed within 1 to 2 months after surgery.

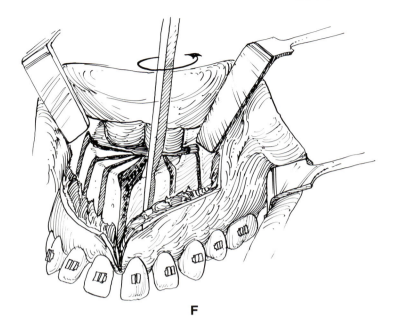

F

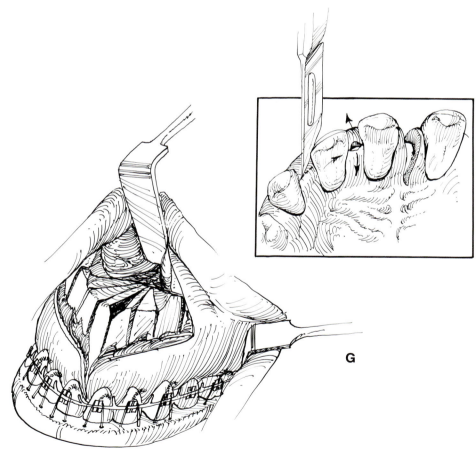

G

Anterior maxillary ostectomy

The anterior maxillary ostectomy is employed primarily to reposition the anterior dento-osseous segment posteriorly but can be used to move it superiorly or inferiorly as indicated. When utilized for the correction of maxillary protrusion it provides excellent esthetic and functional results. Other indications for performing an anterior maxillary osteotomy or ostectomy are correction of bimaxillary protrusion where the anterior maxillary ostectomy is utilized in conjunction with an anterior mandibular subapical ostectomy, to correct unusual open-bite deformities, and to superiorly reposition the anterior dento-osseous segment when a reverse curve of Spee exists in the maxilla. It is often misused when employed for the correction of class II malocclusions that are a result of vertical maxillary excess or true mandibular deficiency.

Several basic surgical techniques have been advocated for performing the anterior maxillary ostectomy. The technique described has some advantages over other commonly used techniques: (1) it is technically simple, (2) provides direct access to the nasal crest of the maxilla and associated nasal septal structures, which permits simultaneous correction of a deviated nasal septum and prevents buckling of the cartilaginous nasal septum when the anterior maxilla is superiorly repositioned, (3) permits removal of the necessary midpalatal bone via direct visualization, and (4) provides an excellent vascular pedicle.

The basic procedure that we have utilized for performing the anterior maxillary ostectomy is described and illustrated.

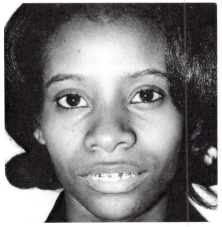 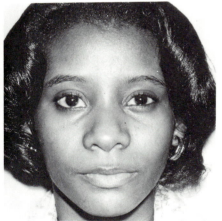

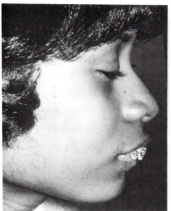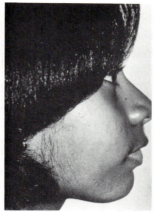

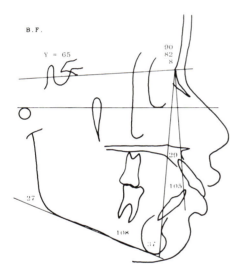

B.F.

Y = 65

90
82
8

29

105

27

108

37

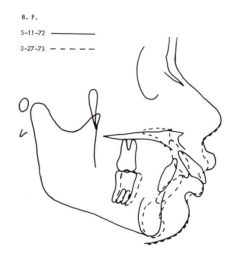

B.F.

5-11-72 ——————

3-27-73 — — — —

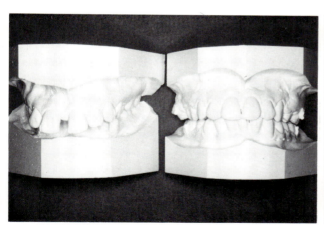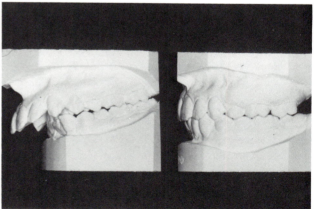

ANTERIOR MAXILLARY OSTECTOMY

Plate 7-4

A. The illustrated case demonstrates a true anterior maxillary protrusion, class II malocclusion, a missing maxillary right first molar, and an excessive curve of Spee in the maxilla. Presurgical orthodontics have aligned and leveled the lower arch. Segmental orthodontics have been done in the upper arch in preparation for an anterior maxillary ostectomy as outlined.

The surgery will consist of extraction of the left maxillary first premolar and an anterior maxillary ostectomy to reposition the anterior maxilla posteriorly and slightly superiorly through the left premolar extraction site and the missing right first molar space.

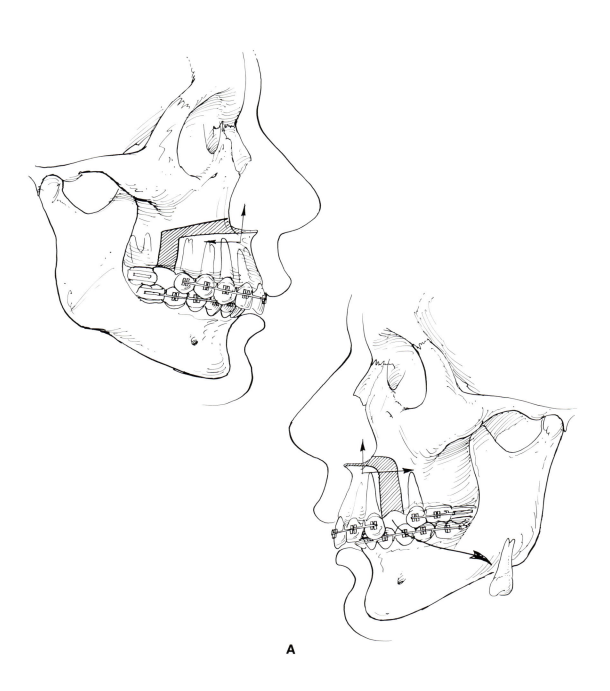

A

ANTERIOR MAXILLARY OSTECTOMY

Plate 7-4

B. The left first premolar is removed, and a horizontal incision is made with a diathermy knife high in the labial vestibule at a level just above the apices of the teeth. The incision extends from the second premolar area on the left to the second molar area on the right. The mucoperiosteum is elevated superiorly to expose the anterior walls of the maxilla, the anterior nasal spine, and the piriform rims of the nose. Careful dissection of the nasal mucoperiosteum from the anterior nasal floor and piriform rims is readily accomplished without tearing of the nasal mucoperiosteum or hemorrhage.

In edentulous areas that are being closed an incision between adjacent teeth is made through the mucoperiosteum on the crest of the ridge. The palatal and buccal gingiva is then slightly reflected to permit closure of the space without soft-tissue interference.

C. Calipers are utilized to measure about 5 mm above the cuspid apices (approximately 34 mm above the cuspid cusp tip) to where the horizontal bone cut will be made. Generally it is impossible to accurately identify the location of tooth root apices at surgery; therefore direct measurement is utilized to determine the level at which to safely make the subapical cuts, thus preventing inadvertent root-tip amputation.

A periosteal elevator is inserted along the lateral nasal wall beneath the nasal mucoperiosteum to elevate and protect it when the osteotomy is carried through the anterior aspect of the lateral nasal wall. The horizontal osteotomy is completed through the anterior maxillary wall into the maxillary sinus from the piriform aperture posteriorly to the location where the vertical interdental ostectomy is to be done. In this case the horizontal osteotomy will extend from the piriform rim to the distal aspect of the missing first molar area on the right.

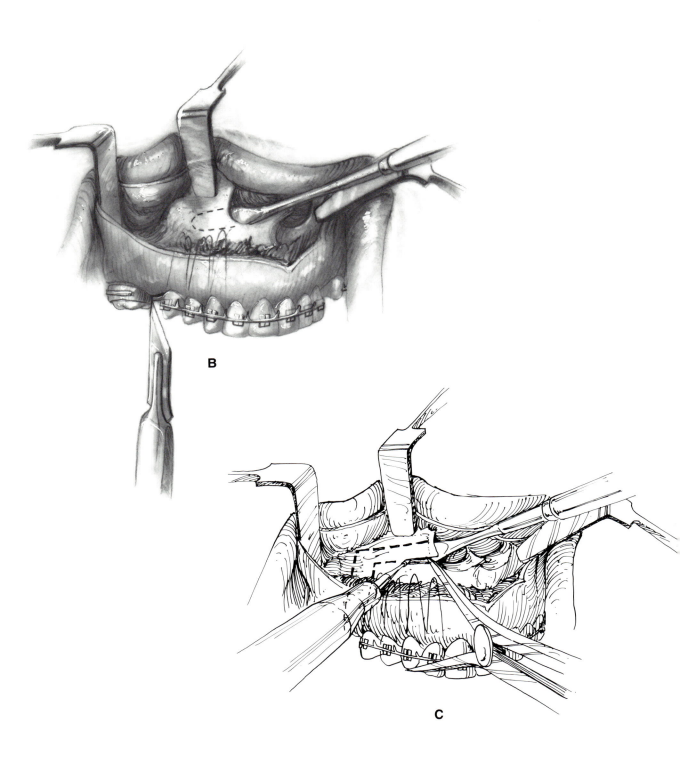

B

C

ANTERIOR MAXILLARY OSTECTOMY
Plate 7-4

D. The buccal mucoperiosteum is carefully elevated overlying the interdental area, which is to be ostectomized. When mobilizing the soft tissues in these areas it is best, if necessary, to reflect the mucoperiosteum distally (from the stable segment) to maintain the maximum amount of attachment of the soft-tissue flap to the anterior segment (mobilized segment).

A small retractor is used to provide access to the interdental bone and protect the buccal mucoperiosteal flap. The vertical interdental ostectomy is marked with a bur. The amount of bone to be removed is accurately pre-determined from the model surgery. The vertical interdental ostectomy is carried through to the palatal aspect of the dentoalveolus while a finger is maintained on the palatal mucosa to detect the bur as it perforates the palatal bone so as not to excessively lacerate the palatal mucoperiosteum. *It is important to make the ostectomies through the dentoalveolus toward the ostectomy site on the opposite side.* This makes completion of the transpalatal ostectomies easier.

The same basic procedure is completed on the left side. The horizontal osteotomy is completed to the distal aspect of the first premolar and the vertical osteotomy through the dentoalveolus as described for the right side. At this time the palatal bone is mostly intact, and no attempt is made to ''blindly'' complete the entire transpalatal ostectomy.

E. If a midline split of the anterior maxilla is indicated to expand the maxillary arch, as determined by the model surgery, *the midpalatal osteotomy is made prior to mobilization of the anterior maxilla.* This ostectomy is readily achieved with an osteotome while the maxilla is stable rather than after it is mobilized.

A sharp thin osteotome is malleted between the central incisors while a finger is placed on the palatal aspect to detect the osteotome as it perforates the palatoalveolar cortical plate. The osteotome is first directed at about 45° through the alveolar bone and then at 90° through the midpalatal bone. If a vertical osteotomy is to be done a bur is used to make the cuts through the dentoalveolar portion, and this bone is removed. It is important to remove less bone in the midline than determined by the workup because there is a tendency to remove more bone than necessary.

The nasal septal osteotome can then be used to separate the nasal septum from the anterior maxilla. The osteotome is inserted and angled slightly inferiorly. A finger is placed on the palate to help with orientation. There is a tendency for the nasal septal osteotome to be directed superiorly or to ride up the superior aspect of the nasal crest of the maxilla and vomer. Therefore angling the osteotome slightly inferiorly will minimize this problem. The osteotome should be malleted posteriorly only to the area of the planned transverse palatal ostectomy.

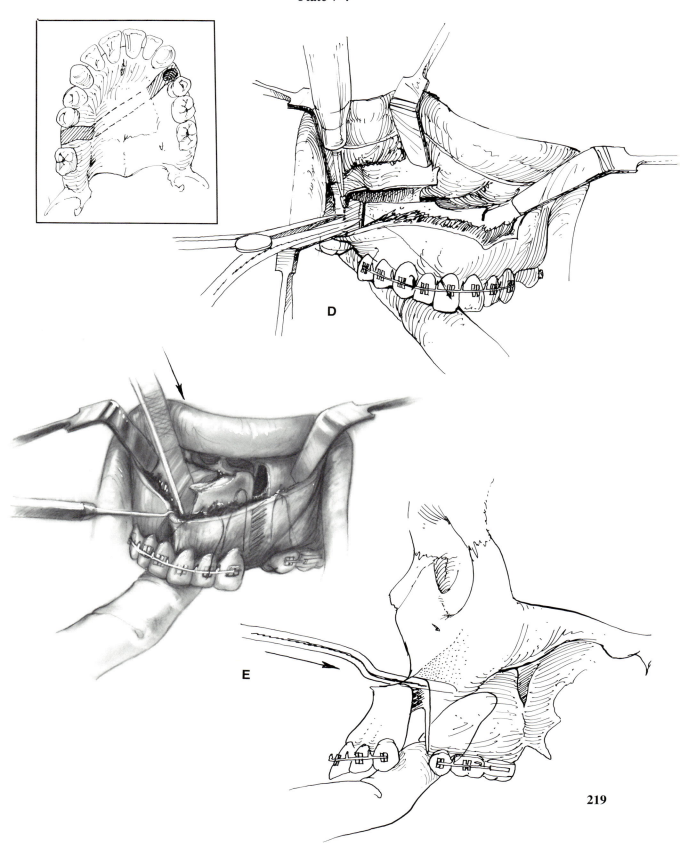

D

E

219

ANTERIOR MAXILLARY OSTECTOMY
Plate 7-4

F. The transpalatal *osteotomy* is completed with an osteotome through one of the dentoalveolar ostectomy sites. In this instance it is done through the premolar ostectomy site, because this site permits the osteotome to be more easily directed to meet the transverse cut through the first molar area on the opposite side. A finger is maintained on the palatal mucosa to prevent the osteotome from lacerating it excessively and thereby compromising its value as a vascular pedicle to the anterior dento-osseous segments.

The insert illustrates the proposed transpalatal ostectomy and the osteotome completing only the osteotomy at this time.

G. After completion of the transpalatal osteotomy the anterior maxilla is down-fractured with finger pressure. If the bone cuts are complete there should be little resistance to its inferior movement. If significant resistance is encountered all bone cuts are rechecked for completeness.

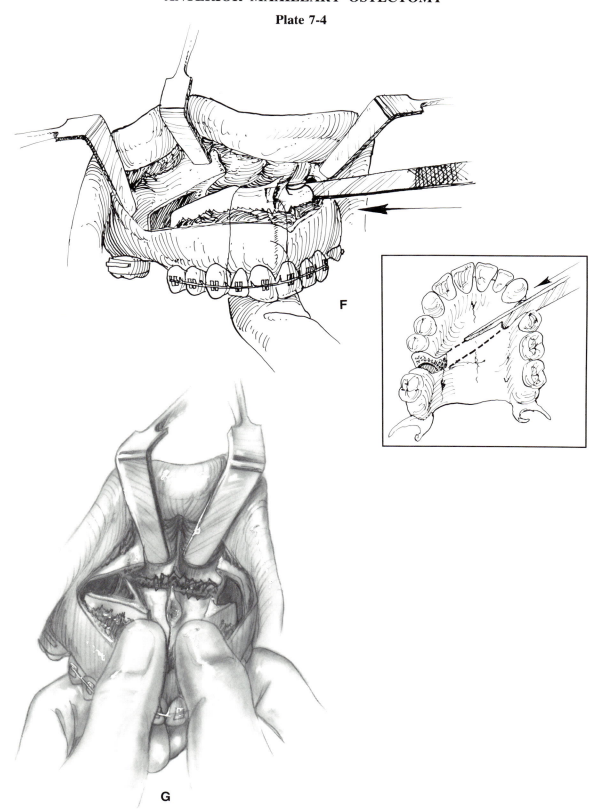

F

G

ANTERIOR MAXILLARY OSTECTOMY

Plate 7-4

H. Following down-fracturing of the anterior maxilla the nasal crest of the maxilla is removed to prevent deviation of the cartilaginous nasal septum when the segments are repositioned. This is readily done with a large bone bur. If necessary, and as dictated by the amount of superior movement of the anterior maxilla, the midline of the nasal floor can be grooved to further accommodate the nasal septum, or a portion of the inferior aspect of the nasal septum can be removed.

I. The palatal mucoperiosteum is now carefully reflected from the stable palate (posteriorly) with a periosteal elevator so that the necessary transpalatal ostectomy can be completed to move the anterior maxilla posteriorly. While completing this ostectomy retractors are placed superiorly to protect the nasal mucoperiosteum and a periosteal elevator is placed inferiorly to protect the palatal mucoperiosteum.

   If the interdental ostectomies are properly done, only the predetermined amount of bone of the horizontal portion of the palate remains to be removed.

J. After the indicated amount of bone is removed in all areas the occlusal splint is inserted and an attempt is made to place the anterior segment into its predetermined position. If the anterior segments do not fit into position the ostectomy sites are examined under direct visualization to identify the specific areas of bony interference that are preventing its proper replacement, and these are selectively removed until the segment can be properly repositioned. If the nasal septal cartilage will be deviated with the repositioning of the anterior segment a portion of it is resected to prevent this.

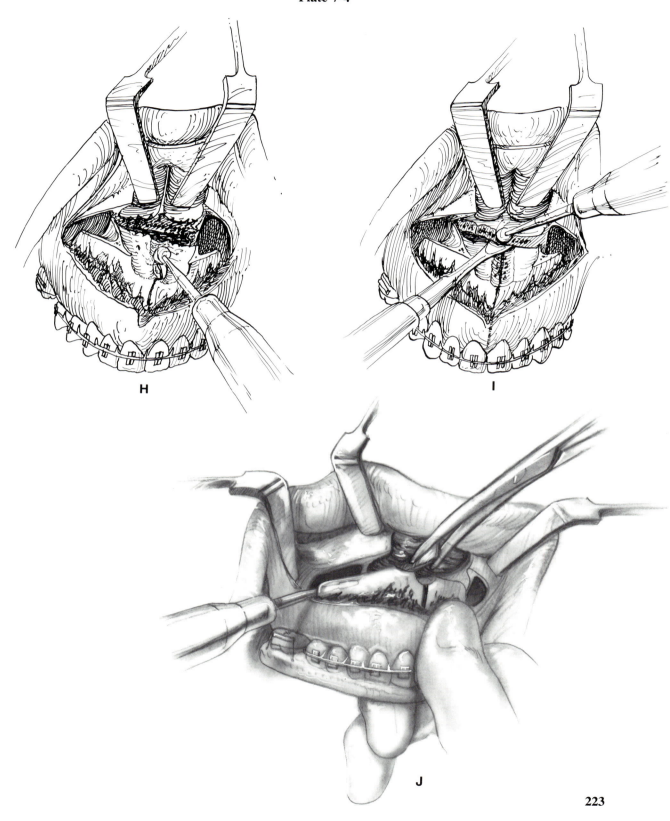

H

I

J

223

ANTERIOR MAXILLARY OSTECTOMY

Plate 7-4

K. After placement of the segments in the splint, they are stabilized by direct wiring of the splint to the teeth. Vertical stability of the anterior segment, especially if it extends posteriorly to the molar areas, is enhanced with piriform rim suspension wires. These are inserted by placing an interosseous hole through the piriform rim above the level of the horizontal osteotomy and passing a 24-gauge wire through it to the occlusal splint. To avoid impingement on the gingiva the wire coming from inside the piriform rim is passed through the gingiva and then brought over the edge of the splint. The wire on the outside of the piriform rim is passed through the hole in the flange of the splint. The wire is tightened until the anterior maxilla is supported sufficiently vertically that the mandibular dentition fits properly into the splint.

The horizontal vestibular incision is closed with absorbable sutures, taking only small bits of tissue in the incision line to minimize the degree that the lip will be shortened. The larger the portions of tissue taken when suturing this incision, the more the upper lip will shorten by rolling the lip inward, with exposure of less vermilion. Generally no intermaxillary fixation is necessary for this procedure. The occlusal splint is maintained for approximately 4 to 6 weeks and the anterior segments tested for stability. If they are unstable the splint is rewired for an additional few weeks; if they are stable it is worn at night for an additional few weeks as a retainer.

ANTERIOR MAXILLARY OSTECTOMY

Plate 7-4

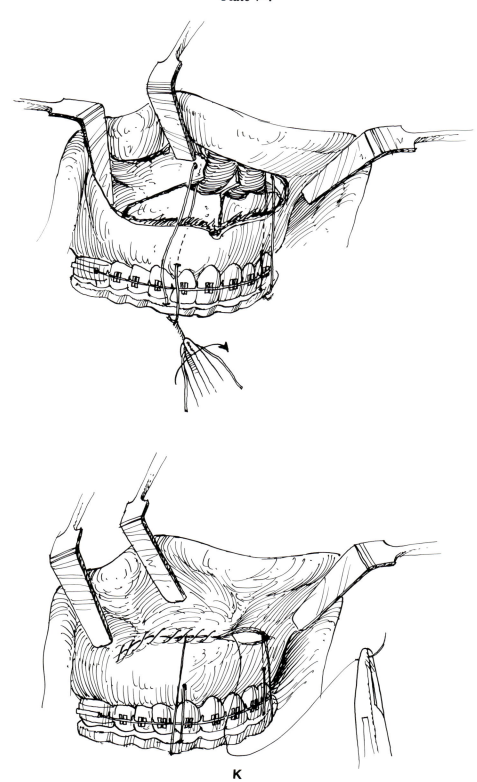

K

225

Posterior maxillary ostectomy

The unilateral or bilateral posterior maxillary osteotomy or ostectomy provides a means of surgically correcting a wide variety of occlusal and dentofacial deformities. The relative indications for this procedure are:

1. To alter the transverse position of the posterior maxilla (i.e., to correct crossbite)
2. To superiorly reposition a supraerupted posterior segment
3. To inferiorly reposition a posterior maxillary segment to close a posterior open bite
4. To move a posterior segment forward to close an edentulous space

In most instances some degree of simultaneous vertical, anteroposterior, and transverse movements of the posterior maxillary segments is effected.

Numerous technical approaches to the posterior maxillary ostectomy have been advocated. Regardless of the specific technique utilized, principles of surgical technique as they apply to the repositioning of dento-osseous segments with this operation do not differ from those advocated for all other segmental procedures, as discussed earlier in this chapter.

The procedure to be described here accomplishes the basic surgical objectives. It is an extension of the principle of the down-fracture in maxillary surgery first put forth by me. This principle is applicable to the anterior maxillary ostectomy as previously described and illustrated, the posterior maxillary ostectomy illustrated here, and the total maxillary osteotomy discussed in Chapter 8. In this regard the procedure described and illustrated is versatile in that virtually all of the deformities of the posterior maxillary dentoalveolus can be corrected via this single operative approach.

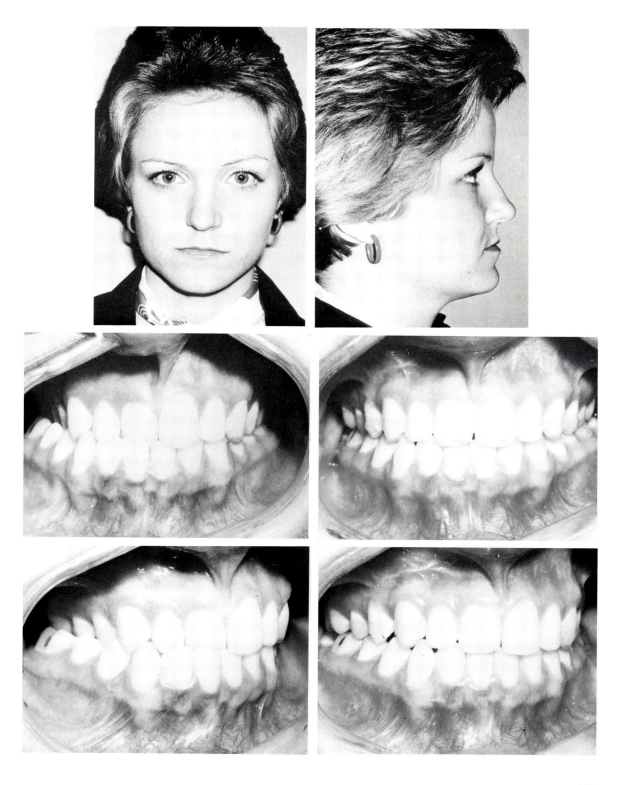

227

POSTERIOR MAXILLARY OSTECTOMY

Plate 7-5

A. The illustrated case demonstrates a class I malocclusion, unilateral posterior buccal crossbite, and a missing maxillary second premolar. Presurgically the lower arch has been leveled and aligned, and segmental orthodontics have been used in the maxilla in preparation for the proposed posterior maxillary ostectomy. The indicated surgical procedure is designed to move the posterior segment slightly superiorly and medially to correct the posterior crossbite and to move the segment anteriorly to close the edentulous second premolar space.

The wider the lateral maxillary ostectomy and the higher the palatal vault, the easier it is to make the palatal osteotomy or ostectomy transantrally. In the illustrated case there is only a small horizontal ostectomy in the lateral maxillary wall and a relatively low arched palate. The segment is to be repositioned medially, which requires a palatal ostectomy, as shown in the insert. Occasionally in this type of case it may be advantageous to utilize a palatal incision to complete the palatal cut, although this is generally not necessary, as will be illustrated.

B. Access for the osseous cuts is made through a horizontal incision high in the buccal vestibule, extending from the distal aspect of the first molar area forward to the distal aspect of the cuspid. This incision then becomes vertical and passes through the papillae one tooth anterior to the proposed interdental ostectomy. The mucoperiosteum is reflected posteriorly to expose the edentulous interdental area. The mucoperiosteum is reflected superiorly to expose the lateral maxillary wall and posteriorly to the pterygoid plate area. If an impacted third molar is present it is ignored at this point, because it will be removed readily later in the procedure.

Calipers are used to measure approximately 5 mm above the apices of the posterior teeth to determine the level of the horizontal osteotomy. As the horizontal subapical osteotomy extends distal to the second molar, it is tapered inferiorly. This portion of the osteotomy can be done with either the bur or curved osteotome. When the posterior osteotomy is tapered in this manner, separation of the pterygoid plates from the posterior maxilla is considerably simplified.

228

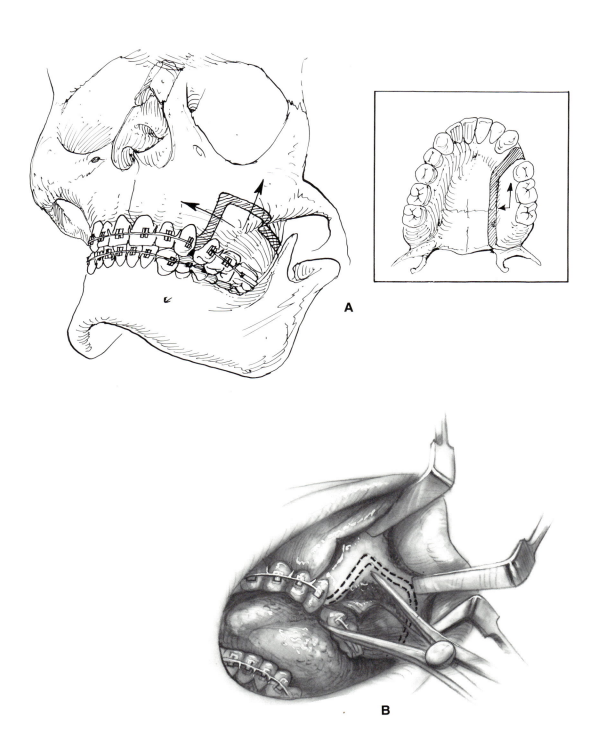

A

B

POSTERIOR MAXILLARY OSTECTOMY

Plate 7-5

C. A predetermined amount of bone (as determined by the model surgery) is removed from the lateral maxillary wall. The interdental alveolar ostectomy is next completed from the buccal aspect through the dentoalveolus and carried toward the palatal midline while maintaining a finger on the palatal mucosa to detect the bur as it perforates the palatal bone. As this ostectomy is being done the alveolar portion of the bone is first removed. This permits much better access for direct visualization while the ostectomy is being extended medially toward the midline of the palate. This ostectomy generally needs to extend only onto the horizontal palatal shelf and not the entire way to the midpalatal suture.

D. After completion of the horizontal and alveolar ostectomies a small curved osteotome is inserted transantrally through the anterior aspect of the horizontal ostectomy so as to cut through the palate at about the junction between its vertical and horizontal shelves and above the palatal apices of the posterior teeth. A finger is placed on the palate to detect the osteotome as it perforates the palatal bone to prevent tearing of the palatal mucosa.

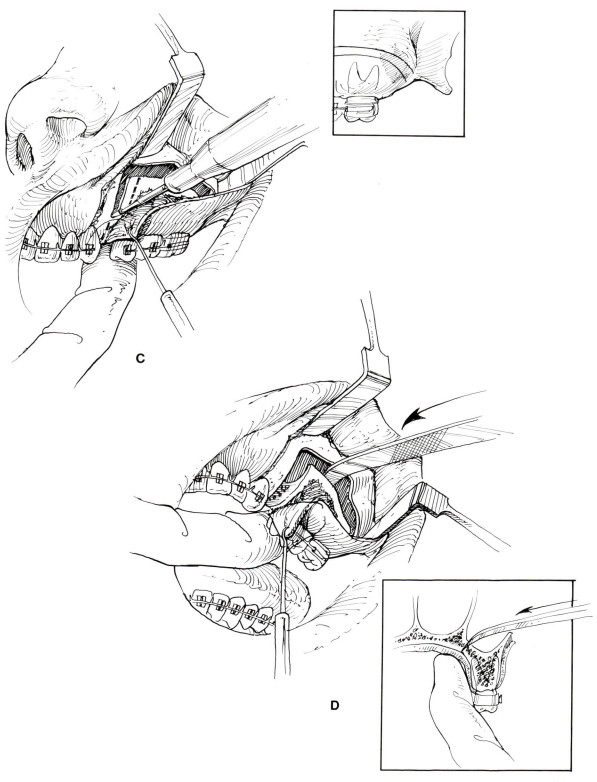

C

D

POSTERIOR MAXILLARY OSTECTOMY

Plate 7-5

E. If only an osteotomy or small osteotomy is indicated through the lateral maxillary wall, it is generally difficult to perform the transantral osteotomy without damaging the lateral maxillary wall. In these cases there are two alternatives: (1) complete the palatal osteotomy with a curved osteotome through the vertical ostectomy or osteotomy site (this is our preferred approach and is illustrated) or (2) make a palatal incision medial to the osteotomy, reflect the mucoperiosteum laterally, and complete the osteotomy or ostectomy from the direct palatal approach. When there is no interdental ostectomy or subapical ostectomy a palatal incision may be required or preferred to complete the palatal cut. In these instances a midpalatal incision with lateral mucoperiosteal reflection to the area where the vertical and horizontal palatal shelves meet is done. The palatal bone osteotomy or ostectomy is then made, into the maxillary sinus and extending posteriorly just medial to the existing greater palatal neurovascular bundle.

F. At this point the posterior maxillary segment can generally be down-fractured with the aid of an osteotome placed in the osteotomy and levered inferiorly. If the segment cannot be mobilized at this time the small curved osteotome is used to separate the pterygomaxillary junction.

   Once the segment is initially mobilized via down-fracturing, any palatal bone that must be removed to accomplish medial movement can be done under direct visualization. To accomplish this the palatal mucoperiosteum is reflected medially from the stable palate to enhance mobility and help avoid compressing it when the segment is repositioned.

232

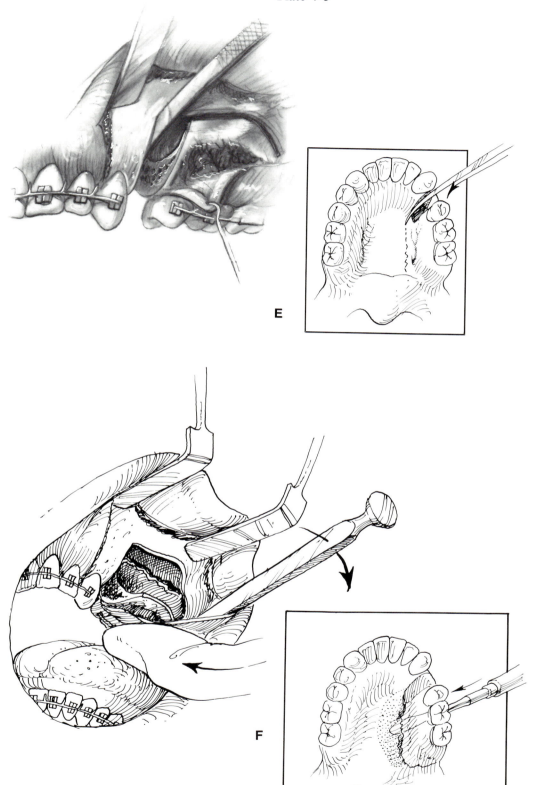

E

F

POSTERIOR MAXILLARY OSTECTOMY

Plate 7-5

G. The palatal bone is removed sufficiently to permit the posterior segment to be moved medially. In the posteromedial aspect of the palate the greater palatine neurovascular bundle is generally identifiable on down-fracturing the segment. Most often bone can be removed medially or laterally to this, and it can be pressured. If necessary it can be electrocoagulated. When the posterior segment is in the down-fractured position, impacted third molar, if present, can be readily removed from its superior aspect.

After the segment is well mobilized and the planned ostectomies completed the preformed occlusal acrylic splint is placed to check for completeness of the ostectomies. If the segment cannot be placed in the splint the ostectomy areas are reinspected and additional areas of bony interference removed.

H. The teeth are wired into the splint, and a buttress suspension wire is generally placed to stabilize the posterior segment in its proper vertical position. Generally no intermaxillary fixation is used. The splint is retained for about 6 weeks, removed, and the segment tested for stability. At this time finishing orthodontics can generally be done.

234

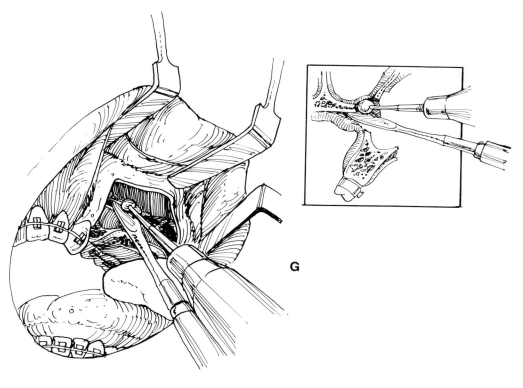

G

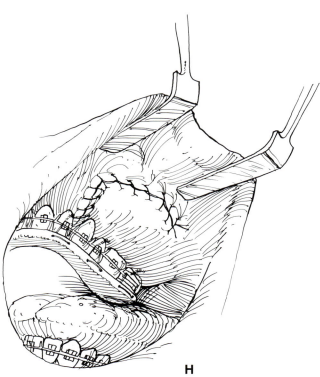

H

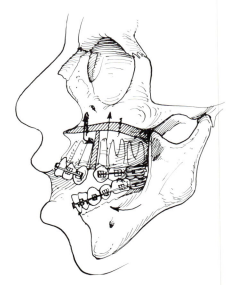

SUPERIOR REPOSITIONING OF MAXILLA

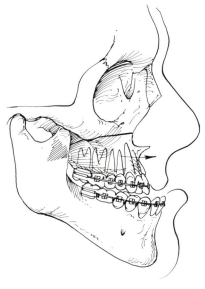

ADVANCEMENT OF MAXILLA

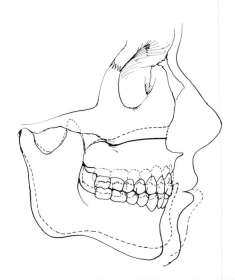

INFERIOR REPOSITIONING OF MAXILLA

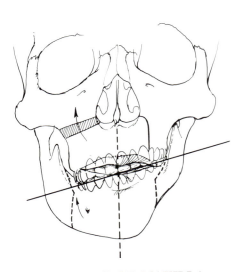

LEVELING OF MAXILLA

CHAPTER 8

Total maxillary surgery

The indications are common for surgical repositioning of the total maxilla superiorly, inferiorly, anteriorly, and posteriorly while simultaneously segmentalizing it to widen, narrow, level, or improve arch symmetry. Indeed with the development of the surgical capabilities and biologic knowledge accompanying repositioning of the total maxilla, the prospects for the definitive surgical correction of maxillary deformities have flourished during the past decade. With this recent interest in total maxillary surgery, technical advances have occurred that have made the surgery easier and safer and the results more predictable.

In this chapter are discussed and illustrated those specific surgical approaches that we have developed, modified, or utilized for total maxillary repositioning and have found to be technically easy, biologically sound, and predictable. Surgical procedures for superior repositioning of the maxilla, advancement of the maxilla, inferior repositioning of the maxilla, and leveling of the total maxilla are presented in sequence.

Superior repositioning of maxilla

The indications for superior repositioning of the maxilla include basically those conditions in which all or part of the maxilla or maxillary dentoalveolus is *excessive* in a vertical dimension. These conditions are generally clinically evident by excessive vertical exposure of the anterior maxillary teeth and lip incompetence. Additionally there are usually coexisting deformities of the maxilla or mandible or both, including an anteroposterior deformity (generally class II), a transverse deformity (posterior crossbite), and a vertical component (open bite).

The unique and exciting aspect of total maxillary surgery is that it generally permits the simultaneous correction of the vertical deformity, the anteroposterior deformity, and the transverse deformities via appropriate repositioning and segmentalization of the total maxilla. However, unlike mandibular surgery where the maxillary dentition serves as a stable referent to which the mandible is aligned and stabilized, at the time of surgery *there is no stable occlusal referent* in total maxillary surgery. Therefore these cases require more careful treatment planning if the desired results are to be achieved. In most instances treatment planning involves performing accurate model surgery on dental models mounted on an anatomic articulator via a face bow transfer and carefully completing cephalometric prediction tracings.

There are two basic operative approaches for superior repositioning of the maxilla: (1) superior repositioning of the maxilla leaving the nasal floor unaltered and (2) superior repositioning of the entire maxilla. With either procedure the maxilla can be repositioned as a single unit or segmentalized into two, three, or four separate dento-osseous units. The relative indications for each of these procedures are as follows:

1. Superior repositioning of the maxilla leaving the nasal floor intact
   a. Superior movement of 5 to 15 mm (major movement)
   b. Preexisting decreased nasal airway function not related to nasal septal deviation or excessively large inferior turbinates
   c. Segmentalization of the maxilla into three to four pieces with considerable movement of the individual segments
2. Superior repositioning of the entire maxilla
   a. Superior movement of less than 5 mm (minor movement)
   b. Existing functional nasal septal deviation or excessively large inferior turbinates
   c. Movement of the maxilla as a single unit or minor movement of multiple segments

These two procedures are separately illustrated and described.

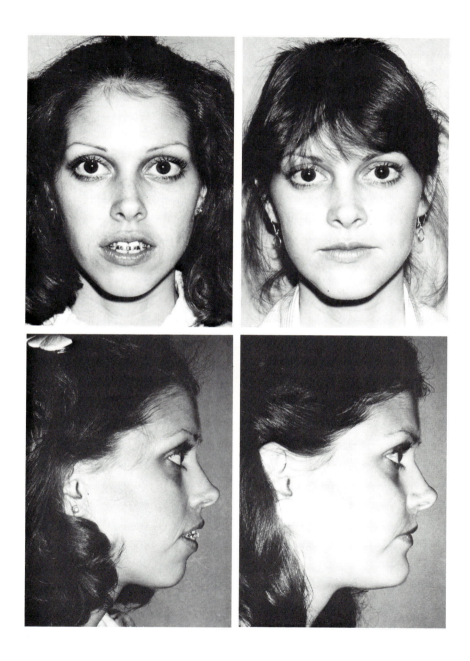

239

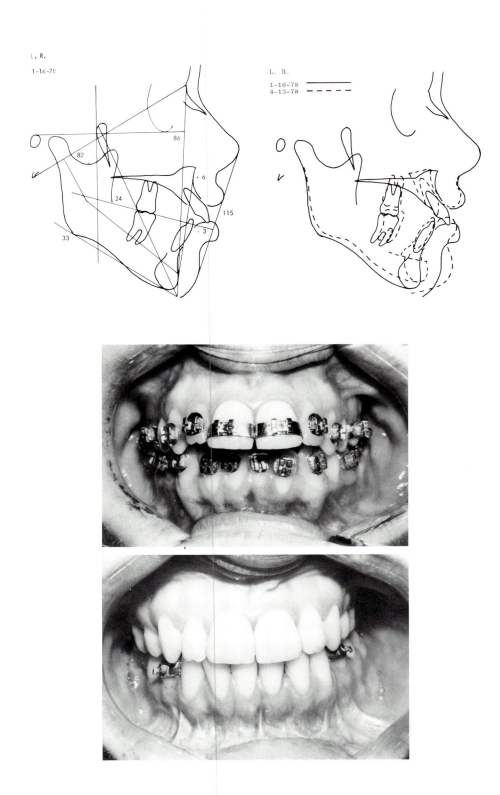

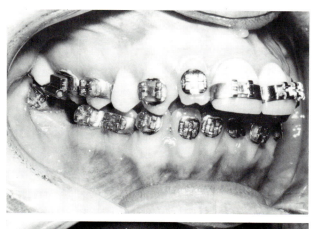

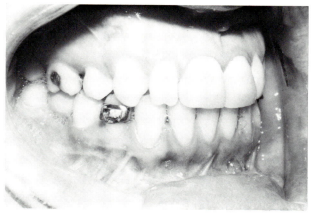

SUPERIOR REPOSITIONING OF MAXILLA LEAVING
NASAL FLOOR INTACT

Plate 8-1

A. The illustrated case in a skeletal class II open-bite deformity to be corrected by superior and posterior repositioning of the maxilla in three segments with a resultant autorotation forward and upward of the mandible. Orthodontic preparation has consisted of four premolar extractions and continuous arch orthodontics in the lower arch and segmental orthodontics in the maxilla. Segmental orthodontics is often indicated in open-bite deformities because it essentially eliminates any *potential postsurgical orthodontic* relapse that otherwise would occur when a continuous arch wire is used.

The amount of superior repositioning is usually determined by planning to reposition the anterior maxillary segment superiorly so that the maxillary central incisors are exposed 2 to 4 mm below the inferiormost portion of the upper lip when the lips are in repose. A careful clinical examination, face bow transferred models mounted on an anatomic articulator, accurate model surgery, and a carefully done prediction tracing will determine the amount of bone indicated for removal in the piriform aperture and molar areas as well as anteroposterior and transverse movements of the various maxillary segments. *The actual amount of bone to be removed in the various locations of the lateral maxillary wall is generally different from the clinically determined amount of superior incisor movement because of independent movement of the various segments.* These predetermined values for removal of bone are recorded and duplicated at surgery.

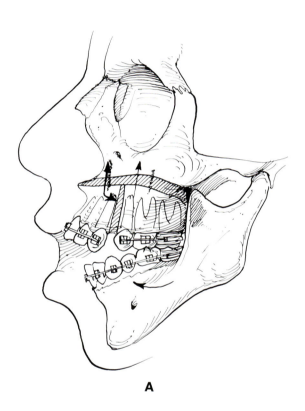

A

SUPERIOR REPOSITIONING OF MAXILLA LEAVING
NASAL FLOOR INTACT

Plate 8-1

B. A circumvestibular incision is made on one side from the region of the zygomaticoalveolar crest to the opposite piriform aperture, just above the level of the root apices. This provides maximal labial soft-tissue attachment (vascular pedicle) to those portions of the maxilla to be mobilized. By stopping the soft-tissue incision at the zygomaticoalveolar crest region and undermining posteriorly to the pterygomaxillary junction, the buccal fat pad can be avoided and a good width-to-length soft-tissue pedicle ratio is maintained to the mobilized anterior segments. Anteriorly the nasal mucoperiosteum is elevated from the lateral nasal wall beginning at the piriform aperture and extending 10 to 15 mm posteriorly. The mucoperiosteum is elevated from the anterior aspect of the nasal floor and the anterior aspect of the cartilaginous nasal septum is reflected from the vomerine groove with a periosteal elevator, exposing the anterior floor of the nose.

Vertical referent lines are inscribed on the bone in the cuspid and molar regions to assure proper anteroposterior movements of the segments when repositioned, as predetermined by the model surgery. Calipers are used to mark a point about 4 mm above the cuspid apex (approximately 34 mm superior to the cuspid cusp tip) and first molar apex (25 mm). These points determine the position of the inferior lateral maxillary wall osteotomy. Calipers are used to measure the amount of bone to be removed from the lateral maxillary wall in the piriform aperture and molar area as precisely predetermined from the model surgery and prediction tracing.

C. A periosteal elevator is inserted along the lateral nasal wall beneath the nasal mucoperiosteum to protect it from being cut with the bur when the horizontal ostectomy through the lateral maxillary wall is being made. The anterior aspect of the lateral nasal wall is also ostectomized for approximately 1 to $1\frac{1}{2}$ cm posteriorly. The measured amount of bone is removed from the lateral wall of the maxilla from the piriform aperture to the pterygoid plates by first completing the inferior horizontal osteotomy and then the superior osteotomy. Once these bone cuts are distal to the maxillary second molar root apices they are curved inferiorly toward the inferior aspect of the pterygomaxillary suture with an osteotome. This tapered cut makes it considerably easier to do an ostectomy in this area when the maxilla is to be repositioned posteriorly. The ostectomized bone is then removed. The identical procedure is then completed on the opposite side of the maxilla.

SUPERIOR REPOSITIONING OF MAXILLA LEAVING
NASAL FLOOR INTACT

Plate 8-1

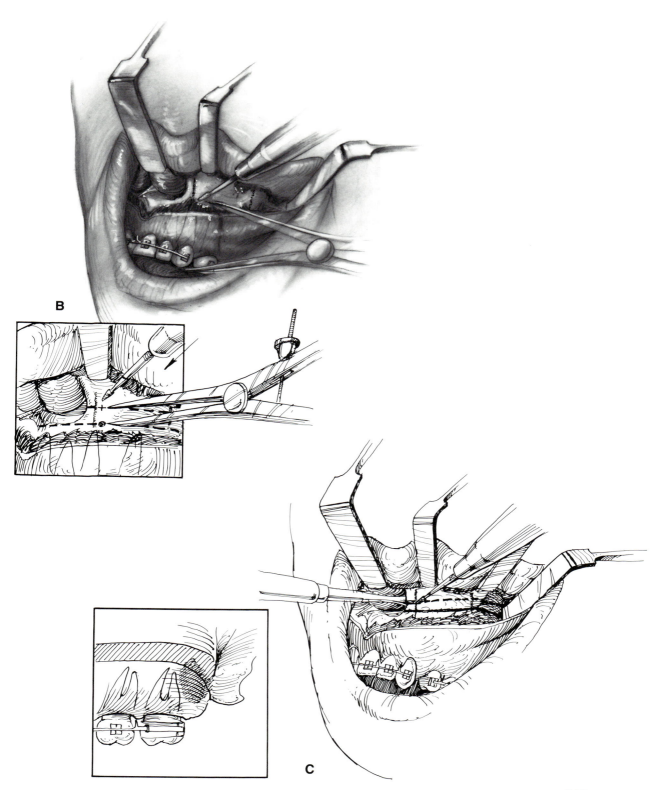

B

C

245

SUPERIOR REPOSITIONING OF MAXILLA LEAVING NASAL FLOOR INTACT

Plate 8-1

D. The mucoperiosteum overlying the alveolus between the cuspid and first premolar, or in the extraction area if a tooth is to be removed, is carefully elevated and gently retracted. Excessive elevation of the mucoperiosteum off the dentoalveolus anteriorly and posteriorly is avoided, as this decreases the vascular pedicle to these dento-osseous segments. A finger is placed on the palatal aspect of the alveolar mucosa to detect the bur as it perforates the cortical palatal bone to avoid excessive damage to this tissue and thereby maintain a good palatal vascular supply to the anterior maxillary segment(s). The vertical alveolar interdental osteotomy or ostectomy is completed through the alveolar portion *only at this time, with no attempt to complete the ostectomy to the palatal midline.* The same procedure is completed on the opposite side.

E. The cartilaginous nasal septum has been previously separated from the anterior aspect of the vomerine groove and is now retracted superiorly to permit good direct access to the anterior nasal floor. The anterior portion of the nasal crest of the maxilla is removed extending about 10 to 15 mm posteriorly. This is done by first making a cut in both sides of the nasal crest of the maxilla with a bur that forms a V-shaped wedge in the underlying maxillary bone, keeping at least 4 to 5 mm above the apices of the central incisors. The vertical dimension of the wedge being removed should at least equal the amount of vertical repositioning of the maxilla.

F. This V-shaped bone resection of the nasal crest of the maxilla is removed from the anterior nasal floor to accommodate the cartilaginous nasal septum and prevent its deviation when the maxilla is superiorly repositioned. If the indicated amount of bone cannot be removed because of the location of the central incisor tooth apices, a resection of the inferior aspect of septal cartilage is performed. When a considerable vertical distance exists between the anterior nasal floor and the apices of the anterior teeth an ostectomy can be performed below the level of the nasal floor. Removal of this bone further minimizes any reduction of the anterior nasal airway, which can occur with superior repositioning of the maxilla. This ostectomy also makes the subsequent transnasal palatal osteotomy easier by decreasing the thickness of the palatal bone anteriorly.

SUPERIOR REPOSITIONING OF MAXILLA LEAVING
NASAL FLOOR INTACT

Plate 8-1

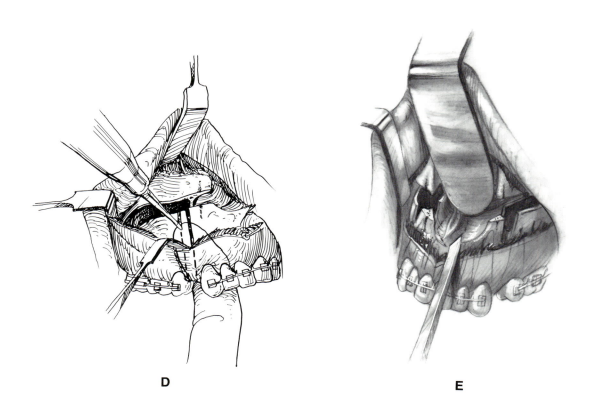

D

E

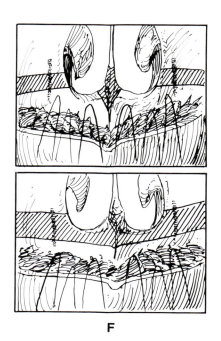

F

247

SUPERIOR REPOSITIONING OF MAXILLA LEAVING
NASAL FLOOR INTACT

Plate 8-1

G. A sharp curved osteotome or a fissured bur is used to begin the transnasal osteotomy through the palate. Generally a small curved osteotome is used; however, when the cephalometric radiography reveals that the anterior palatal bone is excessively thick, this anterior osteotomy is more easily made with a bur. A finger is maintained on the palate to detect the osteotome or bur as it perforates the palatal cortex. This cut is systematically made beginning anteriorly in the nasal floor and progressing in a lateral and posterior direction into the medial aspect of the antral floor as illustrated.

H. As the transpalatal cut progresses posteriorly it enters the maxillary sinus. Once into the maxillary sinus the cut is directed through the inferior aspect of the medial sinus wall, above the molar palatal root apices but just below the level of the nasal floor so that the cut will finish on the oral side of the palate and not into the nose.

I. The transantral cut generally needs to extend posteriorly only to the first molar area, thus avoiding injury to the greater palatine neurovascular bundle. Posterior to the first molar the palatal bone is relatively thin and will easily fracture along the palatomaxillary and pterygomaxillary suture areas when the maxilla is mobilized. When it is fractured in this manner the actual fracture occurs either through or just lateral to the greater palatine foramen.

Plate 8-1

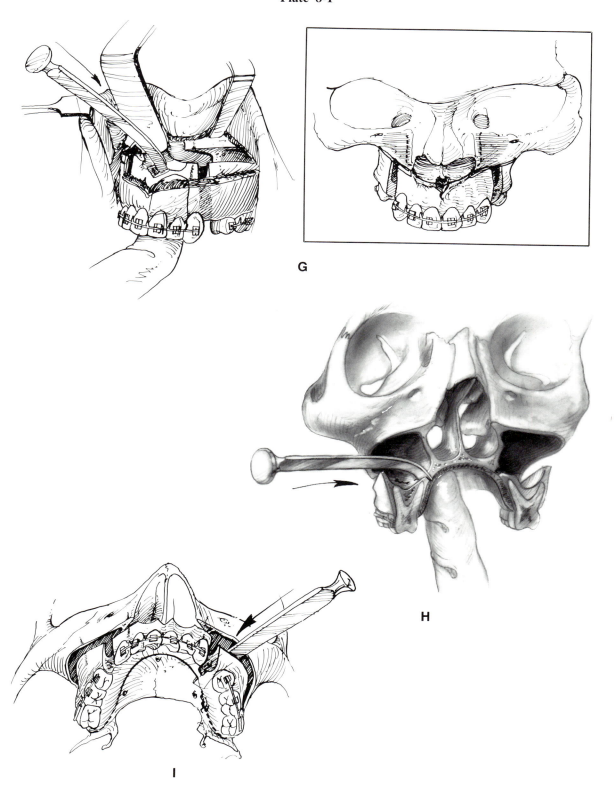

G

H

I

SUPERIOR REPOSITIONING OF MAXILLA LEAVING
NASAL FLOOR INTACT
Plate 8-1

J. Next the maxilla is down-fractured, exclusive of the nasal floor. This can be accomplished with manual manipulation by standing above the patient's head and placing the thumbs in each cuspid area and pushing down forcibly. Or one or two osteotomes can be inserted into the transnasal portion of the palatal osteotomy, between the stable nasal floor and the portion of the maxillary dentoalveolus to be mobilized, and the dentoalveolus forced inferiorly. When the maxilla is segmentalized as in the illustrated case, either maneuver generally mobilizes only the anterior portion of the maxilla, and the posterior segments are then individually sequentially mobilized in an identical fashion. When the maxilla is not segmentalized the initial maneuver with the two osteotomes will mobilize the entire maxillary dentoalveolar segment inferiorly, exclusive of the nasal floor.

K. When the maxilla is to be segmentalized into four pieces and major superior repositioning attempted (8 to 10 mm), it is usually best to retain an additional labial soft-tissue vascular pedicle to the anterior segments to assure that an adequate vascular supply is maintained. The illustrated labial pedicle does not significantly interfere with the access and helps supply both anterior segments.

L. If the posterior maxillary segments cannot be mobilized via down-fracturing with one of these maneuvers, the palatal cuts are all checked for completeness. If they are found to be complete a small curved osteotome is utilized to section the pterygomaxillary junction, as this is the only possible area preventing mobilization. When this area is to be sectioned it is best to use a small curved osteotome directed medially and slightly anteriorly.

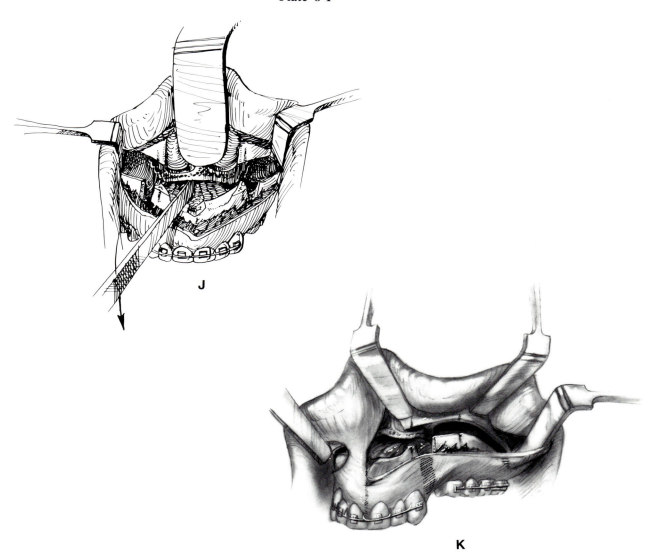

J

K

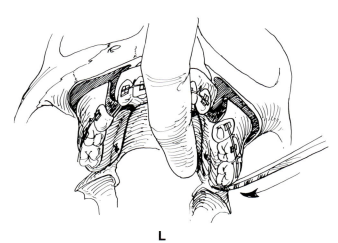

L

251

SUPERIOR REPOSITIONING OF MAXILLA LEAVING
NASAL FLOOR INTACT
Plate 8-1

M. As mobilization of the maxilla proceeds via down-fracturing, the palatal mucoperiosteum is liberally elevated from the stable portion of the palate. This step allows the mobilized segment or segments to be more easily repositioned without crimping, tearing, or inadvertently elevating the palatal mucoperiosteum from the mobilized segments as they are being laterally or superiorly repositioned, *thereby improving the blood supply to the segments.*

N. To reposition the maxillary segments directly superiorly or posteriorly, bone must be removed from the anterior and lateral aspects of the stable palate and the retromolar areas of the maxillary segments. Beginning anteriorly on the stable portion of the palate, bone removal is readily accomplished with a bone bur or rongeur while the maxillary dentoalveolar segments are retracted inferiorly. When the maxillary segments are to be moved superiorly and anteriorly this bone removal is usually not necessary.

O. Proceeding posteriorly, additional areas of bony interference are removed. Depending on the anatomy, specific location of the transantral cut, and direction of movement of the posterior maxillary segments, bone may or may not need to be removed from the lateral aspect of the stable palate. When the posterior maxillary segments are to be moved laterally to correct a posterior crossbite, generally no bone removal is required from the lateral aspect of the stable palate. When the segments are to be moved straight superiorly or medially, bone is removed from either the stable palatal portion, as illustrated, or carefully from the medial aspect of the palatoalveolar border on the mobilized dento-osseous segments.

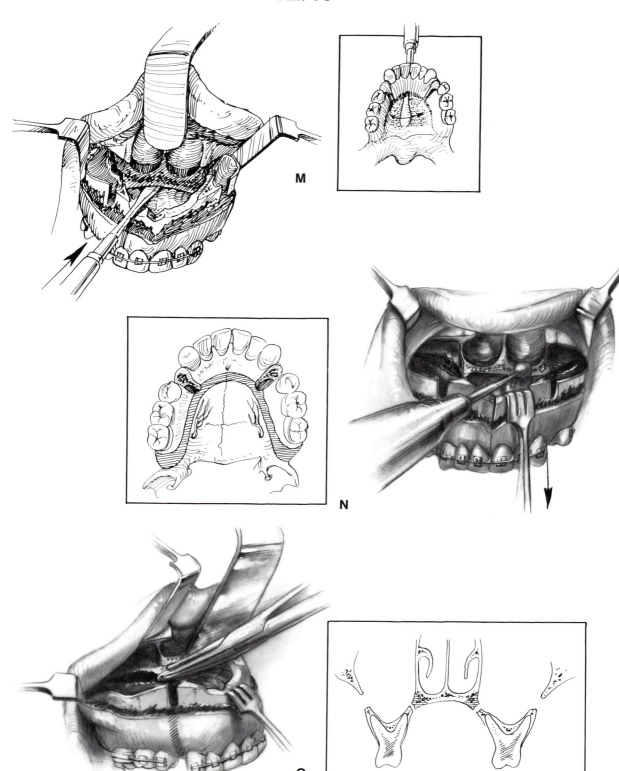

M

N

O

SUPERIOR REPOSITIONING OF MAXILLA LEAVING
NASAL FLOOR INTACT
Plate 8-1

P. If an impacted maxillary third molar is present it is removed through the floor of the maxillary sinus while the maxilla is retracted inferiorly. Care is taken not to incise or tear the lateral mucoperiosteum overlying the third molar, because this is the primary vascular source for the soft-tissue buccal pedicle flap of the mobilized dento-osseous segments.

Q. Generally 5 to 7 mm of posterior maxillary tuberosity can be removed to facilitate posterior movement of the maxilla without injury to the maxillary second molar. This bone is readily removed laterally while the maxillary segments are retracted anteriorly and inferiorly. The bone can be removed by using a fissure bur to initiate a vertical osteotomy through the tuberosity just posterior to the second molar and fracturing the tuberosity off in a posterior direction. Also an osteotome can be used to make the same cut. As the osteotomy proceeds medially, care must be exercised in an attempt to preserve the descending palatine neurovascular bundle. This can generally be accomplished, as it is visible and can be protected. If need be it can be ligated, but this is usually not necessary.

R. An occlusal splint is attached to the maxillary teeth with 26-gauge wire. This stabilizes and consolidates the various segments of the maxilla into a single unit. Temporary intermaxillary fixation is placed and the maxillary-mandibular complex rotated superiorly, being sure that the condyles remain in the fossa. Any bony interferences remaining are removed until the complex can be passively rotated into its new position. Since the maxilla is to be moved posteriorly, circumzygomatic suspension wires can be used. When the maxillary segments are to be repositioned superiorly and anteriorly, infraorbital wires are placed. Two 24-gauge wires are then passed through the loop formed from the 22-gauge circumzygomatic wire and attached to the occlusal splint in the molar and cuspid areas to provide stabilization.

Generally no intermaxillary fixation is used; however, during suspension the teeth are temporarily placed into intermaxillary fixation, primarily to prevent rotation and torquing of the maxillary segments. *The vertical referent line changes must correspond with those recorded from the model surgery and prediction tracings.* Postsurgically interarch elastics are often used to assure accurate and complete closure of the mandible into the splint. At about 3 weeks postoperatively the suspension wires are loosened and the occlusal splint removed, and the segments generally exhibit sufficient stability so that finishing orthodontics can be instituted.

254

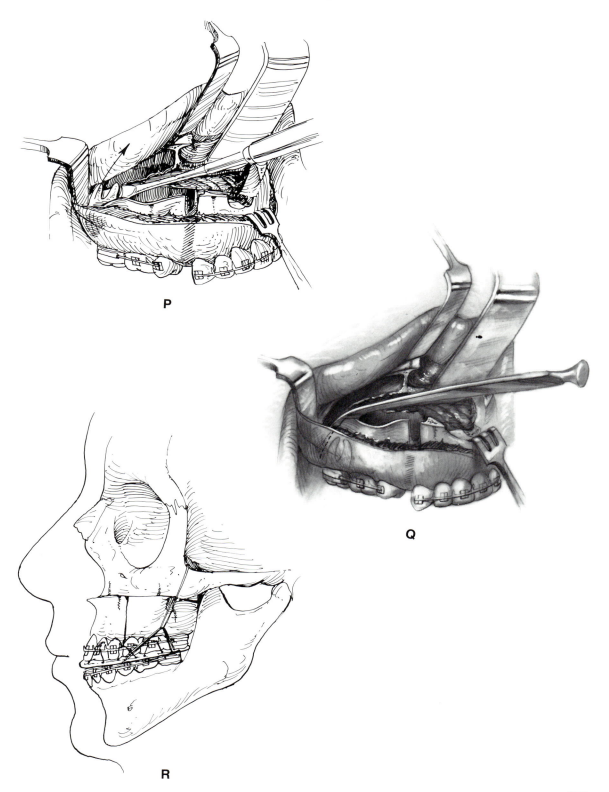

P

Q

R

SUPERIOR REPOSITIONING OF ENTIRE MAXILLA

Plate 8-2

A. In this patient with vertical maxillary excess without open-bite deformity and class II malocclusion the entire maxilla is to be superiorly repositioned about 5 mm. In order to simultaneously correct the class II malocclusion the maxilla will need to be moved posteriorly about 5 mm. Presurgically orthodontic leveling and aligning of both the maxillary and mandibular arches has been achieved.

B. The soft-tissue incisions and dissection are done as described in Plate 8-1, *B*. Because it is usually impossible to accurately visualize the tooth root apices through the bone, calipers are used to determine the location of the inferior cut of the proposed ostectomy on the lateral maxillary wall, about 4 mm above the cuspid and first molar root apices. Vertical referent lines are scored into the maxilla in the cuspid and first molar areas so that precise repositioning of the maxilla in the posterior direction can be achieved at surgery to correspond accurately with the model surgery and prediction tracing.

C. The lateral maxillary wall ostectomy is made from the piriform aperture of the nasal cavity to the pterygoid plates. A periosteal elevator is inserted along the lateral nasal wall to protect the nasal mucoperiosteum. Anteriorly the ostectomy is carried through the anterior portion of the lateral nasal wall. The ostectomy is tapered inferiorly once it passes the second molar root apices, toward the inferior junction of the pterygoid plates and posterior maxilla. By tapering the ostectomy in this manner it is seldom necessary to section the pterygomaxillary junction with an osteotome, and when the maxilla is to be moved posteriorly less bone needs to be removed in the retromolar area. The identical soft-tissue dissection and ostectomy sequence is completed on the opposite side.

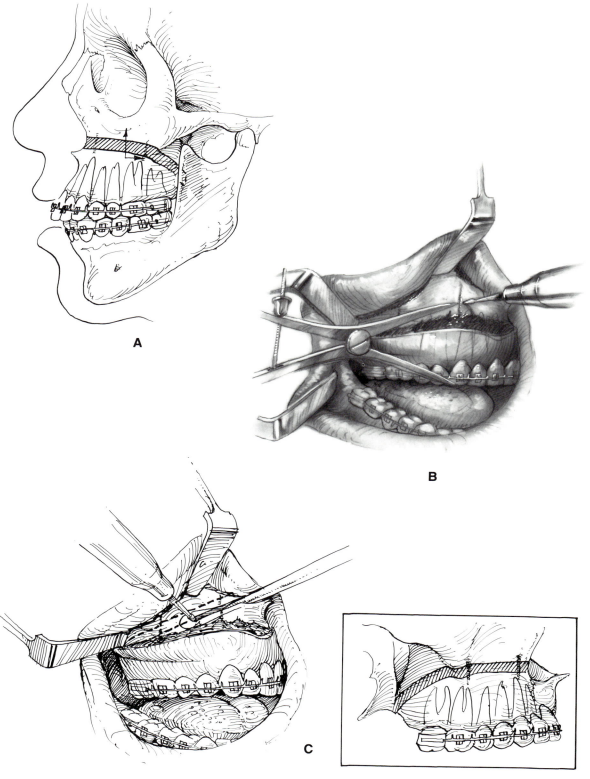

A

B

C

SUPERIOR REPOSITIONING OF ENTIRE MAXILLA

Plate 8-2

D. If the maxilla is to be segmentalized the mucoperiosteal tissues overlying the alveolus in the areas to be osteotomized or ostectomized are carefully undermined to about the alveolar crest. The indicated interdental osteotomies or ostectomies are then completed through the dentoalveolus only, with *no attempt to carry the ostectomy to the midline of the palate*. By not extending the ostectomy across the palate the maxilla can be downfractured in one piece, and the palatal osteotomies can then be completed from the superior aspect under direct visualization.

E. Next the anterior aspect of the cartilaginous nasal septum is elevated from the vomerine groove in the nasal crest of the maxilla, the mucoperiosteum is elevated off the anterior nasal floor, and a nasal septal osteotome is used to separate the nasal septum from the maxilla. Because the osteotome tends to ride up the vomer, it should be angled slightly downward to initiate the cut. A straight osteotome is used to cut the lateral nasal wall posteriorly to about the first molar area. This will assure that the descending palatine vessels are intact at this stage, and only a small portion of the posterior aspect of the lateral nasal wall remains to be fractured.

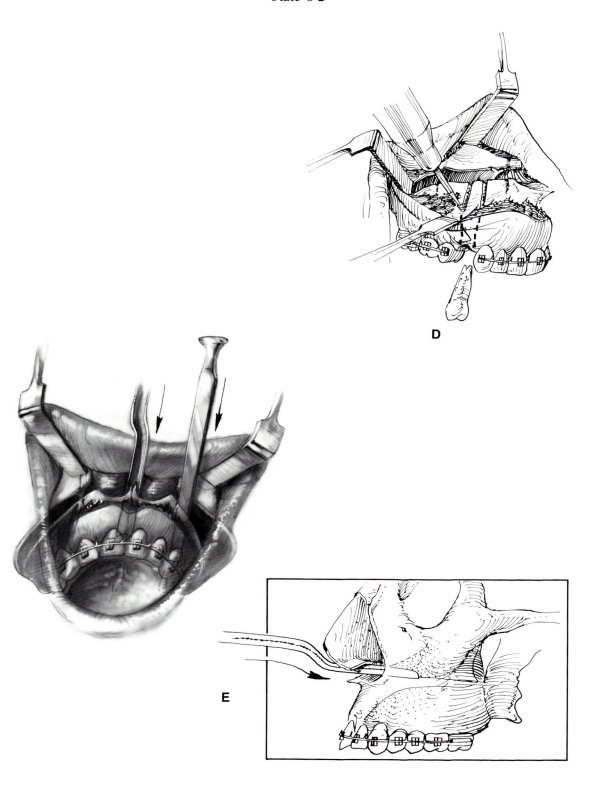

D

E

F. After completion of the nasal septal cut the maxilla is down-fractured with either manual manipulation or maxillary mobilization forceps. If mobilization does not occur, separation of the maxillary tuberosity and pterygoid plates with a small curved osteotome is carried out; however, this is seldom necessary. As the down-fracturing proceeds the nasal mucoperiosteum is progressively elevated from the floor of the nose with a periosteal elevator to the posterior border of the nasal floor or palate.

G. With the maxilla retracted inferiorly, a deep groove is made in the midline the entire length of the superior surface of the maxilla to remove the remaining portion of the vomer and accommodate the nasal septum when the maxilla is superiorly repositioned. Alternatively, or in addition, the inferior portion of the nasal septum may be resected to avoid deviation of the nasal septum when the maxilla is superiorly repositioned. If a functional deviation of the nasal septum preexists, a submucoperiosteal dissection of the nasal septum is done and the septum osteotomized and straightened.

H. The lateral walls of the nose are trimmed with a rongeur to eliminate interferences when the maxilla is superiorly repositioned. The bone of the posterior aspect of the lateral nasal wall is carefully removed so the integrity of the descending palatine artery is maintained. This is usually possible because at this time the neurovascular bundle is readily visible in this area and judicious removal of the bone surrounding it can be achieved.

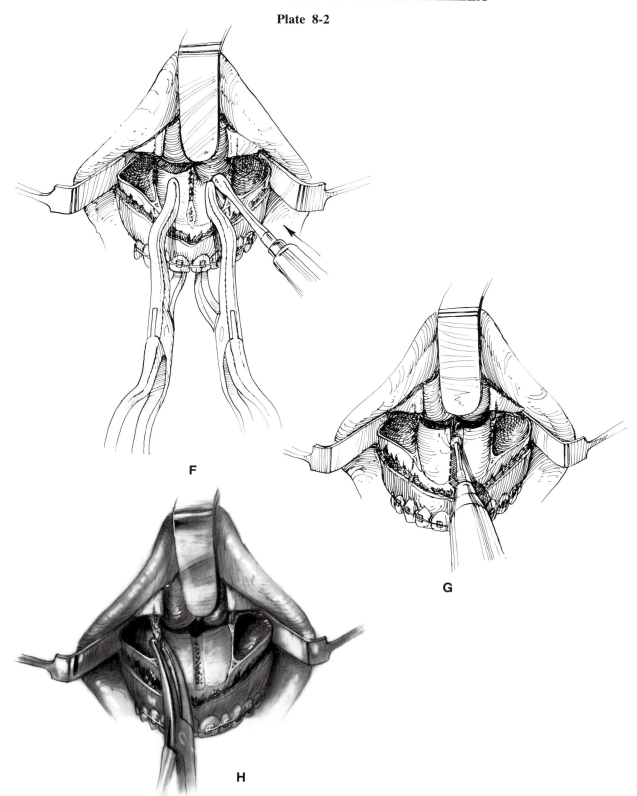

F

G

H

SUPERIOR REPOSITIONING OF ENTIRE MAXILLA

Plate 8-2

I.   If the maxilla is to be segmentalized the vertical interdental osteotomies or ostectomies through the dentoalveolus of the extraction sites will have already been completed, and only the palatal portion of the ostectomies remains to be done. The transverse ostectomy of the palate can easily be done with the maxilla retracted inferiorly. This sequencing of osteotomies and ostectomies proves to simplify this operation because it permits completion of the vertical osteotomies or ostectomies through the dentoalveolus under direct visualization while the maxilla is stable, and completion of the transpalatal osteotomy or ostectomy under direct vision when the maxilla is down-fractured, making these osteotomies much easier.

The posterior maxillary bone is removed in a manner identical to that described and illustrated in Plate 8-1, *P* and *Q*, when the maxilla is to be repositioned posteriorly.

J.   Inferior turbinectomies can be performed as part of this operation if the turbinates are large and obstructing the nasal airway or if they limit superior movement of the maxilla. A long incision is made bilaterally, through the nasal mucoperiosteum from below, to open into the nasal cavity and expose the turbinates. A side-cutting rongeur is then used to resect the turbinates and their overlying mucosa. The resultant soft-tissue raw edges are electrocoagulated to achieve hemostasis.

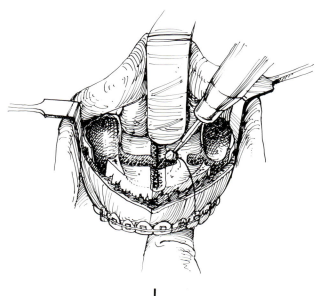

I

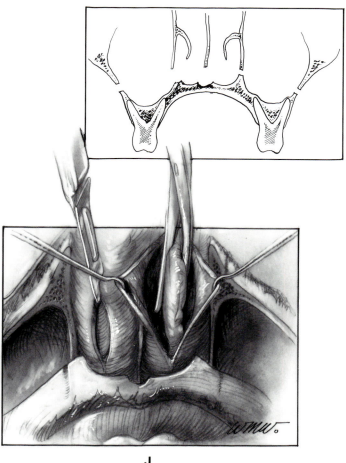

J

K. Suspension and stabilization of the superiorly repositioned maxilla without intermaxillary fixation is as follows. When the maxilla is moved superiorly and posteriorly, circumzygomatic suspension wires usually are used because of their superior and posterior vectors of support. When the maxilla is moved superiorly and anteriorly infraorbital suspension wires are used to provide anterior and superior force vectors. Infraorbital suspension wires are placed through the circumvestibular incision. The dissection is carried up to and over the inferior orbital rim, usually lateral to the infraorbital neurovascular bundle. An interosseous hole is placed through the rim, and a 22-gauge wire is placed through it and brought intraorally and twisted, creating a loop, as illustrated in Plate 8-3, *I*. Two 24-gauge wires are passed through the loop and attached anteriorly in the cuspid area and posteriorly in the molar area. Temporary intermaxillary fixation is used to assure the proper occlusal relationship between the maxilla and mandible, and the complex is then rotated into position. If the complex cannot be passively rotated, any bony interferences are removed. Usually the suspension wires must remain in place longer than when the maxilla is superiorly repositioned and the palate remains unaltered, because that technique usually heals more rapidly as a result of better bony interfaces. Interarch elastics are usually necessary during the postoperative course to assure proper interdigitation of the mandible into the occlusal splint during the healing phase.

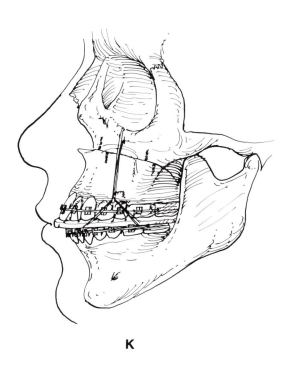

K

Advancement of maxilla

Advancement of the total maxilla can be achieved with highly predictable results and little morbidity. The increased versatility of total maxillary advancement, as opposed to mandibular setback procedures, lies in the fact that simultaneous with advancement the maxilla can be segmentalized and thereby widened or narrowed. Further, the direction of the lateral wall cut can be varied to simultaneously shorten the maxilla and thereby optimize facial esthetics.

The success of treatment results with total maxillary advancement surgery are directly related to several identifiable aspects of the operative procedure: (1) adequate mobilization of the maxilla so that it can be passively repositioned; (2) avoiding inadvertent fracturing of the pterygoid plates and thereby destroying the posterior stop for the bone graft; (3) bone grafting when indicated; (4) proper placement of bone grafts; and (5) proper stabilization of the repositioned maxilla. These technical prerequisites for achieving predictable results with total maxillary advancement surgery are fulfilled in our experience in the following fashion.

Adequate mobilization is well achieved with the down-fracturing technique illustrated, which we advocate as the technique of choice. This permits excellent direct visualization of the entire superior aspect of the maxilla including the nasal septum and the perpendicular plates of the palatine bones. In addition this provides excellent access for segmentation of the maxilla if indicated. In the cleft patient this technique provides good access to manage the soft tissues associated with the alveolar and palatal deformities, as discussed in Chapter 10.

To achieve good mobility of the total maxilla the pterygomaxillary junction must be sectioned. However, in doing so it is equally important not to comminute the maxillary tuberosity or pterygoid plates in this area, because these structures are essential when bone grafting is indicated to stabilize the advanced maxilla. Thus the instrumentation in performing this maneuver is important.

Bone grafting in total maxillary advancement has been a matter of controversy. Recent evaluation by us has resulted in the following recommendations. In all cleft and edentulous patients bone grafting is best accomplished with a cortical cancellous graft placed into the pterygomaxillary gap. When the maxilla is very hypoplastic or atropic and major advancements with or without simultaneous expansion are done, fresh autogenous cancellous grafting to the lateral maxillary walls assures optimal stability. In the cleft patient fresh autogenous cancellous grafting to the alveolar defect will improve stability. In individuals with idiopathic maxillary deficiency stable results are obtainable without bone grafting when the maxilla is advanced 5 to 6 mm or less.

Stabilization of the maxilla is best achieved by the use of infraorbital suspension wires providing an anterosuperior vector of force.

In this section the technique for advancement of the total maxilla is described and illustrated.

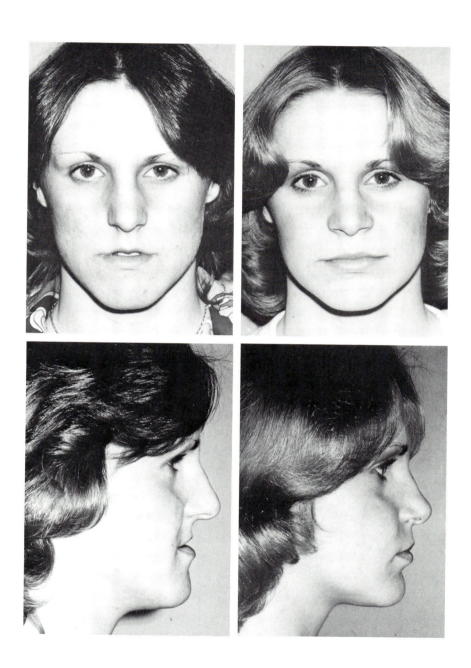

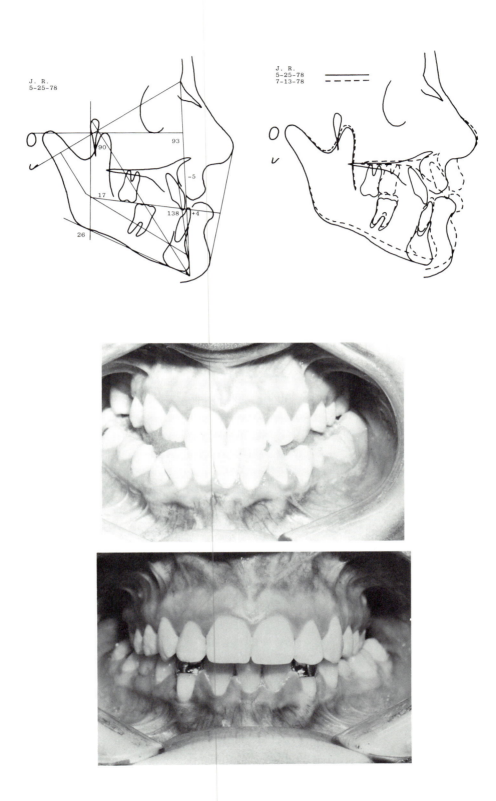

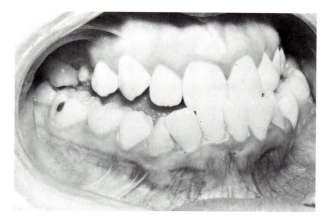

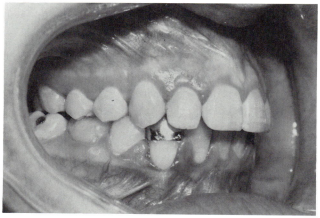

ADVANCEMENT OF MAXILLA

Plate 8-3

A. The maxilla can be advanced as a total unit or in segments. The illustrated case demonstrates advancement of the maxilla as a total unit. This case shows a deficient maxilla (anteroposterior) with a class III malocclusion. The posterior maxillary arch is in bilateral posterior crossbite. The amount of advancement, as determined from dental models and cephalometric prediction tracing, is 11 mm. Therefore bone grafting in the pterygomaxillary areas is indicated.

B. The surgical approach is through a circumvestibular incision made high in the buccal vestibule. The initial incision is made with a diathermy knife, extending from the region of the first molar on one side across the midline to the opposite piriform aperture. Limiting the initial incision to one side, until the osteotomies are completed on that side, minimizes blood loss from the mucoperiosteal incision. The mucoperiosteum is reflected superiorly from the anterior and lateral maxillary walls. This dissection is carried superiorly until the infraorbital nerve is exposed. The subperiosteal dissection extends posteriorly to the junction of the pterygoid plates and the tuberosity of the maxilla. The nasal mucoperiosteum, from the piriform rim and lateral nasal wall, is reflected posteriorly approximately 2 cm.

C. Vertical reference lines are inscribed on the lateral wall of the maxilla in the area of the cuspid and first molar to provide an accurate direct referent for advancement. Utilizing calipers, horizontal reference points are made 4 mm above the root apices of the cuspid and first molar, denoting the level of the proposed horizontal osteotomy.

A periosteal elevator is placed subperiosteally beneath the lateral nasal mucoperiosteum. The horizontal osteotomy is completed from the piriform rim to the pterygoid plates. When bone grafting is to be done between the pterygoid plates and the tuberosity of the maxilla, the horizontal osteotomy is carried straight posteriorly to the pterygoid plates at such a level as to provide a good buttress of bone on the tuberosity of the maxilla for the bone grafting.

If the maxilla is being advanced *without bone grafting,* the lateral osteotomy can be tapered inferiorly toward the inferior aspect of the pterygoid plates posterior to the second molar. This eliminates the necessity of separating the pterygoid plates from the maxilla with an osteotome.

270

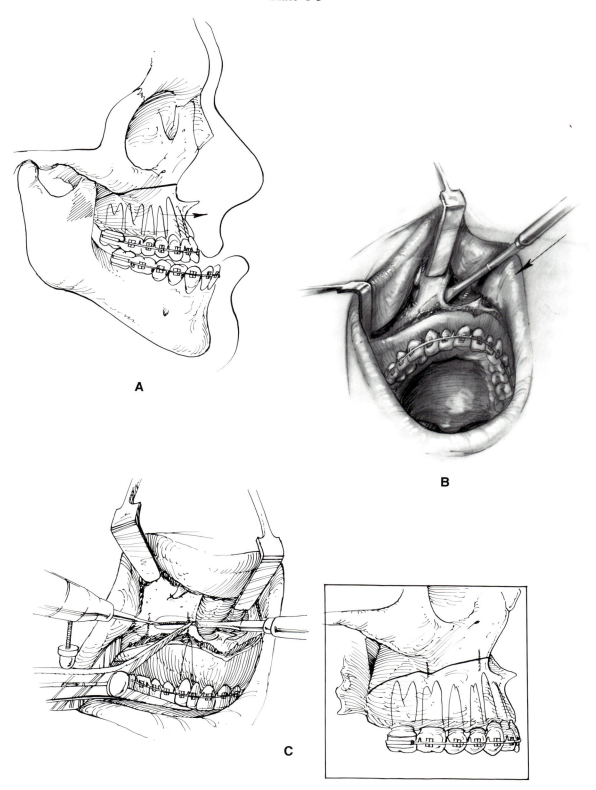

A

B

C

Plate 8-3

D. The soft-tissue incision is completed to the zygomatic buttress on the opposite side, and the same soft-tissue dissection and osteotomies are performed. The mucoperiosteum is elevated from the floor of the nose bilaterally. In doing so the cartilaginous nasal septum is elevated superiorly from
the vomerine groove in the nasal crest of the maxilla, and a nasal septal
osteotome is used to separate the nasal septum from the maxilla.

Care should be taken to direct this osteotome downward toward the palate so that separation of the nasal septum will occur close to the nasal floor
level. The tendency while making this cut is for the osteotome to ride up
the vomer, with the subsequent osteotomy occurring high on the nasal septum posteriorly. A finger at the posterior aspect of the hard palate will help
with orientation during this phase of surgery.

E. A periosteal elevator is inserted subperiosteally to protect the lateral nasal
mucoperiosteum, and the lateral nasal walls are sectioned posteriorly about
3 cm with a thin osteotome. If this cut is carried farther posteriorly the
descending palatine artery can be torn or severed.

A small curved osteotome is used to separate the maxillary tuberosity
from the pterygoid plates. This separation must occur without comminuting
the tuberosity or pterygoid plates so that good bony interfaces remain, between which the bone grafts can be wedged into place. Careless use of a
large osteotome in this area generally causes comminution and makes bone
grafting less useful. The osteotome is directed slightly inferiorly while a
finger is placed on the palatal side of the tuberosity so the cutting edge of
the osteotome can be palpated beneath the mucoperiosteum as the osteotome
completes the separation.

Plate 8-3

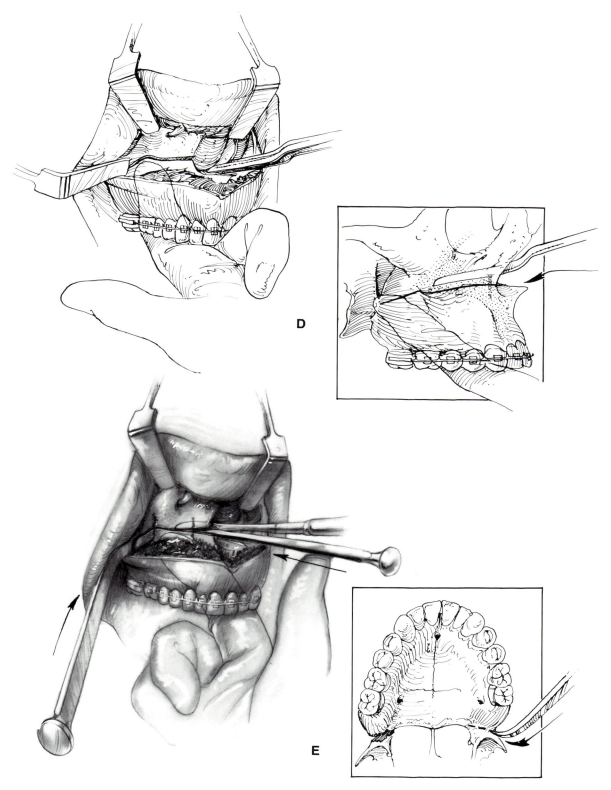

D

E

ADVANCEMENT OF MAXILLA

Plate 8-3

F. The maxilla is now ready for down-fracturing and mobilization. A small piece of gauze is placed on the anterior gingiva, teeth, and orthodontic brackets, and firm downward pressure is applied to the anterior maxilla. Pressure is increased until the maxilla fractures and rotates downward. As down-fracturing proceeds a periosteal elevator is used to elevate the remaining nasal mucoperiosteum from the nasal floor until the posterior border of the hard palate is identified.

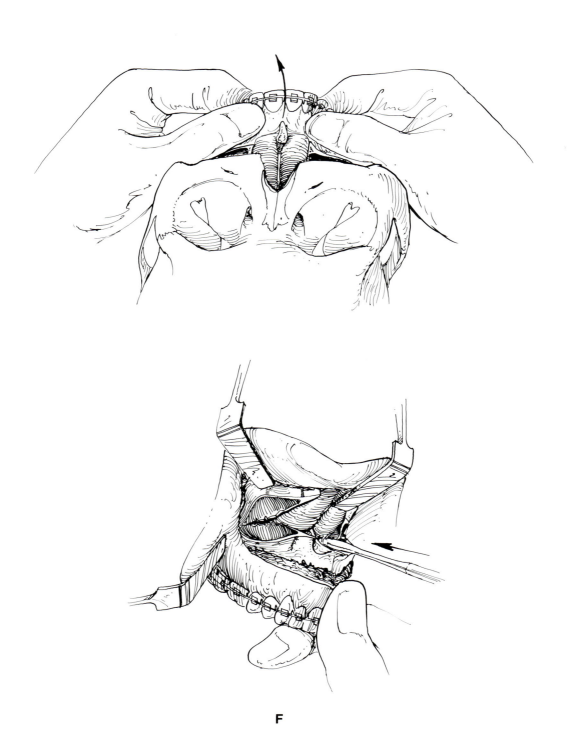

F

G. Anterior mobilization of the total maxilla can be readily achieved with the mobilization forceps. These forceps are designed to engage the hard palate both inferiorly and superiorly yet minimize injury to the palatal mucosa with instrumentation. The lower member of the instrument is placed in the oral aspect of the palate. The upper member of each forceps is placed under the lip and nasal mucoperiosteum on the bone of the nasal floor. One or both members can be used. Gentle continuous forward traction is used to achieve the desired mobilization.

H. A large bone bur is used to remove the residual nasal septum from the superior aspect of the maxilla so that the nasal septum will not be deviated when the maxilla is repositioned. This step must be done even if the maxilla *is not intended to be moved superiorly*.

   If necessary a portion of the inferior aspect of the septum can also be removed. This is best done by making an incision along the inferior portion of the septum, exposing it via a submucous dissection approach and performing the indicated resection. Scissors are used to resect the inferior aspect of the septal cartilage, and a rongeur is used to remove the inferior portion of the bony septum. If the cartilaginous anterior nasal septum is severely deviated a triangular wedge can be removed to straighten the septum.

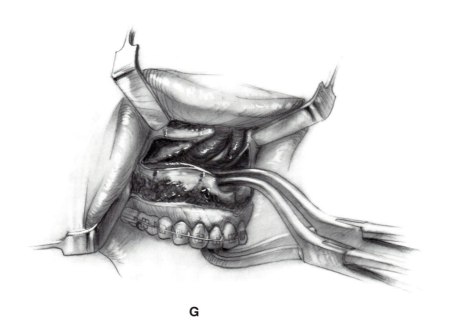

G

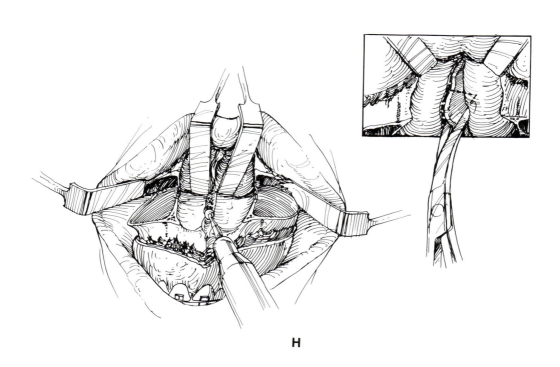

H

ADVANCEMENT OF MAXILLA

Plate 8-3

I. Lateral infraorbital suspension wires are generally used for stabilization of the advanced maxilla because of the anterosuperior traction they can provide. To place these transorally a subperiosteal dissection is extended superiorly to the lateral aspect of the inferior orbital rim, lateral to the exiting infraorbital neurovascular bundle. The dissection is extended over the rim onto the orbital floor. An interosseous hole is placed through the lateral aspect of the rim and a 22-gauge wire passed through it and looped over the rim. This wire is twisted so as to form a loop in the buccal sulcus.

J. The occlusal splint is attached to the maxillary teeth with 26-gauge wire and interdigitated to the mandible via intermaxillary fixation. The vertical inscribed reference lines on the lateral maxillary walls are checked to be certain they correspond to the amount of advancement determined by the model surgery and prediction tracing. Two 24-gauge wires are passed through the 22-gauge wire loop in the buccal sulcus and through holes in the occlusal splint in the second molar and cuspid areas and tightened.

Following stabilization of the maxilla the bone grafting is done. Autogenous or allogenic cortical blocks are placed between the pterygoid plates and tuberosity of the maxilla to provide additional stability to the advanced maxilla by acting as a posterior physical stop. Each block is tapered to facilitate wedging it in place. The bone grafts are firmly wedged between the pterygoid plates and tuberosity of the maxilla. If the bone grafts are too small they will not provide adequate support and therefore will not help prevent relapse. If the grafts are much too large and are wedged tightly into place the maxilla can be inadvertently displaced anteriorly.

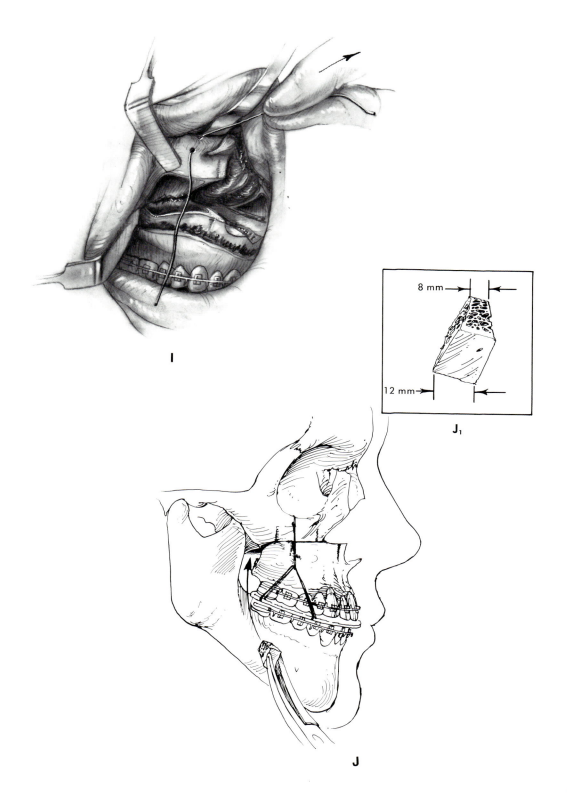

8 mm

12 mm

I

J₁

J

K. Fresh autogenous cancellous strips can be packed anteriorly between the stable anterior maxillary wall and the advanced portion of the anterior maxillary wall and onlayed along the lateral osteotomy site. These will further increase stability as well as promote a more rapid osseous union. With the use of fresh autogenous cancellous bone grafts the maxilla is usually well healed and stable within 3 to 4 weeks. We utilize this form of autogenous bone grafting only in cleft patients, major maxillary advancement cases, or when the ilium is osteotomized to obtain the cortical graft for the posterior stop.

L. The circumvestibular incision is sutured taking small bites of mucosa to minimize decreasing the amount of vermilion that will be exposed clinically. With good execution of the surgical technique, mobilization of the maxilla, and properly placed bone grafts the predictability and stability of results with total maxillary advancement are very good.

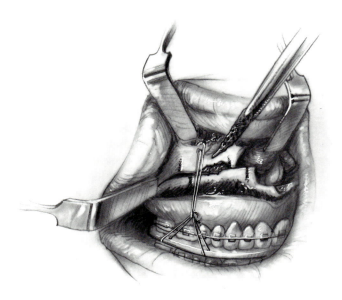

K

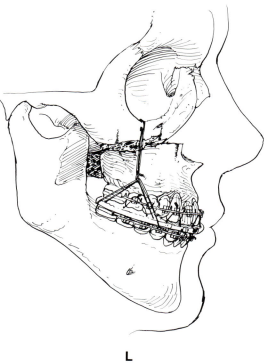

L

SPECIAL CONSIDERATION
ADVANCEMENT OF MAXILLA

Simultaneous expansion of maxilla (Plate 8-4)

A. Expansion of the maxilla is indicated in cases where the maxillary dentition will remain in posterior crossbite after the maxilla is advanced. After the lateral maxillary wall, lateral nasal wall, and nasal septal osteotomies are completed as previously described, a vertical osteotomy in the midline between the central incisors (or where indicated as determined by the model surgery) is made through only the dentoalveolar portion of the maxilla.

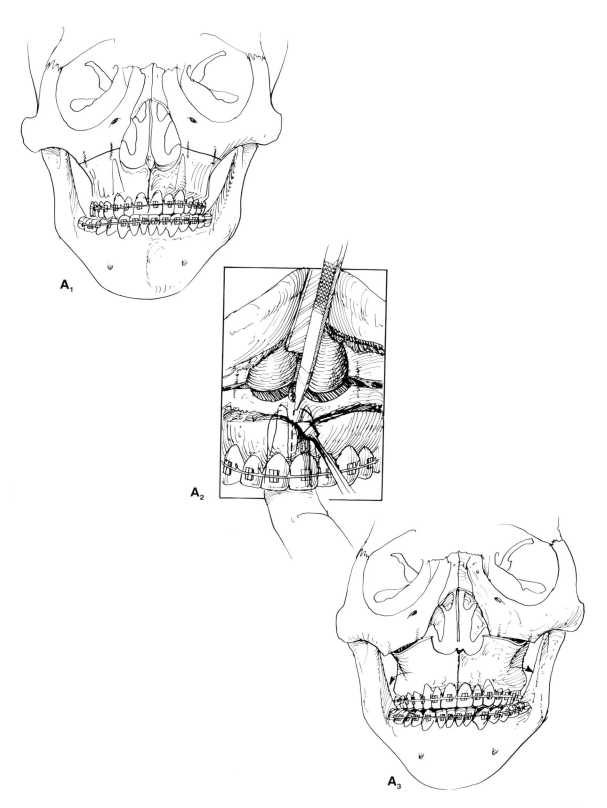

A₁

A₂

A₃

283

ADVANCEMENT OF MAXILLA

Simultaneous expansion of maxilla (Plate 8-4)

B. Following down-fracturing of the maxilla the nasal crest of the maxilla is leveled to the height of the nasal floor with a bone bur. A fissure bur is then used to osteotomize the palate down the midline, with care to maintain the palatal mucoperiosteum intact.

C. The palatal mucoperiosteum is gently reflected from the horizontal aspect of the palate through the osteotomy area. The dissection is extended toward the palatoalveolar junction, with care in the area adjacent to the greater palatine foramen so that the neurovascular bundle is not damaged. This maneuver helps relieve the tension caused by the palatal mucoperiosteum. The palatal mucoperiosteum must remain attached to the dentoalveolus, because this is the primary vascular supply to the maxilla. If a significant amount of midpalatal expansion exists or if the segments are under tension, the defect can be bone grafted to improve stability. The maxilla can usually be expanded up to 6 to 8 mm by this method. Generally bone grafting the palatal defect is not necessary for most expansions that are less than 6 mm.

ADVANCEMENT OF MAXILLA

Simultaneous expansion of maxilla (Plate 8-4)

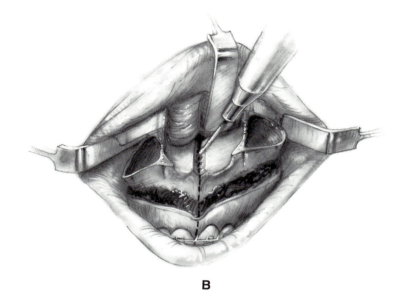

B

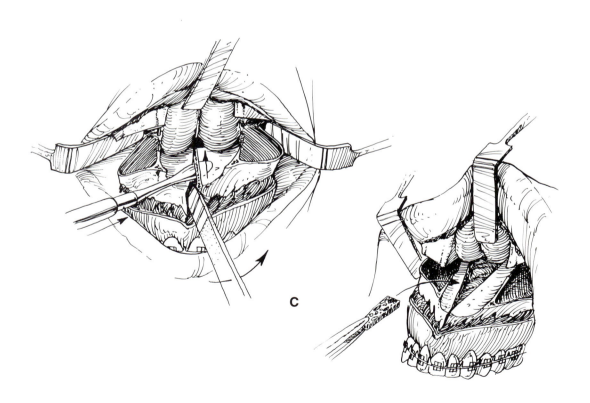

C

ADVANCEMENT OF MAXILLA

Simultaneous expansion of maxilla (Plate 8-4)

D. In rare cases expansion of the maxilla to 10 mm or more may be indicated. The palatal mucoperiosteum usually will not tolerate this much expansion without considerable tension or tearing. If this degree of expansion is necessary it can be dealt with by two methods. The first method, as illustrated here, is to incise the palatal mucoperiosteum down the midline to release the soft-tissue tension. This does not permit simultaneous bone grafting.

E. With this technique it is imperative that the nasal mucoperiosteum remain totally intact without a perforation; otherwise an oronasal fistula may result. Obviously with this technique no grafting of the palatal defect can be done, nor is it necessary. Bone grafting of the lateral maxillary walls with fresh autogenous cancellous bone is indicated to provide stability and bony continuity.

F. If bilateral palatal incisions are made in major expansion cases at the palatoalveolar junction and the midpalatal portion of the palatal mucoperiosteum undermined, adequate lateral relaxation as well as simultaneous midpalatal bone grafting can be done.

When expansion of the maxilla is to be done it is important to add an acrylic palatal bar to the occlusal splint (with at least 3 to 4 mm clearance between the bar and the palatal mucosa) so that good lateral stability is afforded by the splint; otherwise the occlusal splint may be bent medially from the tension of the soft tissues, and some relapse will occur. Also the occlusal splint must be constructed so that the maxillary teeth seat well in it.

ADVANCEMENT OF MAXILLA

Simultaneous expansion of maxilla (Plate 8-4)

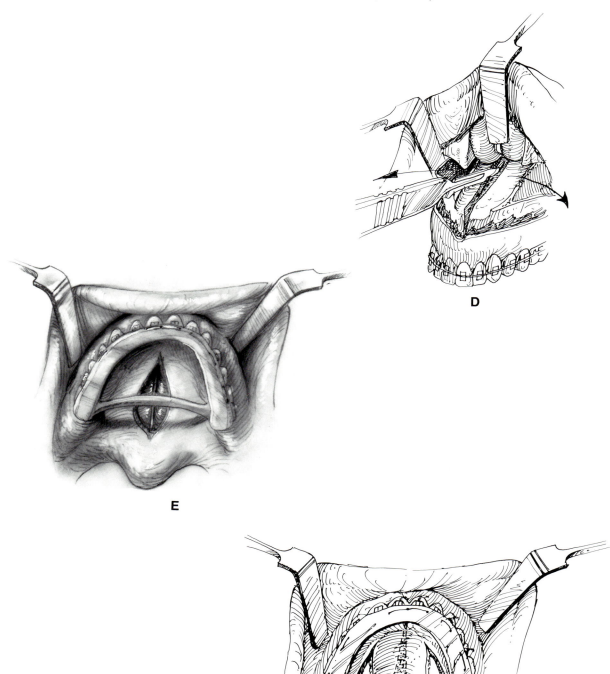

D

E

F

ADVANCEMENT OF MAXILLA

Simultaneous narrowing of maxilla (Plate 8-5)

A. Narrowing of the maxilla as it is advanced is indicated in those cases where the maxillary arch width is such that with the maxillary advancement the maxillary posterior teeth tend toward a buccal crossbite, as illustrated. This problem is seen in patients who initially have a class III malocclusion and normal posterior occlusion. When the maxilla is advanced the posterior teeth are moved into buccal crossbite. This is an indication to narrow the maxilla as it is advanced.

When the maxilla is to be narrowed, prior to down-fracturing, the dentoalveolus is sectioned between the central incisors with a sharp, thin osteotome.

B. The maxilla is then down-fractured by the technique described in detail in Plate 8-4. A wedge ostectomy in the midline of the nasal floor is then done. Utilizing a bur the wedge ostectomy is completed, the width of bone removed having been predetermined by the model surgery. The two lateral maxillary segments are then rotated together, and the palatal mucosa is pushed orally so as not to be entrapped between the two halves of the narrowed maxilla.

C. If necessary an interosseous wire can be placed to facilitate stability, but this usually is not required. The occlusal splint is generally all that is necessary to provide adequate stability. In such cases it is important that the splint be constructed such that the maxillary teeth "key" well into it so as to avoid rotation of either segment.

D. If the medial rotation of the lateral maxillary segments is significant, to where there is minimal bone interface, bone grafting of the anterior and lateral maxillary walls may be indicated for stability, primarily in a vertical direction. The bone taken from the midpalate can be used for this purpose.

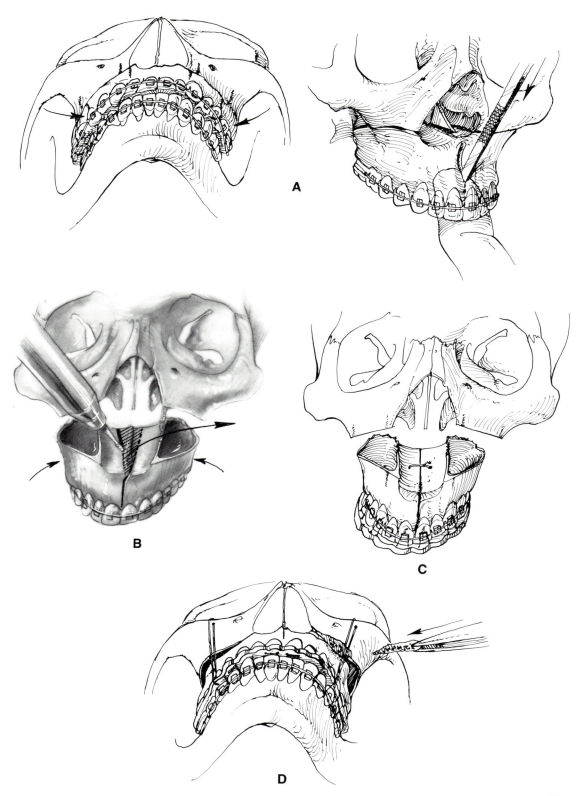

Inferior repositioning of maxilla

The indications for inferior repositioning of the maxilla, in our experience, are far less common than either superior repositioning or advancement of the total maxilla. The specific indication for this procedure is based primarily on the clinical relationship between the upper tooth and upper lip. Normally 1 to 4 mm of maxillary incisor tooth are exposed below the inferiormost aspect of the upper lip when the lips are relaxed. Because individuals with a vertically deficient maxilla generally have vertical overclosure in centric occlusion, the upper-tooth-to-lip relationship is best assessed with the mandible in its clinical rest position. When in this position, if the maxillary incisors are *above* the lip line, a maxillary downgraft procedure may be indicated.

To achieve stable results with this procedure it is essential that the interocclusal space (freeway space) is large enough to tolerate the planned movement and that proper bone grafting is done. Interocclusal space is best determined with a combined clinical and electromyographic approach. It may even be indicated that the patient preoperatively wear an occlusal splint that opens the bite a few millimeters greater than the planned degree of inferior maxillary repositioning to make certain that the masticatory muscles can tolerate the new position of the mandible.

The inferiorly repositioned maxilla is vertically stabilized with cortical bone grafts to the lateral maxillary osteotomy area. Bone grafting must include cortical block grafts that physically stabilize the repositioned segment and fresh autogenous cancellous strips to facilitate rapid bone healing. Freeze-dried bone may be used for the cortical portion of the grafting; however, it is of the utmost importance, to achieve a stable result, that fresh autogenous cancellous strips be overlayed along the lateral osteotomy sites.

Because many of the essential technical aspects of this procedure are identical to those for total maxillary advancement, as described in Plate 8-3, they are not repeated here.

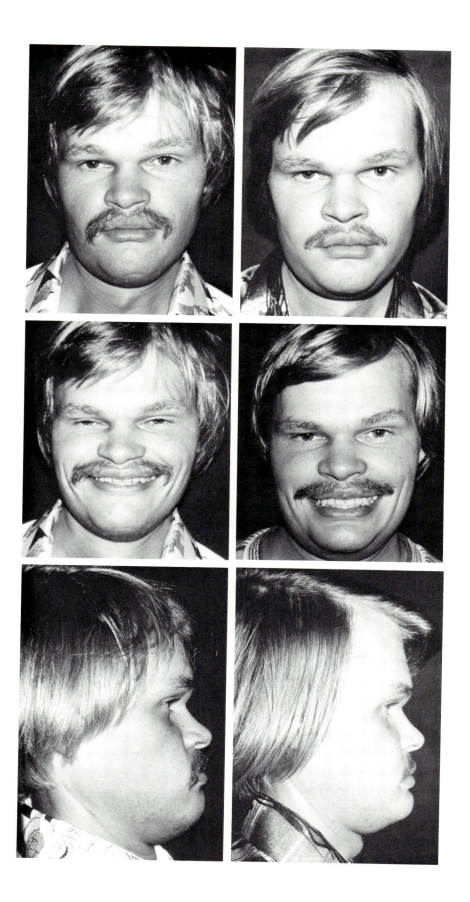

291

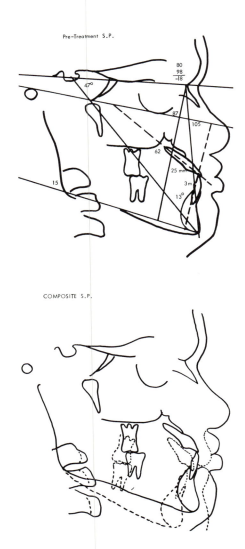

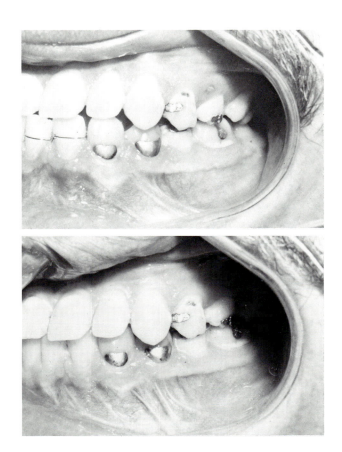

INFERIOR REPOSITIONING OF MAXILLA

Plate 8-6

A. Vertical maxillary deficiency is diagnosed and treatment planned on the basis of the esthetic evaluation of the upper-tooth-to-lip relationship. When the upper incisor teeth are significantly superior to the upper lip line, that is, hidden superiorly beneath the upper lip, and an open-bite deformity is not present, inferior repositioning of the maxilla is to be considered. Correction of this type of deformity from an esthetic standpoint includes establishing a more normal upper-tooth-to-lip relationship and increasing the lower third facial height.

Inferior repositioning of the maxilla is planned so as to reposition the maxilla sufficiently to result in exposure of about 3 mm of maxillary incisor tooth when the lips are in repose. With the inferior repositioning of the maxilla there is autorotation of the mandible downward and backward, which *increases* lower third facial height and *decreases* chin prominence. Depending on the anteroposterior relationship of the chin and upper anterior teeth, the mandible may require simultaneous anterior or posterior repositioning in conjunction with the inferior repositioning of the maxilla. For example, in skeletal class II occlusion with vertical maxillary deficiency the mandible generally must be advanced concomitant with the inferior maxillary repositioning; otherwise considerable posterior repositioning of the maxilla will be required, with subsequent worsening of facial esthetics.

In the illustrated case vertical maxillary deficiency exists with decreased lower third facial height and a class III occlusion. The jaws are opened until the lips just touch, and it is noted that the maxillary incisors are 5 mm superior to the upper lip line. Therefore it is planned that the maxilla be repositioned inferiorly 8 mm to achieve a result in which 3 mm of maxillary incisor tooth are exposed. The model surgery and prediction tracing demonstrate that with inferior repositioning of 8 mm the maxilla will require 2 mm of posterior repositioning to achieve an optimum functional class I occlusal result.

B. The circumvestibular incision provides excellent access for the procedure. A total maxillary osteotomy is performed in the exact manner described in Plate 8-3. However, because of the deficiency in vertical maxillary height, the apices of the maxillary teeth are usually above the level of the palatal plane. Therefore the level of the horizontal osteotomy must be higher, in reference to the piriform aperture, than usual.

The occlusal splint and temporary intermaxillary fixation are applied, and the mandible is autorotated inferiorly and posteriorly. Calipers are used to determine the correct vertical and anteroposterior relationship of the maxilla.

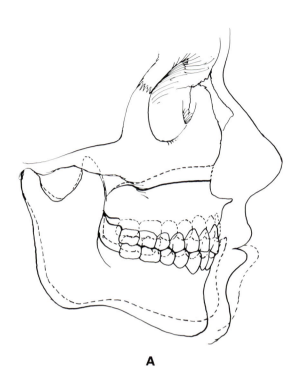

A

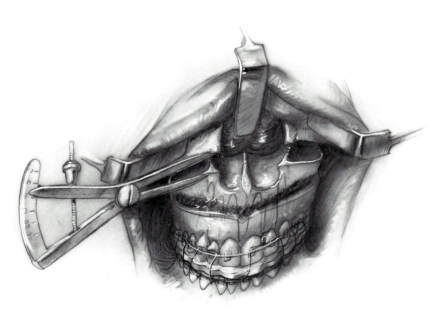

B

Plate 8-6

C. Bone grafts are prepared from cortical or cortical cancellous blocks to fit precisely into the lateral and anterior maxillary wall defects. When preparing these grafts it is advantageous to groove the superior and inferior aspects so that they can be mortised into place. These grafts are directly wired into position to prevent their displacement. It is preferable when placing a cortical cancellous graft to have the medullary aspect facing outward. If the cortex faces outward, multiple holes are placed through it.

After the cortical grafts are stabilized via direct wiring, fresh autogenous cancellous strips are overlayed along each side of the maxilla to promote rapid bony union. If fresh autogenous grafts are not utilized the stability of this procedure is poor.

When only the maxilla has been repositioned and is firmly stabilized the temporary intermaxillary fixation can be released. If the maxilla is very stable at this point no additional stabilization may be required. However, it is often necessary to utilize infraorbital suspension wires that attach to the maxillary splint for additional stability. The occlusion is controlled postoperatively with light elastics. If simultaneous mandibular ramus surgery is done or the stability is questioned, intermaxillary fixation is applied and maintained for an appropriate period.

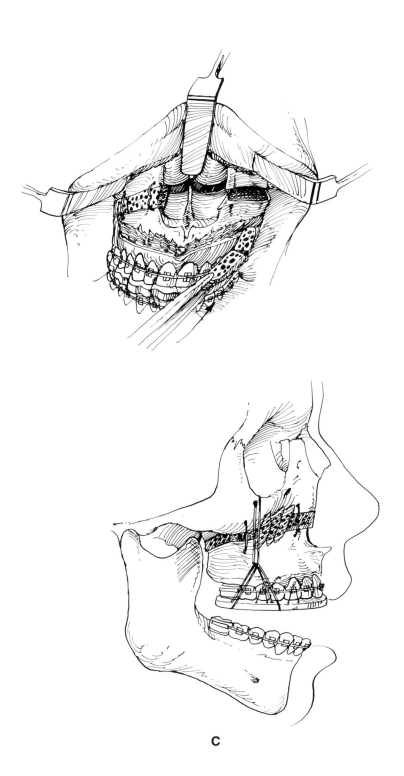

C

Leveling of maxilla

Vertical maxillary asymmetry can occur idiopathically but is more commonly seen in such conditions as hemifacial microsomia, Romberg's disease, condylar hyperplasia, and so on. The occlusal plane in these conditions is canted transversely because of either a lack of vertical growth on one side or excessive vertical growth on the opposite side. The result is an asymmetric maxilla relative to a Frankfort plane or the facial soft tissues, particularly the lips. For optimal esthetics and function in such conditions it is often necessary to level the maxilla.

The basic techniques for leveling the maxilla are: (1) raise one side of the maxilla, (2) lower one side of the maxilla, and (3) simultaneously lower one side and raise the other side of the maxilla. The degree of leveling necessary is determined by the clinical evaluation and the posterior, anterior, and lateral cephalometric analyses. The determining factor for which leveling technique to use depends on the upper-tooth-to-lip relationship. Ideally the end result will be 2 to 3 mm of upper tooth exposed when the lips are relaxed. Therefore, based on the clinical assessment, it can be determined whether to elevate or lower each side of the maxilla to correct the existing asymmetry. *Although these criteria often correlate well with the celphalometric criteria, when they do not the clinical criteria are used to make the treatment planning decisions as to the exact magnitude of leveling.* In this regard the presence of soft-tissue asymmetry must be appreciated in the treatment planning. For example, a patient with hemifacial microsomia often has an associated soft-tissue asymmetry with a canted lip line as well as the canted maxillary plane. In such a case it is better from an esthetic standpoint to correct the occlusal cant relative to the lips and *not* to level the occlusion relative to the cephalometric tracing. It is also noted that as facial asymmetries are corrected, facial soft-tissue distribution is also affected. The side on which the skeletal structures are elevated increases in soft-tissue thickness, and the side opposite has relative thinning of the soft tissues. These soft-tissue changes must be considered in the overall treatment planning, because augmentation procedures to the deficient side may be indicated to provide optimal facial esthetic balance.

In adults it is always necessary to simultaneously reposition the mandible when the maxilla is being leveled. The techniques for mandibular ramus procedures are described in detail in Chapter 2.

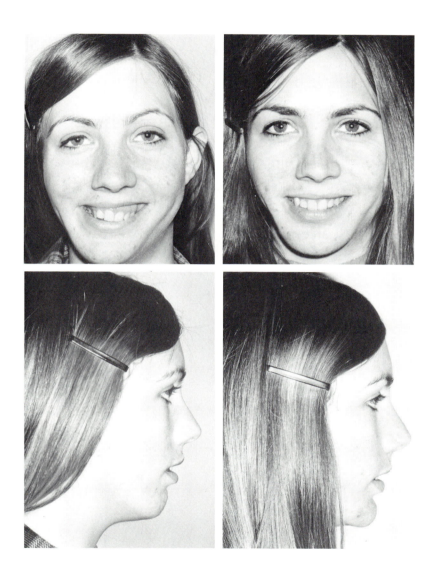

299

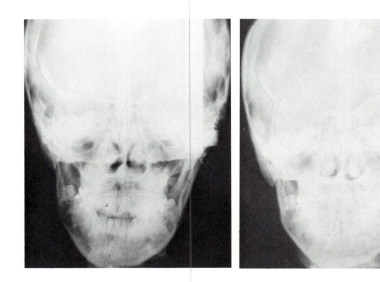

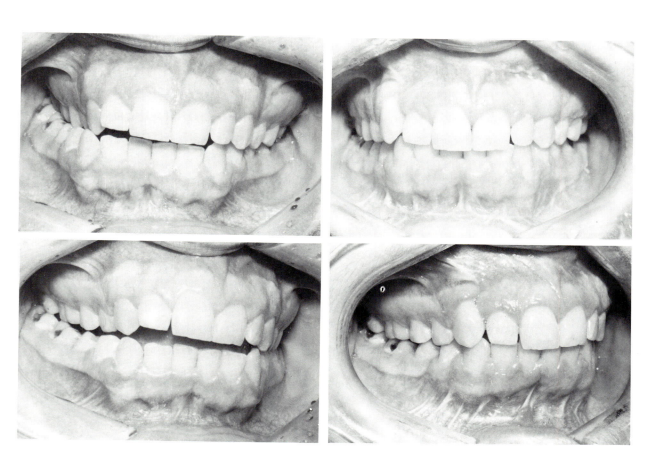

LEVELING OF MAXILLA

Plate 8-7

A. Leveling of the maxilla requires careful clinical assessment to determine the degree of vertical alteration for optimum esthetic results. In this illustrated case of hemifacial microsomia the maxilla is significantly canted. On the right side the cuspid is 8 mm below the lip line and the molars 10 mm below. The left cuspid is judged to be satisfactorily at about 3 mm below the lip line. The mandible is deviated to the left side, and the dental midlines are rotated to the left.

Based on the esthetic evaluation, model surgery, and prediction tracing, it is determined that the right side of the maxilla must be superiorly repositioned 5 mm in the cuspid area and 8 mm in the molar area. This is to be achieved via the outlined maxillary osteotomy and simultaneous bilateral mandibular sagittal ramus osteotomies. The illustrated maxillary osteotomy has an advantage in that a portion of the maxilla remains stable and aids greatly in acting as both a stable referent at surgery and a means of achieving excellent postoperative immobilization.

In instances when both the maxilla and mandible are to be repositioned it is easiest to first complete all the bone cuts for the sagittal ramus osteotomies but not split them, and then to complete the maxillary surgery, including repositioning and stabilization. Finally the mandibular rami are split and the mandible repositioned to the "stable" maxilla.

B. In this case the maxilla is to be leveled via a combined superior movement on one side and a commensurate inferior movement with bone grafting on the other, as outlined. Such movement requires simultaneous bilateral mandibular ramus osteotomies.

C. The surgery, including bone grafting and stabilization, is done exactly as previously described in this chapter.

LEVELING OF MAXILLA

Plate 8-7

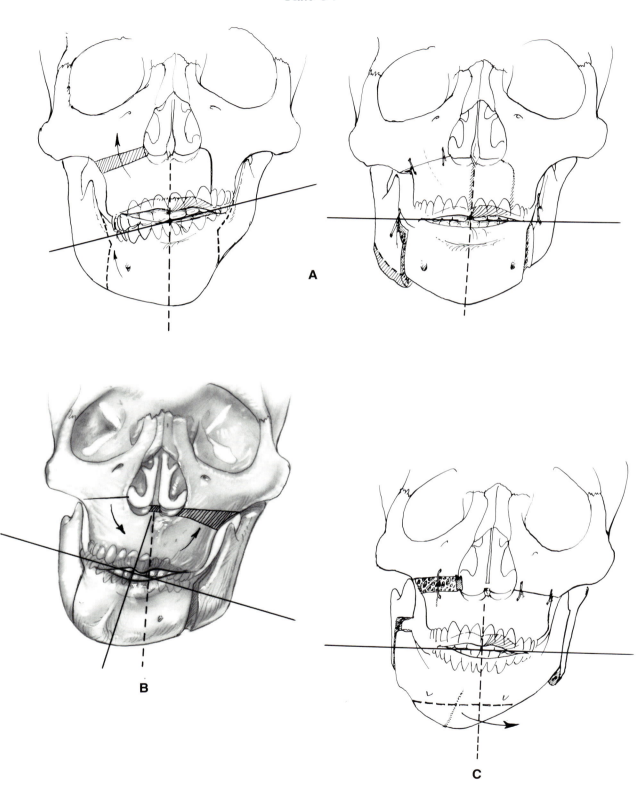

A

B

C

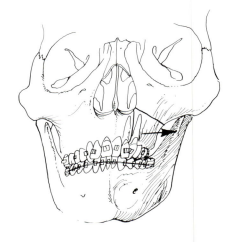

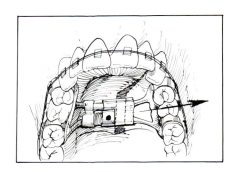

UNILATERAL SURGICAL-ORTHODONTIC EXPANSION OF MAXILLA

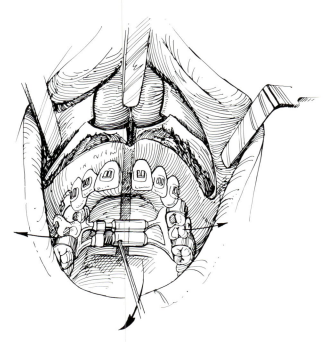

BILATERAL SURGICAL-ORTHODONTIC EXPANSION OF MAXILLA

CHAPTER 9

Surgical-orthodontic expansion of maxilla

In children both unilateral and bilateral transverse maxillary deficiency can usually be treated successfully via orthopedic rapid maxillary expansion. In adults successful orthodontic treatment can be achieved when a minimal bilateral transverse arch width deficiency (5 mm or less) exists or when the deficiency is due primarily to tipping of the teeth. In those instances in which the magnitude of maxillary expansion is to be greater than 5 mm or when the posterior maxillary teeth already exhibit dental compensations, that is, they are already inclined buccally, a combined surgical-orthodontic approach is advocated.

In patients over the age of 16 years attempted orthopedic rapid maxillary expansion is frequently associated with significant difficulties. This is usually the result of fusion of the various craniofacial sutures, which results in a lack of suture opening on expansion. Inability to activate the expansion appliance and expand the maxilla is not uncommon. Tipping of the teeth, bending of the alveolar bone, and movement of the teeth through the buccal cortical plates are common consequences of orthopedic rapid maxillary expansion in adults. Overcorrection to compensate for these undesirable changes is frequently frustrated by unpredictable and uncontrolled relapse after the orthopedic expansion appliance is removed. Subsequent relapse, even with prolonged retention, usually occurs. In addition *treatment of true unilateral transverse maxillary deficiency in adults is not feasible via conventional orthopedic palatal expansion techniques,* because a physiologic centric occlusion cannot be maintained. In such instances the expansion of the maxilla occurs bilaterally and masticatory function worsens.

In this chapter a detailed protocol for the combined use of selected maxillary osteotomies in concert with orthopedic forces to correct both unilateral and bilateral transverse maxillary deficiency are described and illustrated in detail.

305

Unilateral-surgical orthodontic expansion of maxilla

True unilateral transverse maxillary deficiency, previously referred to as posterior crossbite, commonly exists in individuals with unilateral cleft palate and less frequently as an isolated idiopathic entity. When it coexists with an anteroposterior maxillary deficiency or vertical maxillary hyperplasia it is best corrected surgically simultaneously with the correction of the anteroposterior or vertical problem, as discussed in Chapter 8.

Additionally, if surgery alone can optimally correct the existing malocclusion or if the posterior segment must be simultaneously repositioned anteroposteriorly, vertically, or rotated, primary surgical repositioning of the posterior segment may be employed. However, *if any orthodontic treatment is necessary* and the indicated movement of the posterior segment is primarily transverse, there is seldom an advantage to repositioning the posterior segment surgically, because the straight surgical approach requires additional surgery, fixation, immobilization, and retention. Thus in many instances of unilateral posterior crossbite the combination of selected maxillary osteotomies in concert with orthopedic expansion of the maxilla is the treatment of choice. In adults both unilateral or bilateral transverse maxillary deficiency can be successfully corrected via the use of selected maxillary osteotomies utilized in concert with rapid maxillary expansion principles.

The surgical procedure described and illustrated here for the combined surgical-orthodontic correction of unilateral transverse maxillary deficiency has been utilized by us for many years and has proved to be reliable and predictable. In addition there is little morbidity associated with this procedure, and it can be done on an outpatient basis without general anesthesia.

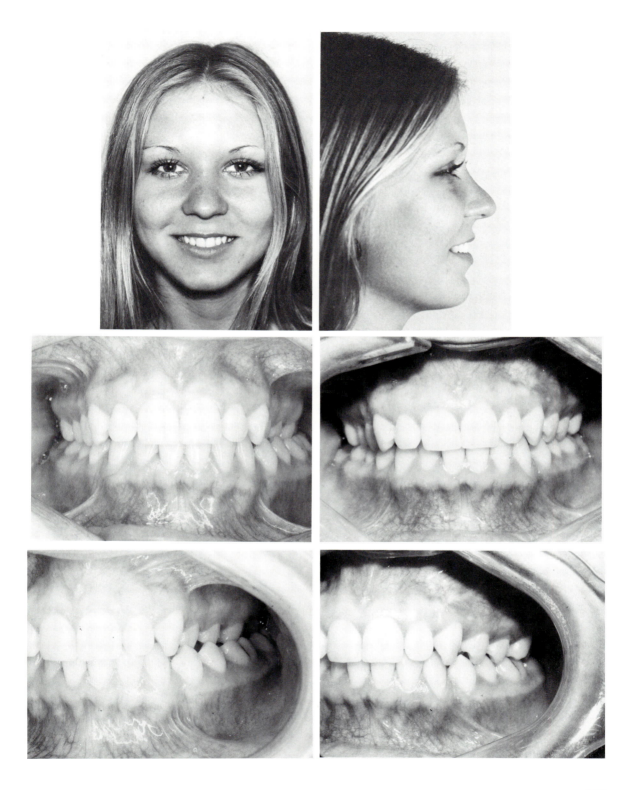

307

UNILATERAL SURGICAL-ORTHODONTIC EXPANSION OF MAXILLA

Plate 9-1

A. The illustrated case is an idiopathic true unilateral transverse maxillary deficiency extending from the left cuspid posteriorly in an 18-year-old patient. It is *not* primarily due to tipping of the teeth, as determined by analysis of the dental models and posteroanterior cephalometric radiograph. Evaluation of the mandibular rest position–centric occlusion relationship demonstrates that this is a true unilateral deformity, because no occlusal shift occurs during closure of the mandible into maximum intercuspation. The measured degree of transverse maxillary deficiency is 7 mm. The segment to be expanded includes the maxillary left cuspid and posterior teeth.

Anteriorly dental crowding and rotations exist, which will be corrected orthodontically simultaneously with the surgical-orthodontic expansion of the maxilla. Therefore the teeth are fully banded, and a palatal expansion appliance is constructed *but not inserted*. The insert schematically illustrates the corrected deformity 3 days following surgery and the type of palatal expansion appliance utilized. At this time the maxillary arch wire is inserted, and correction of the rotated and crowded anterior teeth is instituted.

B. A horizontal incision is made in the depth of the buccal vestibule at about the level of the tooth root apices from the region of the first molar anteriorly to the region of the cuspid. An anterior vertical limb is then made that incises the papillae between the cuspid and lateral incisor. The mucoperiosteum is elevated posteriorly and superiorly to expose the interdental area between the cuspid and lateral incisor, the piriform aperture, and the lateral aspect of the maxilla above the level of the horizontal soft-tissue incision. The periosteum is then undermined posteriorly until the pterygomaxillary junction is identified. The soft-tissue dissection is done so as to maintain the maximum possible amount of buccal mucoperiosteum attached to the posterior maxillary segment, which is to be mobilized.

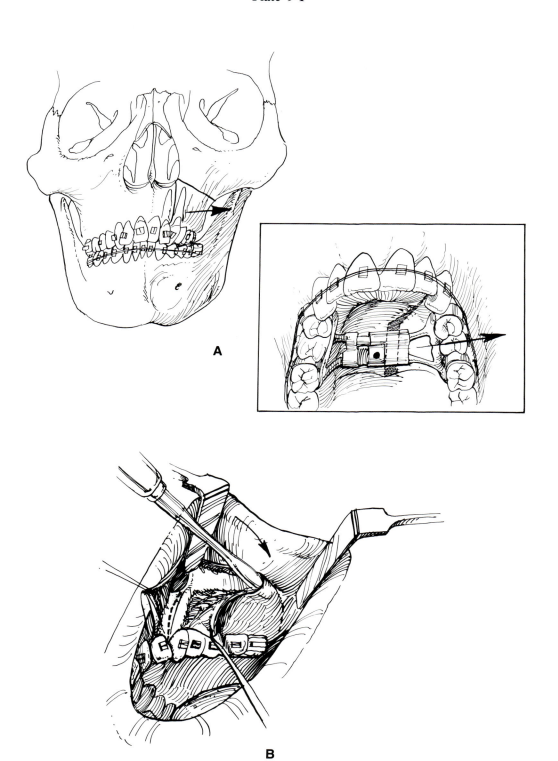

A

B

C. Calipers are used to determine the level of the horizontal subapical osteotomy through the lateral maxillary wall at about 4 mm above the tooth root apices, approximately 34 mm above the cuspid cusp tip, and 25 mm above the first molar cusps. As the horizontal osteotomy extends distal to the second molar root apices it is curved sharply inferiorly so as to terminate at the *inferior aspect of the pterygomaxillary junction.* This distal extent of the horizontal osteotomy is often made with a small curved osteotome. This is accomplished by stopping the horizontal bur cut just digital to the second molar root apices and malleting the curved osteotome distally and inferiorly through the lateral maxillary wall until it reaches the inferior aspect of the pterygoid plates.

D. The vertical interdental osteotomy is made from the piriform aperture with a fine-fissure bur between the cuspid and lateral incisor roots. This osteotomy is made only through the lateral cortex so that it stops about 3 mm short of the alveolar crestal bone. Whenever adjacent tooth roots are in close proximity to one another the interdental ostectomy is made only through the outer cortex with the bur and completed with a fine osteotome.

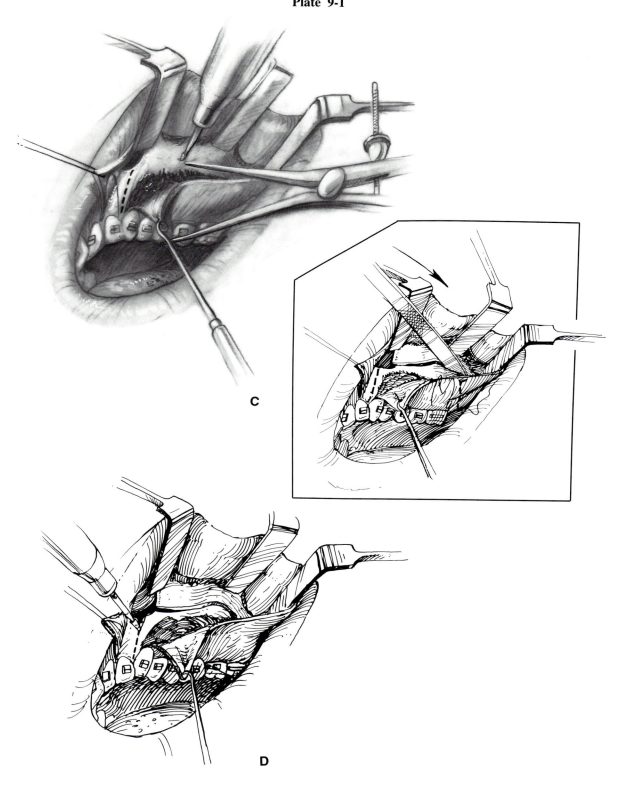

C

D

E. The vertical interdental osteotomy is completed through the alveolar portion with an osteotome while maintaining a finger on the palate to detect it as it perforates the palatal cortex. Next the osteotome is malleted higher across the palate until it reaches the palatal midline.

F. At this time the posterior maxillary segment is torqued downward with the aid of an osteotome inserted into the osteotomy site or with simultaneous downward digital pressure. When this force is applied the posterior maxillary segment will generally down-fracture along the residual pterygomaxillary, palatomaxillary, and midpalatal sutures. In some instances the medial fracture may occur laterally on the hard palate at about the junction of the vertical and horizontal palatal processes. If the posterior segment does not mobilize at this time a small curved osteotome is malleted low in the pterygomaxillary suture area, and mobilization is readily achieved.

Regardless, *it is not necessary to mobilize the segment to the extent that it is completely down-fractured* but simply to assure that all areas of bony resistance are separated so that the posterior maxillary segment can be subsequently moved laterally with the orthopedic force created by the palatal expansion appliance.

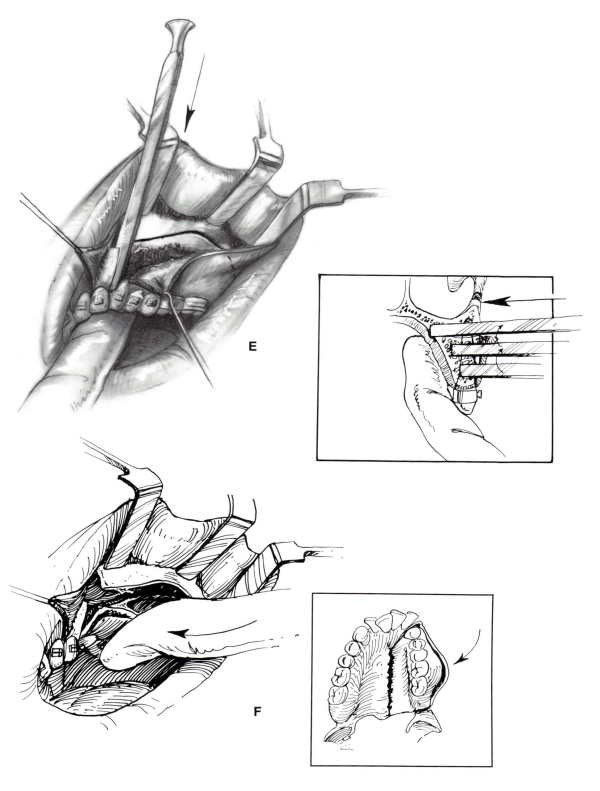

E

F

G. The palatal expansion appliance is inserted and activated. It is most simply inserted by placing the appliance on the osteotomized segment first, because mobility exists in it, and then inserting it on the stable portion of the maxilla. *After it is inserted and cemented it is immediately activated four to six turns to make certain the dento-osseous segment is being orthopedically moved.* This is done while directly observing the lateral wall of the maxilla in the regions of the osteotomies to be certain that lateral movement of the posterior maxillary segment is being accomplished.

The patient is then instructed to activate the appliance so as to complete the expansion within 3 to 6 days. However, *the segment is not to be over-expanded* or it will heal in this position and a permanent buccal crossbite will result because relapse does not occur with this procedure when properly executed.

After the desired degree of expansion is achieved an arch wire is inserted to institute orthodontic correction of the rotations and crowding, and the appliance is maintained in place for at least 6 to 8 weeks to permit good bone healing to occur.

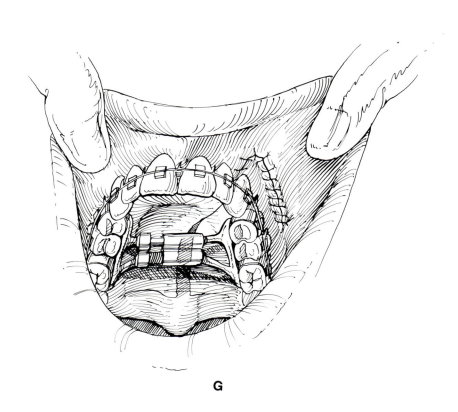

G

UNILATERAL SURGICAL-ORTHODONTIC EXPANSION OF MAXILLA

Unilateral cleft palate deformity (Plate 9-2)

A. A left unilateral complete cleft palate and unilateral transverse maxillary deficiency in an adult is illustrated. A class I occlusion is present. In this instance the maxillary expansion appliance can be inserted prior to surgery, because the palatal cleft will serve as the palatal osteotomy, and therefore the posterior segment will not have to be down-fractured to create this. Optimum treatment of the unilateral cleft is to orthodontically expand the maxilla and secondarily bone graft the alveolus when the patient is about 11 years of age. This approach is described in Chapter 10.

Two options exist for the adult patient with unilateral cleft with a unilateral transverse maxillary deficiency: (1) utilize segmental maxillary arch orthodontics to level and align the deficient posterior maxillary segment and then simultaneously surgically reposition it laterally and bone graft the alveolar defect and (2) utilize a similar approach as described in Plate 9-1 for surgical orthodontic expansion of the maxilla and then permanently retain the expansion by secondarily bone grafting the alveolar defect. The first approach, often preferred, is illustrated and discussed in Chapter 10. Here only the combined surgical-orthodontic expansion is discussed, with respect to several of the unique problems that exist in the combined surgical-orthodontic expansion of the posterior maxilla in the cleft patient.

In order to perform the combined surgical-orthodontic expansion, as opposed to the simultaneous surgical repositioning and alveolar bone grafting, two factors must be considered. First, is there a need, on the basis of stability, periodontal health, planned fixed-bridge construction, or planned orthodontic tooth movement (see Chapter 10), to perform an alveolar bone graft? If not, the combined surgical-orthodontic expansion approach is indicated. Second, are the soft tissues in the area scarred or otherwise damaged such that it would be more predictable to first expand the posterior maxilla and secondarily perform the alveolar graft for one of the above reasons? If so, the combined approach is indicated.

UNILATERAL SURGICAL-ORTHODONTIC EXPANSION OF MAXILLA

Unilateral cleft palate deformity (Plate 9-2)

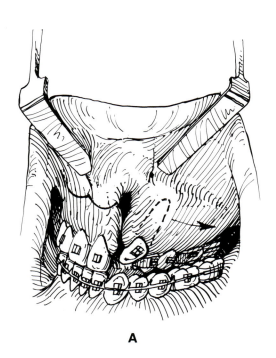

A

UNILATERAL SURGICAL-ORTHODONTIC EXPANSION OF MAXILLA

Unilateral cleft palate deformity (Plate 9-2)

B. Through a horizontal vestibular incision beginning in the area of the cleft the horizontal osteotomy is made about 4 mm above the tooth root apices from the area of the piriform rim above the alveolar cleft, posteriorly to the inferior aspect of the pterygomaxillary suture. Since the alveolar cleft serves as the interdental osteotomy, no vertical osteotomy is required. Similarly the palatal bony cleft serves as the palatal portion of the osteotomy. The pterygomaxillary suture is separated with a small curved osteotome. Next the expansion appliance is activated about 2 mm to directly visualize the orthopedic movement of the lateral segment.

C. Because of the soft tissue scarring that exists in most cleft patients the actual expansion is done at about one half the rate as in those without cleft palate. This permits the soft tissues to stretch and proliferate more readily. In addition, because no areas of bone contact exist palatally or in the anterior alveolus, the segment must be retained longer, or until an alveolar graft is done (as described in Chapter 10), or a fixed or removable appliance is inserted for permanent retention. If expansion is to be greater than it is felt the soft tissues can tolerate, a midline palatal incision can be made directly over the base of the nasal septum and the mucoperiosteum reflected off the nasal septum on the cleft side to release the soft-tissue tension and allow the segment to move laterally much easier.

UNILATERAL SURGICAL-ORTHODONTIC EXPANSION OF MAXILLA

Unilateral cleft palate deformity (Plate 9-2)

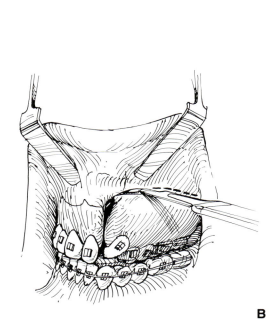

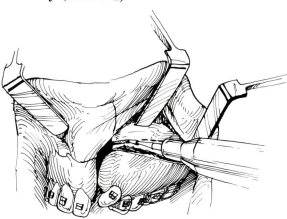

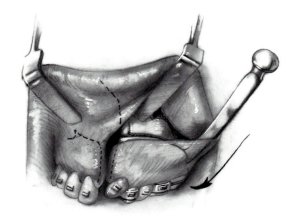

B

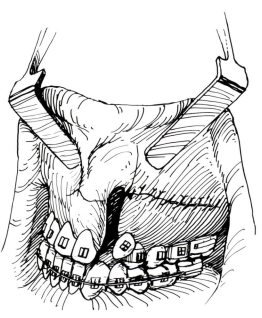

C

Bilateral surgical-orthodontic expansion of maxilla

Bilateral or complete transverse maxillary deficiency is a more commonly occurring deformity than unilateral transverse maxillary deficiency. This entity frequently exists in individuals with mandibular retrognathism, mandibular prognathism, class II skeletal open bite, class III skeletal open bite, maxillary retrognathism, and bilateral cleft lip-palate deformity. In the patient over the age of 16 years its stable correction generally requires either a primary surgical approach or a combined surgical-orthodontic approach. When total maxillary surgery is being done for any reason, the transverse deformity is routinely corrected as part of the maxillary surgery by simultaneously segmentalizing the maxilla as described in Chapter 8.

In cases where the primary skeletal deformity in the maxilla is bilateral transverse maxillary deficiency, expansion of the maxilla by a combined surgical-orthodontic approach is indicated.

Various types of maxillary osteotomies have been empirically proposed to facilitate lateral movement of the maxilla via palatal expansion appliances in adults. Historically the midpalatine suture was implicated as the primary problematic area; that is, in cases resistant to mechanical expansion its fusion was stated to be the cause. Based on this thesis midpalatal osteotomies have been performed to aid in maxillary expansion. However, others have postulated that the midpalatal suture and the zygomaticomaxillary buttress are both problematic areas. Accordingly they have used a combination of lateral maxillary and palatal osteotomies. Still others have sectioned virtually all of the maxillary bone articulations.

The thesis of this section is how selected maxillary osteotomies can be used in concert with rapid maxillary expansion appliances to achieve correction of bilateral transverse maxillary deficiency in the adult. The techniques reported are based on research implicating the zygomaticomaxillary and pterygomaxillary articulations in addition to the midpalatal suture as the primary anatomic sites of resistance to lateral movement of the maxilla by rapid maxillary expansion appliances. Our clinical use of the techniques described has confirmed their feasibility and success. The recommended techniques and the rationale for their use are described and illustrated.

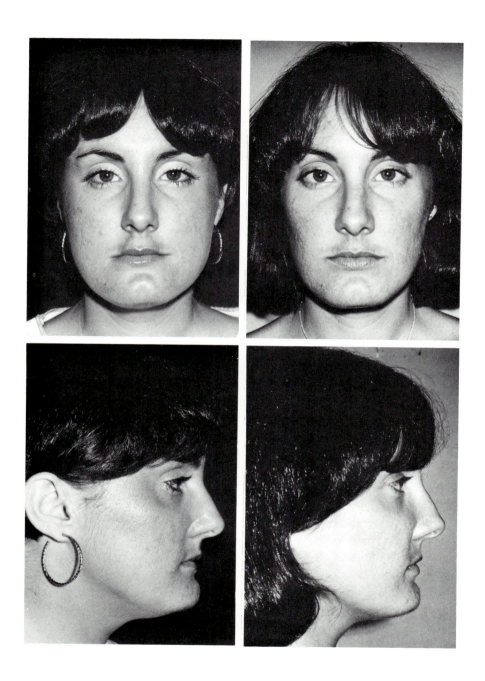

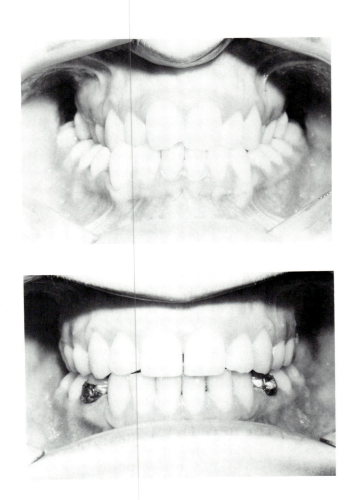

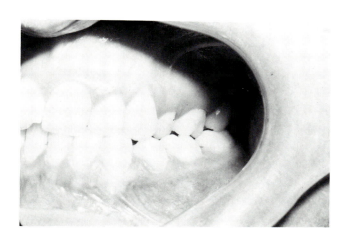

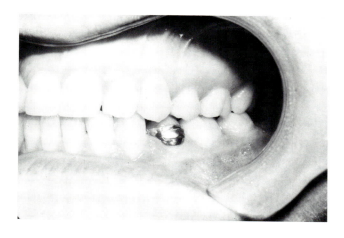

BILATERAL SURGICAL-ORTHODONTIC EXPANSION OF MAXILLA

Plate 9-3

A. The illustrated case exhibits a slight class III tendency with complete bilateral transverse maxillary deficiency in a 20-year-old patient who previously had orthodontic treatment with relapse.

   The treatment will consist of preliminary orthodontics in the mandibular arch to begin uprighting the posterior teeth, leveling the arch, and correcting the crowding and rotations. No orthodontic expansion of the maxillary arch will be done at this time.

B. The preparatory orthodontics have been done in the mandibular arch and have increased the magnitude of the actual transverse maxillary deficiency, making it about 10 to 12 mm. The maxillary teeth are banded, and the palatal expansion appliance is in place. A high circumvestibular incision is made from above the first molar region on one side to the same location on the opposite side. The soft tissues are reflected from the lateral wall of the maxilla, and the piriform apertures are exposed bilaterally. The mucoperiosteum is then carefully reflected from the lateral wall and floor of the nose anteriorly. On the lateral aspect of the maxilla the mucoperiosteal flap is undermined to the pterygomaxillary junction, and retractors are inserted in preparation for the osteotomies.

   A horizontal osteotomy is made about 4 mm above the tooth root apices from the piriform aperture to the pterygoid plates. The anterior portion of this osteotomy is completed through the anterior aspect of the lateral nasal wall, while a periosteal elevator protects the nasal mucoperiosteum. Once the osteotomy is distal to the second molar tooth root apices it is tapered inferiorly toward the inferiormost aspect of the pterygomaxillary junction. The same osteotomy is performed on the opposite side.

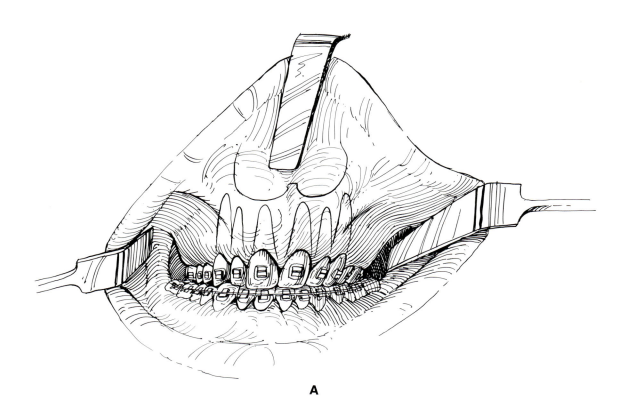

A

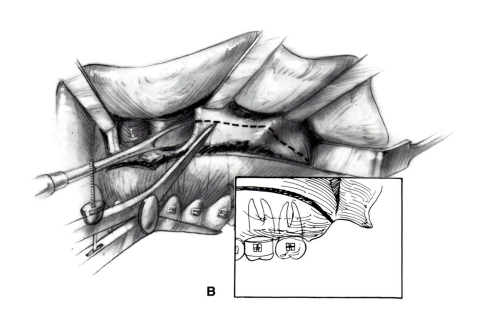

B

C. After completion of the horizontal osteotomies bilaterally a vertical midline osteotomy is done. After undermining the mucosa a fine-fissure bur is used to groove the cortical bone between the central incisors. The midline osteotomy is generally then completed with a fine osteotome. The osteotome is first directed through the alveolus while a finger is placed on the palate to detect its penetration through the palatal bone. Next it is directed straight posteriorly to divide the entire midpalatal suture. Finally it is torqued, while still in place, to test for completion of the midpalatal osteotomy. This maneuver can be done with the maxillary expansion appliance on; however, the torquing must not be excessive.

The nasal septal osteotome may be utilized at this time; however, the anatomy in this area is such that if the midpalatal osteotomy is done as described it is generally not necessary unless the midpalatal osteotomy was performed to one side or the other relative to the nasal septum.

D. Finally the lateral nasal walls are sectioned with an osteotome while the nasal mucoperiosteum is protected with a periosteal elevator. In doing this the osteotome is malleted only about 30 mm posteriorly from the piriform rim so as not to transect the descending palatal neurovascular bundle. The only major bony attachment remaining is the perpendicular plate of the palatine bone.

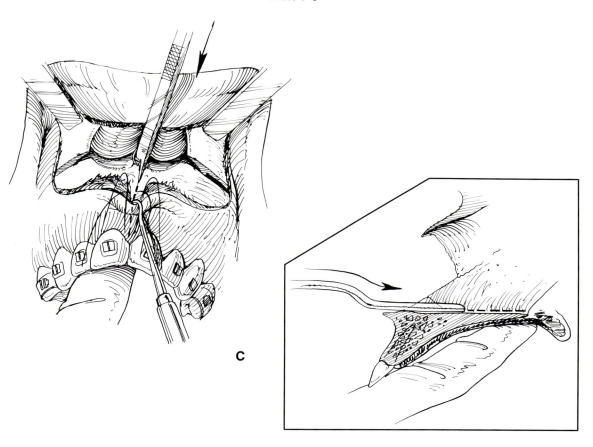

C

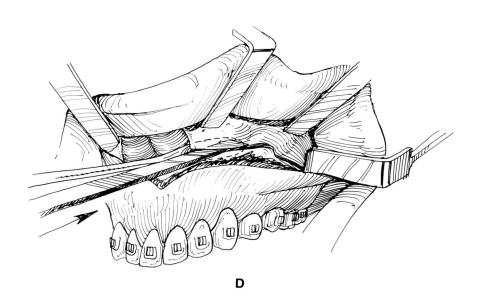

D

E. The maxilla is now judiciously mobilized; however, *no attempt is made to totally down-fracture the maxilla* as this will defeat the purpose of the prescribed approach and will consequently require vertical stabilization with suspension wires. To mobilize the two halves of the maxilla, osteotomes are inserted in the lateral maxillary and midline osteotomy sites and torqued to test for mobility of the maxillary segments. *The most important aspect of mobilization is that the right and left halves are equally mobilized.* If one side is more mobile than the other, when the expansion appliance is activated unilateral expansion will occur. If it appears that there is poor mobility of the maxillary segments the pterygomaxillary areas are osteotomized with a small curved osteotome as previously described.

F. While directly observing the surgical sites the expansion appliance is activated at least 2 to 3 mm to make certain bilateral symmetric orthopedic expansion is occurring. The complete expansion is accomplished over the next 4 to 6 days, depending on the degree of expansion indicated. The expansion appliance is maintained in place for a *minimum of 8 weeks* to permit complete bone healing to occur. With large expansions (greater than 8 to 10 mm) a retainer should be constructed and worn or the expansion appliance left in place for an additional 2 to 3 months to assure good bony healing of the sites and stability of the expansion.

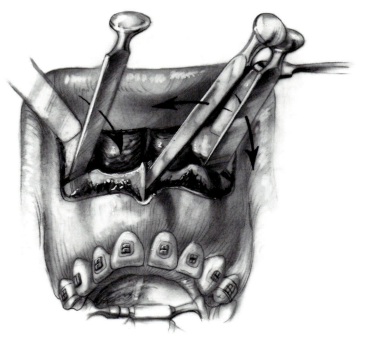

E

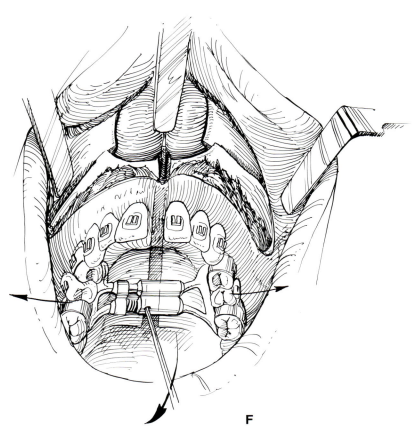

F

329

SPECIAL CONSIDERATION
BILATERAL SURGICAL-ORTHODONTIC EXPANSION OF MAXILLA

Bilateral cleft palate deformity (Plate 9-4)

A. The case illustrated shows a repaired bilateral complete cleft lip-palate and bilateral transverse maxillary deficiency in an adult. Optimum sequential treatment for this patient would have been to orthodontically expand the maxilla bilaterally and secondarily bone graft the alveolar defects at about the age of 11 years. This is discussed in Chapter 10.

This patient has essentially a class I malocclusion with a bilateral transverse maxillary deficiency. There are two primary options to correct this deformity: (1) orthodontically segmentally level and align the posterior maxillary segments and secondarily surgically reposition them laterally with simultaneous bone grafting of the alveolar cleft defects and (2) surgically orthodontically expand the transverse maxillary deformity and retain it, perhaps permanently with a fixed prosthesis, or secondarily graft the existing alveolar bone defects. The first alternative is discussed in Chapter 10; only the combined surgical-orthodontic expansion is discussed here with respect to the unique problems that exist in the patient with bilateral cleft lip-palate.

B. Through a high horizontal vestibular incision the lateral maxillary wall from the piriform rim to the pterygoid plates is exposed. The mucoperiosteum is reflected off the anterior aspect of the lateral nasal wall. A horizontal osteotomy is made from the piriform rim above the alveolar cleft and apices of the teeth to the pterygoid plates. The alveolar clefts serve as the vertical alveolar osteotomies and the palatal bony clefts as the palatal osteotomy. The lateral nasal wall is so thin it seldom needs to be osteotomized to facilitate surgical mobilization of the posterior segments or their subsequent orthopedic expansion. Posterior to the second molar the osteotomy is curved downward toward the inferior aspect of the pterygoid plates, or a small curved osteotome is used to separate the pterygoid plates from the tuberosity of the maxilla. The same procedure is done on the opposite side. The segments can be torqued downward to facilitate some mobility, but *the segments are not down-fractured entirely*.

C. The maxillary expansion appliance is activated about 2 to 3 mm to expand the segments and make certain that they are expanding symmetrically while directly observing them. Because of the scar tissue usually present in cleft patients, the expansion is done at a slower rate than in the noncleft patient so the soft tissues can stretch and proliferate. Following adequate expansion the segments are maintained with the expansion appliance for at least 3 months, and then a removable or fixed prosthesis is immediately inserted so the expansion can be maintained. Bone grafts to the alveolar defects can be done later to stabilize the segments, as described in Chapter 10.

BILATERAL SURGICAL-ORTHODONTIC EXPANSION OF MAXILLA

Bilateral cleft palate deformity (Plate 9-4)

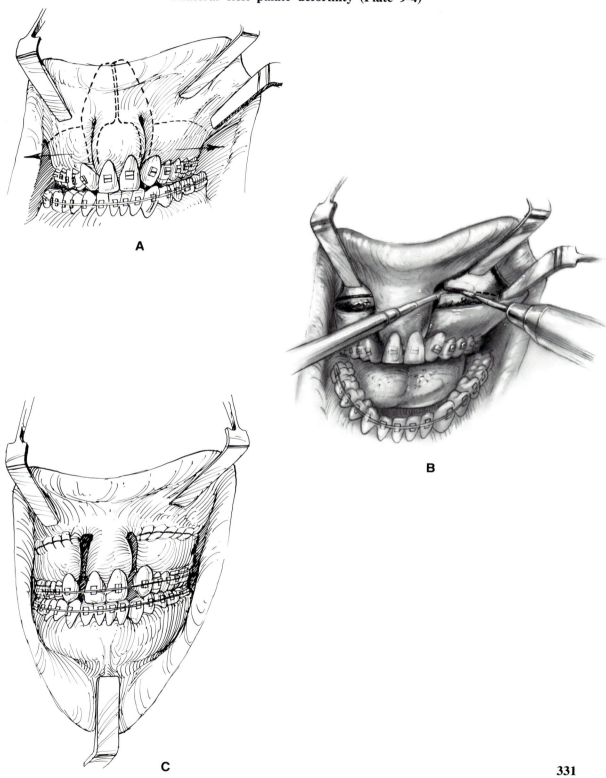

A

B

C

331

CHAPTER 10

Bone grafting of alveolar clefts

Many individuals with cleft lip-palate have a multitude of secondary esthetic and functional disorders of the orofacial region. It is not the intent of this chapter to deal with the entire scope of secondary cleft lip and palate rehabilitation but to discuss the indications, timing, surgical-orthodontic sequencing, and surgical techniques for bone grafting of alveolar clefts.

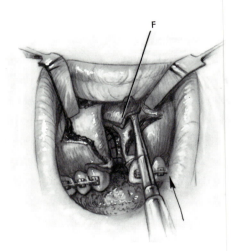

**UNILATERAL CLEFT
ALVEOLAR BONE GRAFTS**

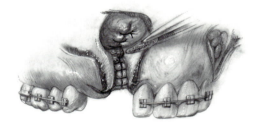

**BILATERAL CLEFT
ALVEOLAR BONE GRAFTS**

Bone grafting of alveolar clefts in patients with unilateral and bilateral cleft is often an integral aspect of their total care. Properly timed and executed alveolar grafting can provide relatively normal alveolar bone continuity, good stabilization for mobilized or expanded maxillary dento-osseous segments, and supporting bone for adjacent teeth to erupt into or be orthodontically moved into and can improve the periodontal health and longevity of teeth adjacent to the cleft. To achieve these objectives grafting must be technically well done and properly timed with respect to age, the stage of tooth development, the existing deformity, and the specific orthodontic needs inherent in each case.

The basic indications for considering alveolar bone grafting in cleft individuals are as follows:

1. Stabilize orthodontically repositioned dento-osseous segments
2. Provide bone continuity in the alveolus for the eruption and orthodontic movement of teeth adjacent to the cleft into their optimal position
3. Prevent periodontal loss of teeth adjacent to the cleft
4. Provide support to the alar bases of the nose

We generally perform bone grafting of alveolar clefts when the patient is between 9 and 12 years of age. At this time the maxilla is expanded orthodontically or orthopedically to the desired width, as dictated by the mandibular arch, and then the alveolar cleft is grafted.

The exact timing is dependent to a large extent on the relationships of the teeth adjacent to the alveolar cleft and their surrounding bone. If the relationship is such that orthodontically the adjacent teeth can be moved into the arch without periodontal compromise, this is done first, and alveolar grafting is generally deferred until about the age of 11 to 12 years. In other cases, after maxillary arch expansion the graft is done at a younger age so that teeth can erupt through the bone graft or orthodontically be moved into the graft site.

In this chapter the specific surgical techniques for alveolar bone grafting in unilateral and bilateral clefts are illustrated and described in context with the aforementioned indications and proper orthodontic sequencing.

Unilateral cleft alveolar bone grafts

Bone grafting of alveolar clefts in the past has met with varying success. Difficulties are usually encountered because of soft-tissue management problems or the bone-grafting techniques utilized. Moreover, the age at which the graft is performed can influence results. Early bone grafting can significantly affect facial growth vertically, anteroposteriorly, and particularly transversely. Therefore the longer the alveolar grafting is deferred the less effect the surgical procedure will have on subsequent facial growth. If alveolar bone grafting is done prior to orthodontic expansion of the maxilla it may be impossible to achieve either an adequate degree of or stable expansion. Consequently maxillary expansion is best completed orthodontically prior to or at the same time as bone grafting of the alveolar cleft.

In unilateral clefts the lesser segment is often in crossbite and can generally be adequately expanded orthodontically in patients up to the age of about 16 years. In adolescent or adult patients it is more predictable and stable to surgically mobilize the lesser segment to expand it and perform an alveolar cleft bone graft at the same time. When a class III malocclusion exists and total maxillary advancement surgery is indicated, the maxilla is advanced and the alveolar cleft simultaneously grafted.

Fresh autogenous cancellous bone from the iliac crest is used for alveolar grafting. Numerous techniques have been described to manage the soft tissues in the cleft area. The basic technique, with several commonly indicated variations, that we have found to be successful for grafting of the unilateral alveolar cleft is described and illustrated here.

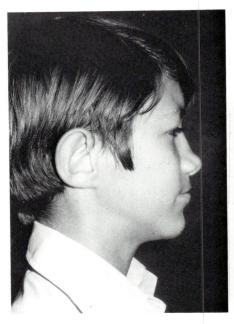
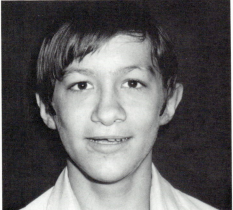

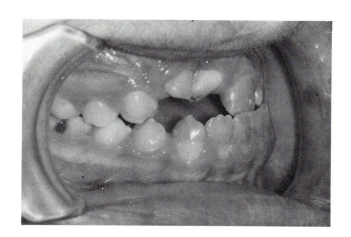

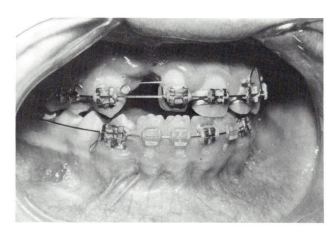

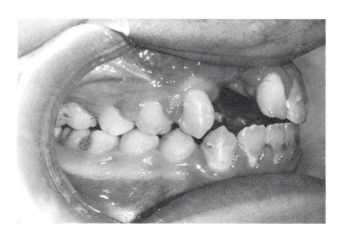

335

UNILATERAL CLEFT ALVEOLAR BONE GRAFTS

Plate 10-1

A. The illustrated case demonstrates a repaired right unilateral cleft lip and palate in a 12-year-old patient. A class I cuspid and molar relationship exists bilaterally, and the maxilla has been orthodontically expanded to correct the previously existing crossbite on the right side. The right maxillary lateral incisor is missing. There is a residual alveolar cleft and an associated oronasal fistula.

   The objective of alveolar grafting in this case is to stabilize the expanded lesser maxillary segment, eliminate the oronasal fistula, create a more favorable periodontal situation for the adjacent teeth, and improve the alveolar ridge anatomy for future prosthetic replacement of the missing tooth.

B. In most cases the palatal aspect of the alveolar cleft can be closed utilizing the tissue lining the cleft. The width of the palatal aspect of the bony alveolar cleft is measured with calipers *(A to A')*; in this case it is 6 mm. Half of the soft tissue needed to close the defect is taken from each side of the alveolar cleft. From point *A* 3 mm are measured to point *B*, extending through the cleft on the greater segment, plus an additional 2 mm to point *C*. The extra 2 mm are added to facilitate soft-tissue closure on the palatal side. The same measurements are done on the lesser segment, labeling the points *A'*, *B'*, and *C'*. Point *D* is the posterior extent of the alveolar cleft.

C. A full-thickness incision is made from point *C* to *D* on the greater segment and from *C'* to *D* on the lesser segment. If possible a collar of attached gingiva is left around the necks of the teeth adjacent to the cleft, as illustrated. This provides tissue to facilitate suturing and results in better periodontal health. Full-thickness mucoperiosteal flaps are elevated and rotated palatally. It may be necessary to reflect the mucoperiosteum from the palatal aspect of the alveolus for several millimeters on each side of the cleft to achieve mobility to facilitate soft-tissue closure.

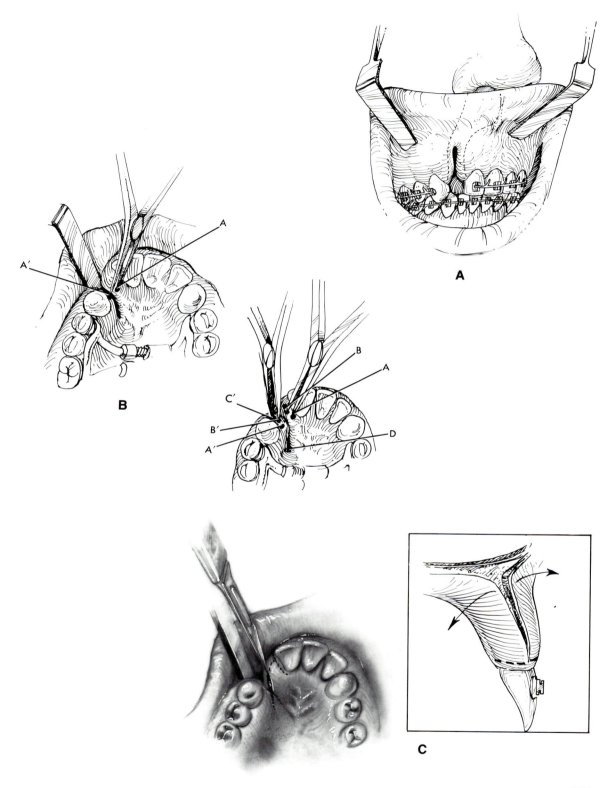

A

B

C

337

D. Interrupted horizontal mattress sutures are used to close the palatal flaps, completing the soft-tissue manipulation on the palatal side. This closure must be complete in order to eliminate oral contaminants and secondary infection of the bone graft.

E. The remainder of the soft tissue in the cleft areas is reflected labially, completely exposing the alveolar bone in the cleft area. A *horizontal incision* approximately 2 cm long is made in the depth of the vestibule extending just above the superior aspect of the oronasal fistula. The horizontal incision is made through the periosteum on the lateral maxillary wall area and anterior nasal spine area; *however, over the area of the alveolar cleft it is extended only down to nasal mucosa.* The mucoperiosteum is reflected superiorly, exposing the piriform rim and anterior nasal spine.

F. The mucoperiosteum from the lateral nasal wall and from the nasal septum is continuous into the cleft area. Therefore to create a soft-tissue nasal floor horizontal incisions are often necessary on the lesser and greater segments just below the nasal floor plane, extending posteriorly into the depth of the cleft. The mucoperiosteum is reflected off the nasal septum and the lateral nasal wall, mobilizing the tissue to aid in closure of the nasal floor. These two flaps *(F to F')* will be used to establish a soft-tissue nasal floor.

G. The flaps are sutured, sealing off the nasal cavity from the alveolar cleft. With careful management of these flaps the nasal floor can be totally closed in this basic step. The alveolar cleft is a pyramidal osseous defect, so at this point two of the three soft-tissue walls have been closed.

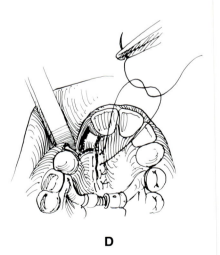

D

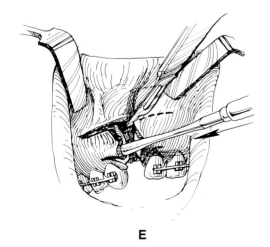

E

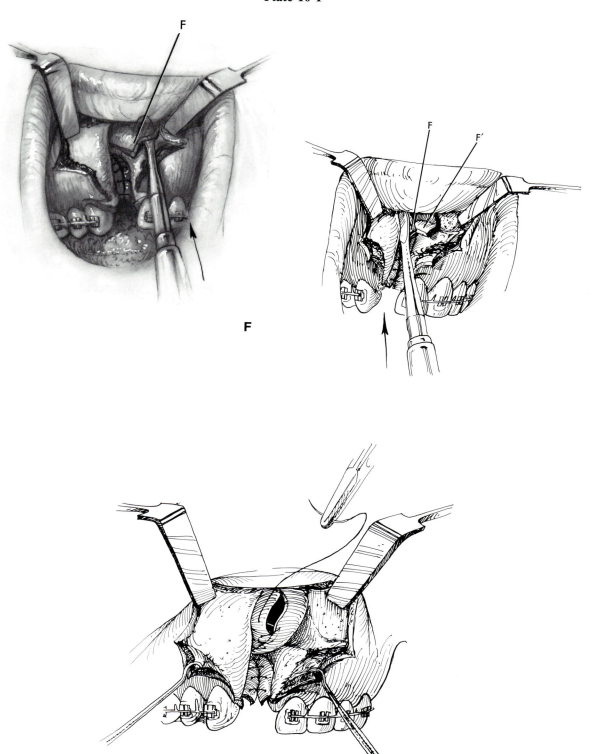

F

G

H. Fresh autogenous cancellous bone from the iliac crest is packed into the alveolar osseous defect. The bone should be packed firmly but not forced into the actual cleft area or the superior or posterior flaps may be torn lose. However, it is advisable to overpack the cleft labially to assure optimal graft take.

Procurement of the cancellous bone is such that it is inserted in the alveolar cleft almost immediately after harvesting. This provides optimally viable bone with the best osteogenic potential.

I. The labial flaps *(E* and *E')* are then sutured. If some additional length of tissue is needed for closure the mucogingival flap can be reflected from around the necks of the adjacent teeth to provide additional length, or a trapezoidal lip flap or pedicled vestibular flap can be used, as illustrated in Plate 10-2, *B* and *C.*

Interrupted horizontal mattress sutures are used to provide a watertight closure over the graft area, and a running suture can be used to close the horizontal vestibular incision. The palatal expansion device is maintained in place for 6 to 8 weeks following grafting to allow sufficient healing of the alveolar bone graft. After this period the alveolar cleft graft provides good stability of the expanded maxilla.

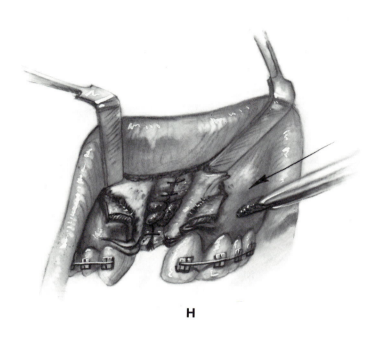

H

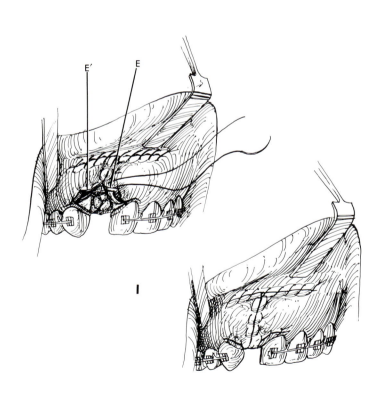

I

341

UNILATERAL CLEFT ALVEOLAR BONE GRAFTS

Wide cleft (Plate 10-2)

A. When the cleft is wide it is often difficult to close the soft-tissue aspect of the cleft on both the palatal and labial sides by utilizing only the soft tissues lining the cleft itself. Therefore other tissue must be used to cover the bone graft.

A cleft defect of 12 mm with a missing lateral incisor and an unerupted cuspid is illustrated. The palatal aspect of wide alveolar clefts can be closed by simply increasing the length of flaps *A* to *C* and *A'* to *C'* with extension, if necessary, on the labial surface of the clefts. The palatal flaps are closed with interrupted horizontal mattress sutures as described in Plate 10-1, *D*. It is desirable, if possible, that a collar of attached gingiva be maintained around the necks of the teeth adjacent to the cleft to enhance periodontal health, *B*. The horizontal vestibular incision is used for exposure of the piriform rim and anterior nasal spine area. The lateral nasal and septal mucoperiosteal flaps are mobilized and sutured, as described in Plate 10-1, *F* and *G,* to create the new nasal floor. The fresh autogenous cancellous bone graft from the iliac crest is inserted. The labial soft-tissue defect can then be closed with a trapezoidal lip flap or a pedicled vestibular flap.

B. The trapezoidal lip flap is made with divergent vertical incisions into the labial vestibule, extending to the depth of the orbicularis oris muscle. The flap is undermined full thickness out into the lip toward the vermilion and advanced over the bone graft. This wide-based flap provides an excellent vascular bed for the flap as well as for the bone graft.

UNILATERAL CLEFT ALVEOLAR BONE GRAFTS

Wide cleft (Plate 10-2)

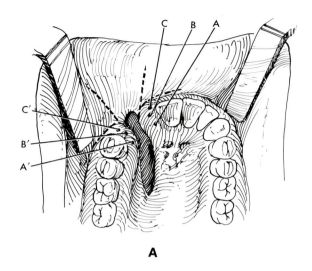

A

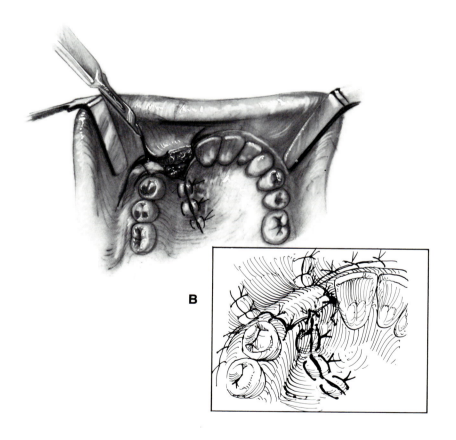

B

UNILATERAL CLEFT ALVEOLAR BONE GRAFTS

Wide cleft (Plate 10-2)

C. As an alternative the vestibular pedicled "finger flap" is a long narrow flap raised from the depth of the vestibule and rotated over the bone graft. The width of this flap should be at least equal to one third of the flap length.

D. This flap is also useful if a soft-tissue void exists on the palatal aspect, as it can be extended over the alveolar cleft to cover any residual palatal soft-tissue defect. It is best to close the flap with interrupted horizontal mattress sutures.

E. The trapezoidal flap and the finger flap provide excellent means by which to mobilize additional tissue to cover the bone graft. However, periodontally the type of loose, unattached mucosa provided by these flaps is not ideal around the adjacent teeth. Therefore following the alveolar bone graft procedure it may be indicated that the tissue be replaced with attached gingiva. This can be done any time after the second month following bone grafting. The trapezoidal lip flap is released *supraperiosteally* and resutured back into the lip at the depth of the vestibule. If the finger flap is used the unattached, mobile tissue is simply excised off the graft area *supraperiosteally*. A split-thickness mucosal graft is taken from the palate and sutured over the periosteum, providing attached gingivae to the grafted area. A periodontal pack can be placed over the mucosal graft for 1 week to help stabilize and protect it while it is healing.

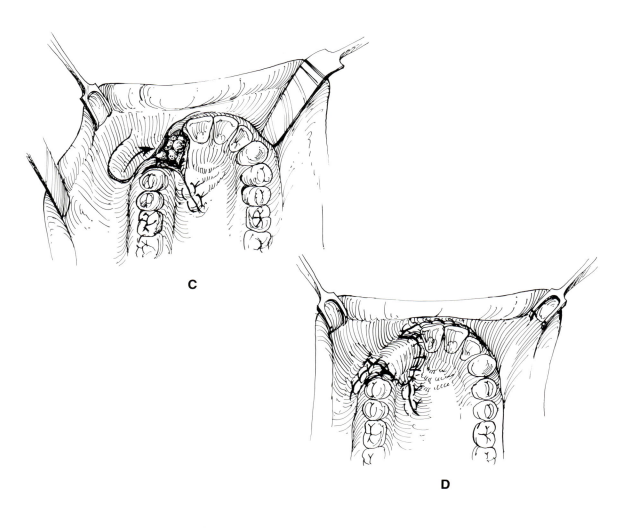

C

D

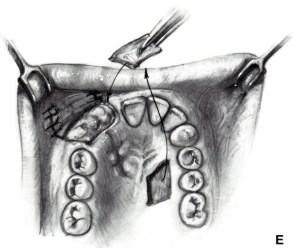

E

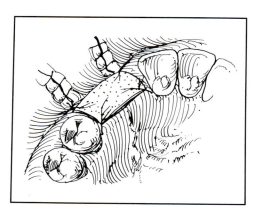

UNILATERAL CLEFT ALVEOLAR BONE GRAFTS

Simultaneous surgical expansion and grafting (Plate 10-3)

A. Frequently in the adult patient the lesser segment is in crossbite and is best surgically repositioned with simultaneous alveolar bone grafting.

   The illustrated case demonstrates a left unilateral repaired cleft lip and palate with a residual alveolar cleft, class I occlusion on the right, a missing lateral incisior on the left, and the left lesser segment collapsed into crossbite. A horizontal vestibular incision is made from the cleft site, extending posteriorly to the first molar area.

B. The mucoperiosteum is elevated from the lateral aspect of the maxilla and the lateral nasal wall and a horizontal osteotomy performed from the piriform rim posteriorly to the pterygoid plates at a level of 4 to 5 mm above the apices of the teeth. Once the osteotomy is posterior to the second molar, it is curved inferiorly toward the base of the pterygomaxillary junction. This simplifies separation of the pterygomaxillary suture and often eliminates the need to mallet an osteotome in this area.

C. The only osseous structure remaining intact is a portion of the lateral nasal wall, and at this time the segment can generally be mobilized by in-fracturing. This is done carefully so that the nasal mucoperiosteum on the lateral nasal wall is not torn.

UNILATERAL CLEFT ALVEOLAR BONE GRAFTS

Simultaneous surgical expansion and grafting (Plate 10-3)

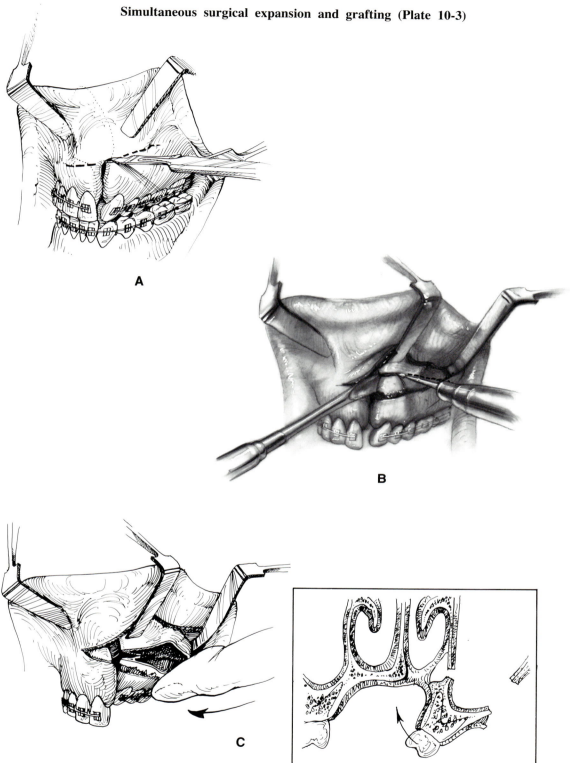

A

B

C

UNILATERAL CLEFT ALVEOLAR BONE GRAFTS

Simultaneous surgical expansion and grafting (Plate 10-3)

D. The palatal tissue flaps are created and managed as described in Plate 10-1, *B* to *D,* to establish soft-tissue coverage on the palatal aspect of the cleft. The lengths of the palatal flaps *(A* to *C* and *A'* to *C')* are determined from the dental model surgery, because the original cleft width will be increased as the crossbite is eliminated. At this time the occlusal splint is tried in position, and the lesser segment should fit passively in the splint. If the segment is difficult to expand, as is often the case, the palatal mucoperiosteum on the greater segment can be elevated from the palate to facilitate expansion of the lesser segment. However, this may be technically difficult to do, and with the soft-tissue scarring usually only a minor degree of soft-tissue relaxation can be achieved.

E. If this does not provide adequate soft-tissue relaxation, there are two alternatives to achieve passive expansion of the lesser segment. The first method is to incise directly over the septum and reflect the mucoperiosteum off the septum carefully so no oral communication is created into the nose. The soft-tissue gap created will granulate in and epithelialize.

F. The second method is to make a releasing incision at the palatoalveolar junction on the greater segment and elevate the mucoperiosteum on the palatal shelf so the palatal tissues can move toward the expanded segment. This creates a soft-tissue gap on the greater segment that subsequently granulates and epithelializes.

G. The occlusal splint is secured in place via direct wiring. When performing expansion it is advisable to construct the occlusal splint with a posterior palatal bar; otherwise the splint will often bend and result in relapse with resultant incomplete expansion of the segment.

  The alveolar bone graft is placed, and the lateral maxillary wall is also grafted to promote rapid healing and stability. The labial soft tissues are closed as indicated with a trapezoidal or finger flap.

  The splint is maintained for at least 6 to 8 weeks until the bone graft has an opportunity to heal well and stabilize the segments. If the trapezoidal or finger flap is used to cover the bone graft a split-thickness palatal mucosal graft may be necessary secondarily to provide attached gingiva in the grafted area.

UNILATERAL CLEFT ALVEOLAR BONE GRAFTS

Simultaneous surgical expansion and grafting (Plate 10-3)

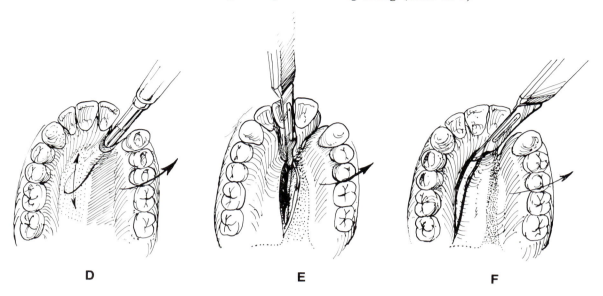

D   E   F

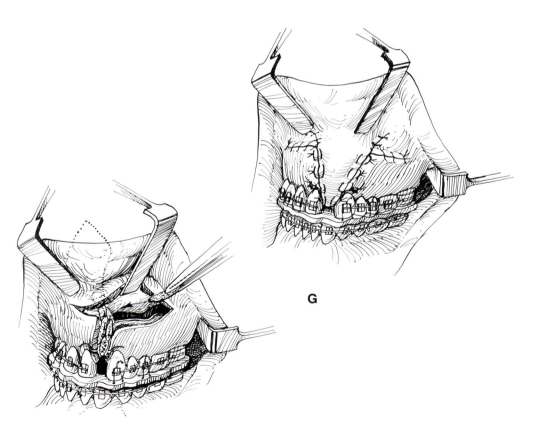

G

349

UNILATERAL CLEFT ALVEOLAR BONE GRAFTS

Simultaneous advancement of maxilla and grafting (Plate 10-4)

A. The maxilla can be advanced, widened, or segmented simultaneously with the alveolar cleft bone grafting procedure. In the illustrated case a maxillary retrusion with transverse deficiency (bilateral posterior crossbite) is present as well as the alveolar cleft. The proposed surgery includes a total maxillary advancement of 8 mm, expansion of the maxilla 5 mm, and simultaneously bone grafting the alveolar cleft.

B. Generally a circumvestibular incision can be used that passes through the oronasal fistula at its most superior aspect. The anterior and lateral maxillary walls are exposed, and the mucoperiosteum is dissected off the lateral nasal wall. The lateral osteotomy is then completed, including the anterior aspect of the lateral nasal wall. Because pterygomaxillary bone grafts are to be used, the horizontal osteotomy is carried straight back to the pterygoid plates. The pterygoid plates and tuberosity of the maxilla are carefully separated with a thin curved osteotome. The same osteotomies are then completed on the opposite side.

   The mucoperiosteum is dissected from the nasal septum on the side of the cleft, and the mucoperiosteum is elevated from the opposite nasal floor. The nasal septum is then separated from the maxilla with an osteotome.

C. When the greater segment must be segmentalized with a small anterior segment it is advisable to maintain an anterior labial pedicle to the anterior segment to assure an adequate vascular supply.

UNILATERAL CLEFT ALVEOLAR BONE GRAFTS

Simultaneous advancement of maxilla and grafting (Plate 10-4)

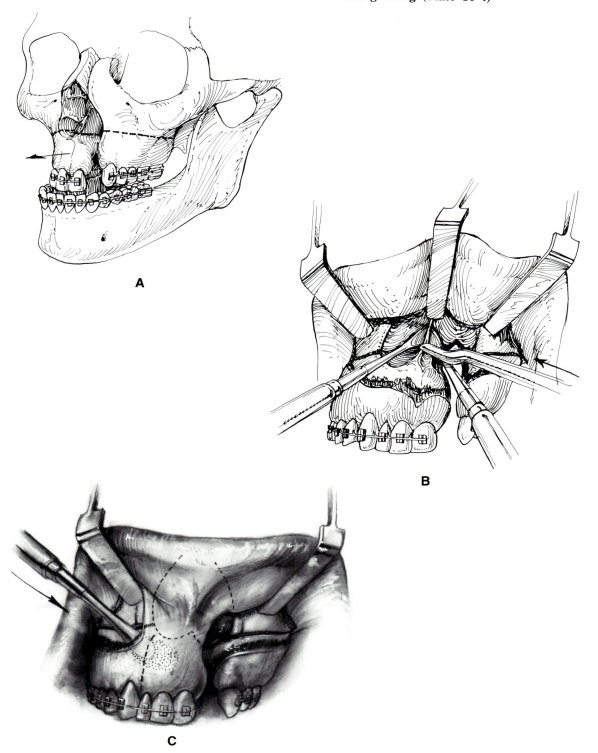

A

B

C

UNILATERAL CLEFT ALVEOLAR BONE GRAFTS

Simultaneous advancement of maxilla and grafting (Plate 10-4)

D. A horizontal incision is made just below the level of the nasal floor in the cleft area to release the lateral nasal mucoperiosteum and nasal septal mucoperiosteum from their continuation into the cleft area. These flaps will later create the nasal floor. *These incisions must be done prior to down-fracturing of the maxilla to avoid tearing of the mucoperiosteum in the cleft area.*

E. The maxillary segments are then down-fractured and mobilized. Each segment can be independently mobilized with or without the mobilization forceps, and the segments can be temporarily placed in the occlusal splint to make certain they can be properly repositioned passively as a unit.

The nasal floor is closed by suturing the mucoperiosteal flaps from the lateral nasal wall and nasal septum.

The splint is removed while the palatal soft-tissue flaps are closed, as described in Plate 10-1, *C* to *E*.

UNILATERAL CLEFT ALVEOLAR BONE GRAFTS

Simultaneous advancement of maxilla and grafting (Plate 10-4)

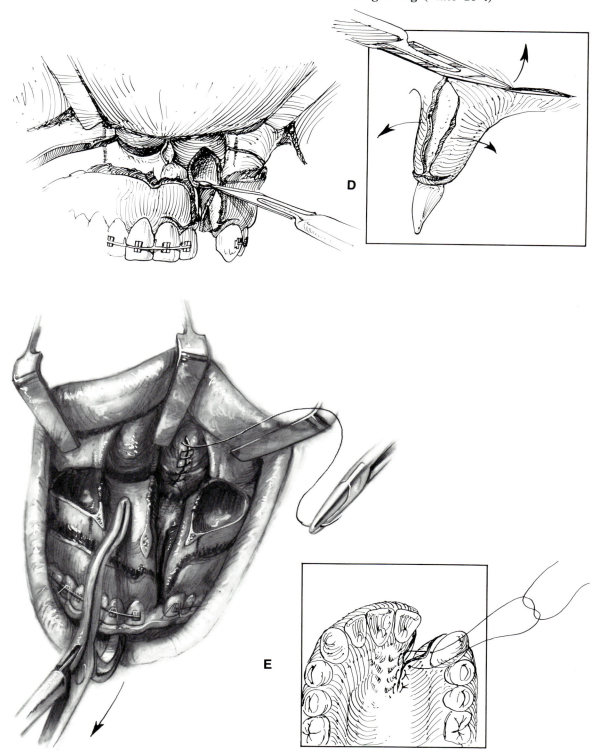

UNILATERAL CLEFT ALVEOLAR BONE GRAFTS

Simultaneous advancement of maxilla and grafting (Plate 10-4)

F. The occlusal splint is inserted and secured to the maxillary segments. Intermaxillary fixation is applied as well as infraorbital suspension wires. Fresh autogenous cancellous bone from the iliac crest is placed in the alveolar cleft area. Similarly cortical bone grafts are placed between the tuberosities and pterygoid plates and cancellous grafts onlayed along the lateral maxillary wall osteotomy sites.

G. The residual tissue from the alveolar cleft can be used to close the labial aspect of the cleft if sufficient tissue remains. If not, a trapezoidal lip flap or finger flap can be advanced over the bone graft, as described in Plate 10-2, *B* and *C*.

H. Intermaxillary fixation is maintained for about 6 weeks, and on release the stability of the maxilla is carefully evaluated. Generally after about 6 weeks light interarch vertical or class III elastics can be used to control the occlusion for an additional 2 to 3 weeks. During this time they are used for progressively fewer hours per day, while carefully observing the occlusion to make certain relapse is not occurring.

UNILATERAL CLEFT ALVEOLAR BONE GRAFTS

Simultaneous advancement of maxilla and grafting (Plate 10-4)

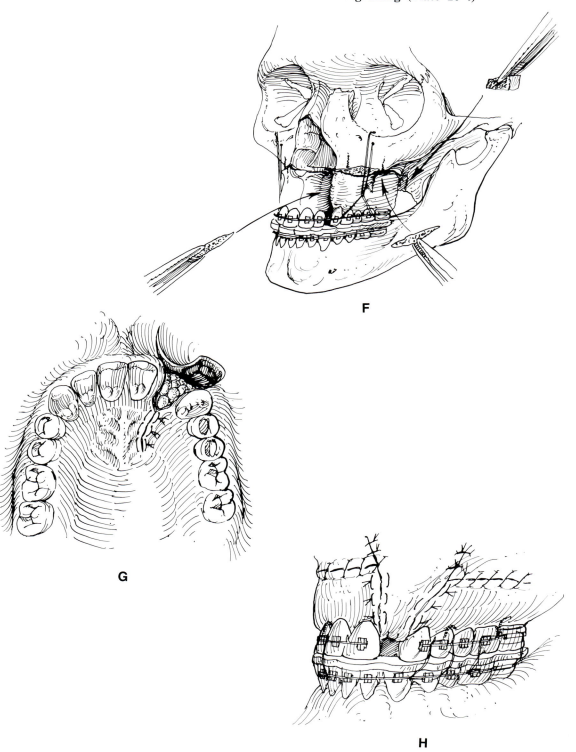

F

G

H

Bilateral cleft alveolar bone grafts

Bone grafting of bilateral alveolar clefts is understandably more complex than unilateral alveolar clefts, primarily because the soft-tissue flaps are more difficult to develop. They become even more difficult if the premaxilla is to be mobilized simultaneously. The indications for bone grafting of the bilateral alveolar cleft are as follows:

1. Stabilize the premaxilla
2. Provide alveolar bone for tooth eruption or orthodontic tooth movements
3. Provide stabilization for maxillary expansion

As in unilateral cleft, the maxilla must be adequately expanded prior to bone grafting of bilateral alveolar clefts. If grafting is done prior to expansion it will be extremely difficult to orthodontically eliminate an existing crossbite. However, the maxilla is relatively easy to expand prior to bone grafting. If the alveolar bone grafting is done before the patient is 9 years of age maxillary growth may be significantly impeded, with subsequent worsening of the dento-facial and occlusal deformities. In bilateral alveolar cleft, often the premaxilla is semimobile, being attached primarily to the vomer and cartilaginous nasal septum. The premaxilla and incisors frequently are quite vertical in orientation relative to the long axes of the teeth. The premaxilla can be simultaneously repositioned and the alveolar cleft defects bone grafted. With careful preparation and dissection of the soft-tissue flaps the three dento-osseous segments (premaxilla and the two posterior segments) can be mobilized and repositioned and the alveolar clefts bone grafted simultaneously. Most often the indications for repositioning of the premaxilla are the following:

1. Anteroposterior malposition
2. Excessive vertical orientation
3. Excessive anterior deep bite

Indications for repositioning of the posterior segments generally are as follows:

1. Posterior crossbite
2. Posterior open bite
3. Anteroposterior malposition

Reflection of soft tissue off the premaxilla must be done with extreme care, because the blood supply to the premaxilla is provided primarily from the nasal septal mucoperiosteum and vestibular aspect of the upper lip.

In this section are discussed and illustrated our surgical approaches to bone grafting of bilateral alveolar clefts with and without simultaneous mobilization of the various maxillary segments.

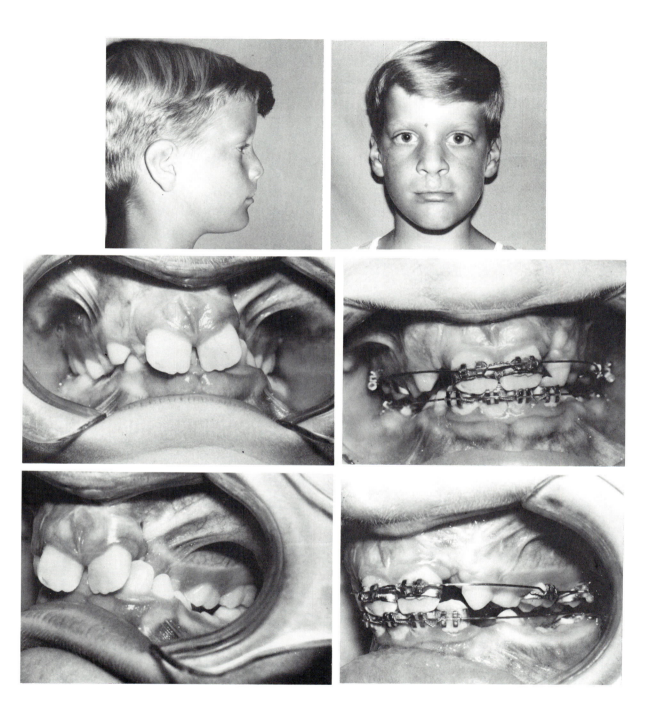

BILATERAL CLEFT ALVEOLAR BONE GRAFTS

Plate 10-5

A. The illustrated case demonstrates residual bilateral alveolar clefts and oro-nasal communications in a 12-year-old patient. There is a class I molar relationship. The permanent maxillary cuspids are erupting toward the alveolar clefts but are not yet clinically visible. Orthodontics have been completed to align the maxillary incisors and expand the posterior segments. The premaxilla is mobile because it is attached only to the anterior portion of the vomer and cartilaginous nasal septum.

The reasons for performing alveolar grafting in this case are to stabilize the premaxilla, provide good alveolar bone for subsequent eruption and orthodontic alignment of the cuspids, and stabilize the previously expanded posterior segments.

B. The soft tissues are prepared in a manner similar to that in which they are prepared for the unilateral cleft, but extreme care must be exercised when the flap preparation is being done on the premaxilla so that the vascular supply to this segment is not jeopardized. For this reason, if the cleft is wide the majority of the soft tissue to cover the palatal aspect of the cleft must come from the posterior segment.

The cleft width is measured with calipers to determine the amount of tissue needed to close the palatal aspect. Generally on the premaxilla point *C* should *not* extend onto the labial aspect of the premaxilla. The majority of tissue to cover the palatal aspect of the cleft *must* come from the posterior segment. Therefore the distance from *A* to *C* is usually less than from *A'* to *C'*. A vertical incision is made in the cleft area of the premaxilla, paralleling the palatal aspect of the cleft up to the level of the palatal plane and extending to the posterior aspect of the alveolar cleft (point *D*). The mucoperiosteal flaps are carefully reflected palatally and labially, exposing only the bone in the cleft. The amount of tissue necessary for closure of the palatal soft-tissue defect plus an additional 2 mm are measured from the posterior segment (point *A'* to *C'*), and a similar vertical incision is made and that flap rotated palatally.

Plate 10-5

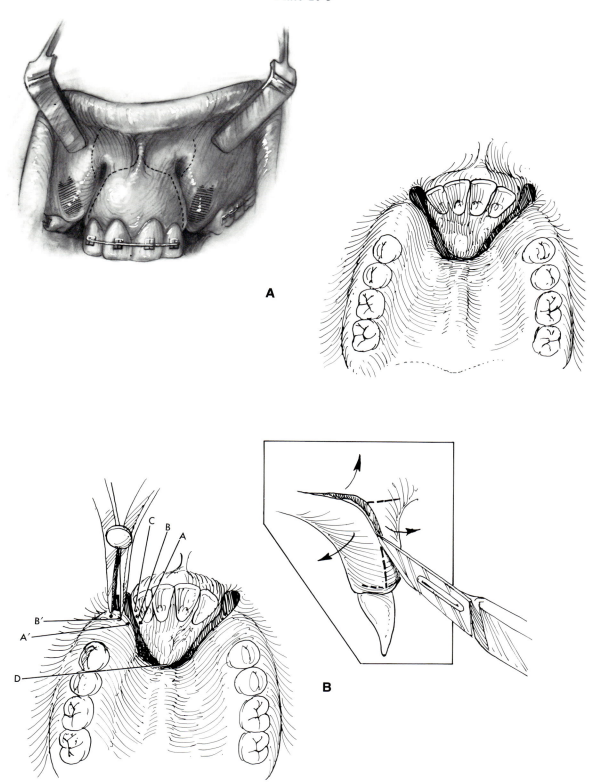

A

B

C. Horizontal mattress sutures are placed to close the soft tissues on the palatal aspect of the cleft. Horizontal vestibular incisions are then made extending from just superior to the oronasal fistula, posteriorly 2 cm to provide good exposure of the operative area. *No horizontal incisions are made anterior to the alveolar cleft*. The lateral nasal mucoperiosteum is elevated off the lateral nasal wall, and the mucoperiosteum is reflected off the nasal septum (flaps *F* and *F'*). An anterior vertical incision is sometimes necessary to adequately mobilize this flap. These flaps are then rotated together and sutured to create the nasal floor.

It must be remembered that with these flap designs *the vascular supply to the premaxilla is totally dependent on the remaining labial flap. No soft tissues can be reflected off the anterior aspect of the premaxilla*. The same soft-tissue procedures are done on the opposite side.

D. Two of the three soft-tissue walls of the clefts are now closed. Fresh autogenous cancellous bone is obtained from the iliac crest and placed in the alveolar defect. Procurement of the bone graft should be coordinated so it will be as fresh as possible when placed in the recipient site for optimal osteogenic potential.

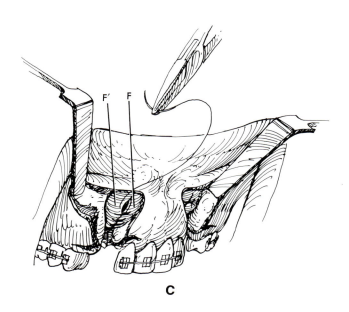

C

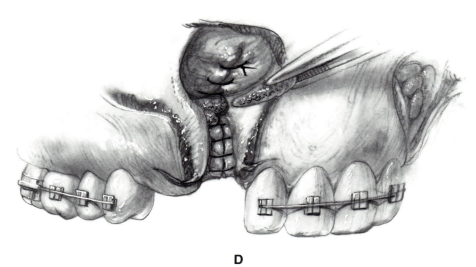

D

BILATERAL CLEFT ALVEOLAR BONE GRAFTS

Plate 10-5

E. If sufficient tissue is available adjacent to the cleft it is mobilized, primarily off the posterior segment, and advanced over the bone graft and sutured.

F. If the cleft is wide or if insufficient tissue is available to directly close over the bone graft, an advancement flap procedure is indicated. A trapezoidal flap, as described and illustrated in Plate 10-2, *B,* can be advanced over the bone graft and sutured.

G. A finger flap can also be used to close the soft-tissue defect on the labial aspect of the cleft. When either of these flaps is employed a secondary gingival graft procedure may be indicated on the alveolar bone graft area to provide attached gingiva, as described in Plate 10-2, *E*.

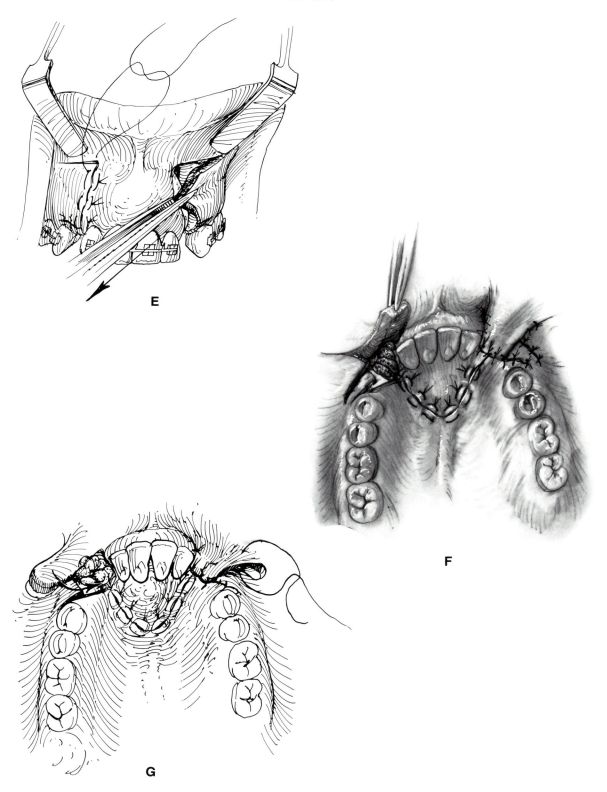

E

F

G

BILATERAL CLEFT ALVEOLAR BONE GRAFTS

Simultaneous mobilization of premaxilla and grafting (Plate 10-6)

A. In this illustrated case the premaxilla is protrusive with an excessive deep bite anteriorly. The premaxilla is to be moved superiorly and posteriorly to decrease the deep bite and to improve incisor angulation, with simultaneous bilateral alveolar bone grafting.

B. The soft-tissue flap design for closure of the alveolar clefts is the same as described for unilateral cleft alveolar bone grafts. It is generally easier to create the palatal and labial flaps off the premaxilla while it is still semistable prior to mobilization of it. With a protrusive premaxilla usually a portion of the vomer is seen intraorally between the posterior segments and the premaxilla. From the palatal aspect a midline vomerine incision is made. The mucoperiosteum is reflected from the nasal septum on both sides with a periosteal elevator. A vertical osteotomy is completed through the vomer to the level of the cartilaginous septum with a curved osteotome or bur.

BILATERAL CLEFT ALVEOLAR BONE GRAFTS

Simultaneous mobilization of premaxilla and grafting (Plate 10-6)

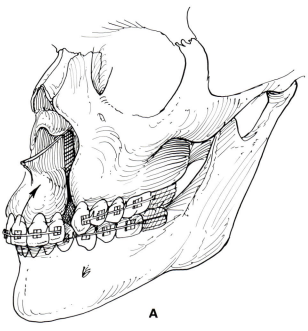

A

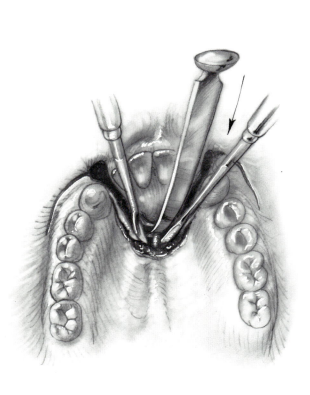

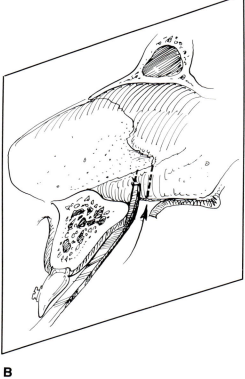

B

BILATERAL CLEFT ALVEOLAR BONE GRAFTS

Simultaneous mobilization of premaxilla and grafting (Plate 10-6)

C. The premaxilla is then out-fractured, pedicled to the labial mucoperiosteal flap. While out-fractured, adequate vomerine bone is removed with a rongeur or a bone bur, and a portion of cartilaginous nasal septum is resected, if necessary, to allow the premaxilla to be passively repositioned superiorly and posteriorly.

D. The occlusal splint is next tried in place to assure that the premaxilla can be passively repositioned as desired. The soft tissues of the palatal aspect and the mucoperiosteum of the nasal floor are closed as described in Plate 10-5, *B* and *C*. The occlusal splint is inserted and secured to the maxillary teeth with 26-gauge stainless steel wire, and fresh autogenous cancellous iliac bone grafts are placed bilaterally. The procurement of the bone from the iliac crest should be coordinated so that the grafts are as fresh as possible when inserted into the alveolar cleft to the osteogenic potential.

E. Because the premaxilla is repositioned posteriorly, usually the labial aspect of the cleft can be closed with a gingival flap as illustrated here. If adequate tissue is not present an advancement lip flap is used to provide adequate coverage for each of the bone grafts, as described in Plate 10-2, *B* to *D*. The splint is maintained for about 6 weeks and then removed. If an advancement flap is used it is generally released after 2 months and a split-thickness gingival graft done to provide attached gingiva over the alveolar graft area, as described in Plate 10-2, *E*.

BILATERAL CLEFT ALVEOLAR BONE GRAFTS

Simultaneous mobilization of premaxilla and grafting (Plate 10-6)

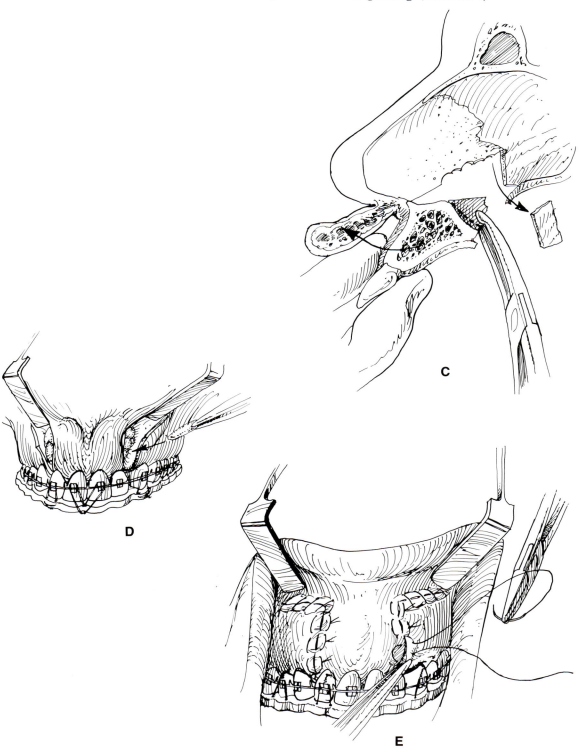

C

D

E

SPECIAL CONSIDERATION
BILATERAL CLEFT ALVEOLAR BONE GRAFTS

Simultaneous advancement of maxilla and grafting (Plate 10-7)

A. In this illustrated case a class III occlusal relationship exists with bilateral posterior crossbite. The surgery to be performed will consist of mobilizing the three segments of the maxilla for advancement of the entire maxilla with simultaneous expansion of the posterior segments and bilateral alveolar bone grafting.

The incisions for closure of the palatal soft-tissue aspect and anterior nasal floor are done in the manner described in Plate 10-5, *B* to *D*. The amount of tissue necessary to close the palatal aspect of the clefts is determined from the dental model surgery. These flaps are usually easier to develop prior to mobilization of the segments. The premaxilla is mobilized by out-fracturing as described and illustrated in Plate 10-6, *B* and *C*.

B. Next the posterior segments are mobilized through horizontal incisions extending from the oronasal fistulas posteriorly to the zygomatic buttress area. The anterior and lateral maxillary walls are exposed. The nasal mucoperiosteum is elevated off the lateral nasal wall. A horizontal osteotomy of the anterior and lateral maxillary wall is completed from the nasal piriform rim posteriorly to the pterygoid plates at a level 4 to 5 mm above the apices of the teeth. Since the total maxilla is being advanced, requiring bone grafting, the horizontal osteotomy is taken straight back to the pterygoid plates. A curved osteotome is used to separate the pterygoid plates from the tuberosity of the maxilla. A small straight osteotome can be used to section the anterior aspect of the lateral nasal wall. The same osteotomies are performed on the opposite side. Each posterior segment is independently mobilized by torquing the segment palatally, which fractures the remaining lateral nasal wall. In patients with bilateral cleft there is generally no osseous connection between the palatal shelves or to the nasal septum; therefore each segment can be readily independently mobilized.

C. Through the cleft area the mucoperiosteum is reflected from the nasal septum and lateral nasal walls to facilitate mobilization of the maxillary segments for the advancement.

Generally in bilateral clefts there are no osseous connections between the alveolus and nasal septum, that is, no interconnecting palatal shelves. However, to further facilitate mobilization it is often helpful to section the vomer slightly higher than usual so the inferior aspect of the vomer is advanced with the palatal mucosa, allowing the palatal mucosa to advance with the posterior segments.

This technique is adequate if no or only moderate expansion is necessary.

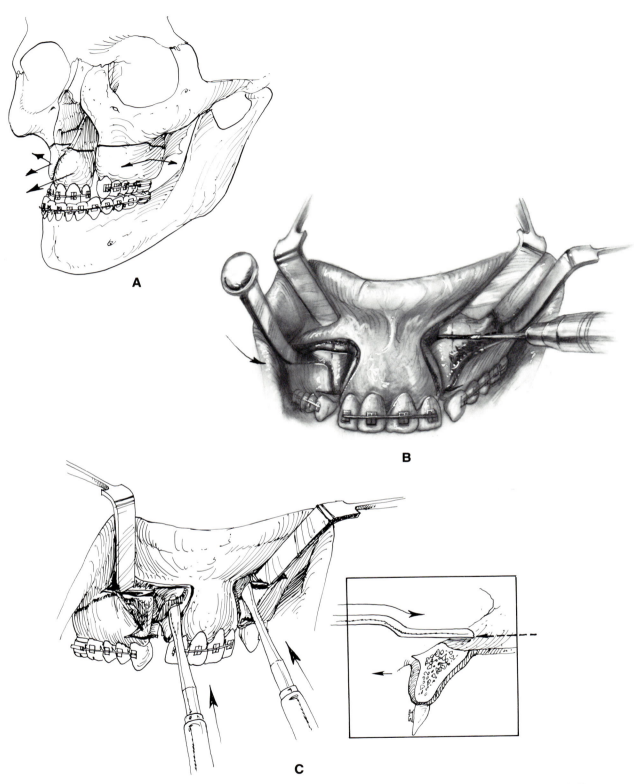

A

B

C

BILATERAL CLEFT ALVEOLAR BONE GRAFTS

Simultaneous advancement of maxilla and grafting (Plate 10-7)

D. When significant expansion is necessary, as in this illustrated case, a midline palatal incision is made directly over the vomer, and the septal mucoperiosteum is reflected from both sides of the vomer. This allows significant expansion yet maintains separation between the oral and nasal cavities.

E. The palatal flaps of the cleft alveolus are then sutured, the occlusal splint inserted, and the anterior nasal floor sutured as described in Plate 10-5, *C* and *D*. Suspension wires are inserted for stabilization of the segments. Inferior orbital rim and zygomatic suspension wires can be used. *However, inferior orbital suspension wires are sometimes difficult to insert, because the amount of retraction necessary for adequate exposure to insert them may pull the labial soft-tissue pedicle off to the premaxilla,* resulting in an avascular osseous segment. Therefore piriform aperture and zygomatic buttress wires are preferable, as illustrated here. Bone grafts are inserted in the alveolar clefts, pterygoid maxillary areas, and along the anterior maxillary walls to provide bony continuity, stabilize the segments, and promote more rapid healing.

F. The appropriate flaps are used to close the labial soft tissues over the alveolar bone grafts. Because the alveolar cleft width is often decreased by properly aligning the segments, labial gingival flaps can usually be used to cover the bone grafts. If adequate tissue is not available, bilateral trapezoidal flaps or finger flaps are used to cover the bone grafts, as shown in Plate 10-5, *F* and *G*. The occlusal splint is usually maintained for 6 weeks. With wide expansion the vomer is evident at surgery through the palatal midline dissection. This will granulate and epithelialize during the healing phase. If pedicle flaps are used, after 2 months they are released supraperiosteally and palatal split-thickness grafts placed to provide attached gingiva in the grafted area.

BILATERAL CLEFT ALVEOLAR BONE GRAFTS

Simultaneous advancement of maxilla and grafting (Plate 10-7)

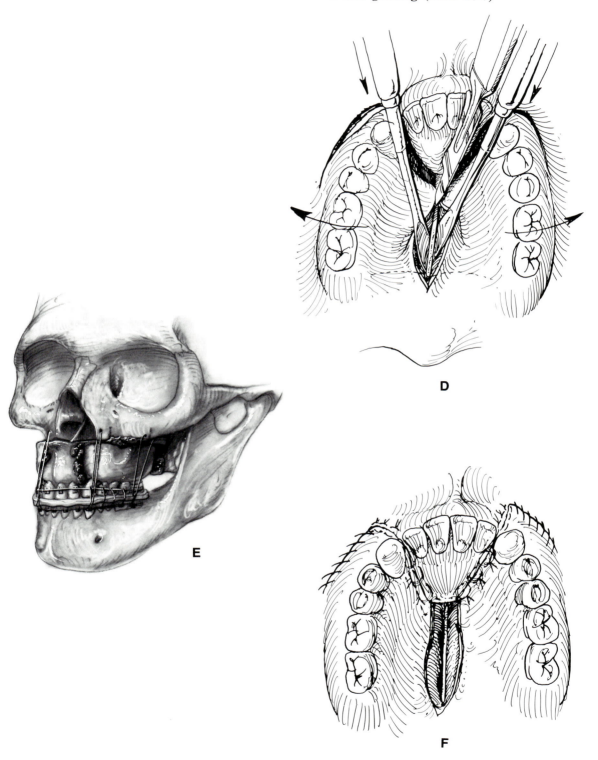

D

E

F

PART THREE

MIDFACE SURGERY

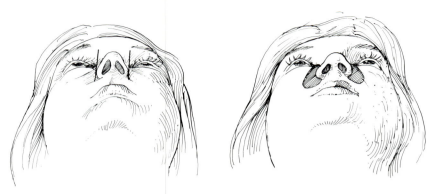

PARANASAL AUGMENTATION

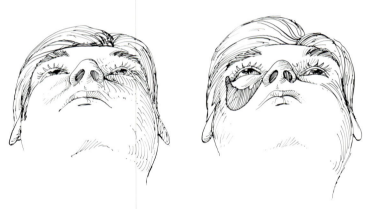

MALAR AUGMENTATION

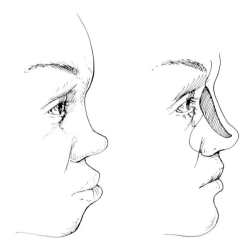

NASAL AUGMENTATION

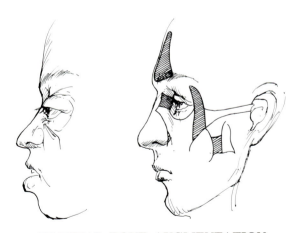

FRONTAL BONE AUGMENTATION

CHAPTER 11

Midface augmentation

There are numerous indications for augmentation of the various anatomic areas of the upper and middle third face such as the paranasal areas, malar bones, infraorbital rims, nasal dorsum, supraorbital rims, and frontal bone. In some instances augmentation of these structures is done as an independent operation in concert with the surgical correction of mandibular deformities, for example, mandibular prognathism. However, these procedures are more commonly indicated coincident with the various middle third face osteotomies to be described and illustrated in Chapter 12. For example, in certain instances a LeFort III midface advancement results in incomplete correction of the severely hypoplastic and retrusive infraorbital and malar areas and existing exophthalmos. When this situation arises two basic decisions must be made: (1) whether to perform augmentation surgery simultaneously with the primary surgery or as a secondary operation and (2) what material to use for the proposed augmentation. In general we prefer to perform these adjunctive augmentation procedures in concert with the primary operation. However, to do so requires careful preoperative planning, especially with respect to the actual sequencing of the operation. This topic is covered in considerable detail in this and the following chapter. The material preferred for augmentation varies with the situation and includes autogenous bone graft, autogenous cartilage graft, allogenic bone graft, allogenic cartilage graft, and alloplasts.

In this chapter the timing, techniques, and specific materials used for midface augmentation—specifically paranasal, malar (infraorbital rim), nasal, and frontal bone (supraorbital rim) augmentation—are discussed.

The techniques that we have employed to augment the various structures of the midface, both as independent and simultaneous procedures, are illustrated and discussed in detail.

Paranasal augmentation

In our experience paranasal augmentation is most commonly done as an adjunctive procedure to correct paranasal deficiency when mandibular surgery is being done (such as with the correction of mandibular prognathism), in secondary cleft repair, and in idiopathic entities. Patients to be considered for paranasal augmentation exhibit depressions in the alar base area relative to the cheeks and upper lip. Clinically an accentuated depression can be palpated at the junction of the maxillary alveolus and maxilla at about the level of the apices of the teeth, adjacent to the alar bases. Clinically the alar bases are narrow, the nasal dorsum may appear somewhat prominent, and the paranasal areas are recessive. Therefore the esthetic facial characteristics associated with paranasal or anterior maxillary hypoplasia or retrusion are evident both frontally and in profile.

When paranasal augmentation is properly done it results in widening of the alar bases, decrease of the paranasal recessiveness, and a relative decrease in the nasal prominence. These esthetic changes are important because, for example, if widening of the alar bases is not deemed esthetically desirable, regardless of profile esthetic findings, the use of this procedure must be carefully considered.

Paranasal depressions are usually present bilaterally; however, they can exist unilaterally, as in the patient with unilateral cleft lip-palate. In these individuals this deformity can be corrected by "overpacking" at the time of alveolar bone grafting, as described and illustrated in Chapter 10. In most other cases we prefer alloplastic augmentation as the method of choice because of the predictability of results and technical ease of performing the surgery. If, however, paranasal augmentation is being done simultaneously with maxillary procedures requiring bone grafting (that is, alveolar bone grafting in a patient with unilateral cleft lip-palate or total maxillary advancement surgery), additional bone can be harvested and used for paranasal augmentation by onlaying it to the paranasal areas. Both methods of paranasal augmentation are best approached via an intraoral route.

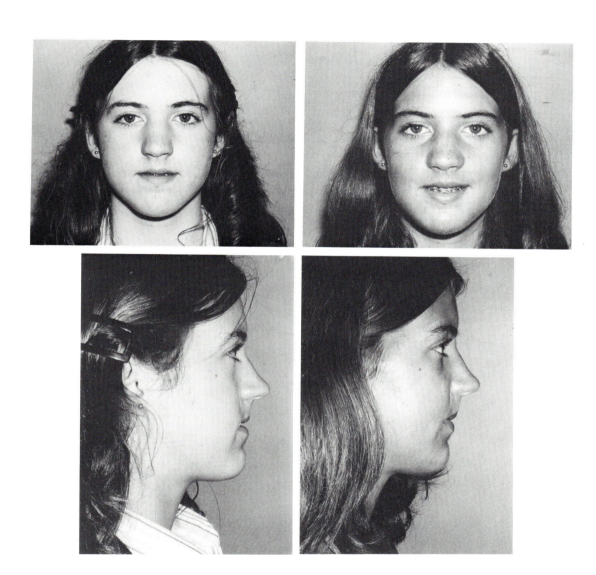

PARANASAL AUGMENTATION
Plate 11-1

A. The illustrated case demonstrates an individual with narrow alar bases and depression in the paranasal areas with true mandibular prognathism. This patient will simultaneously undergo bilateral mandibular ramus osteotomies for mandibular setback and alloplastic paranasal augmentation. When simultaneous mandibular surgery and paranasal augmentation procedures are done, *we perform the augmentation as the final operative procedure*.

Following alloplastic paranasal augmentation the nasal esthetics and balance with the remainder of the face will be improved, especially the alar base width.

B. On completion of the mandibular ramus osteotomies, placing the jaws in intermaxillary fixation and closing the mandibular surgical sites, the paranasal augmentation is done. The surgical approach is via a horizontal incision in the depth of the anterior maxillary vestibule made with a diathermy knife. The mucoperiosteum is elevated from the anterior and lateral walls of the maxilla, identifying and dissecting out the anterior nasal spine and inferior and lateral nasal rims (piriform apertures of the nose). The nasal mucoperiosteum is carefully mobilized from the piriform apertures of the nose bilaterally, extending posteriorly 5 to 10 mm so holes can be drilled through the piriform apertures and wires placed to stabilize the implants. Great care is taken not to tear the nasal mucoperiosteum during this part of the dissection to avoid nasal contamination with the implant. If a tear occurs during the dissection it must be repaired to prevent infection.

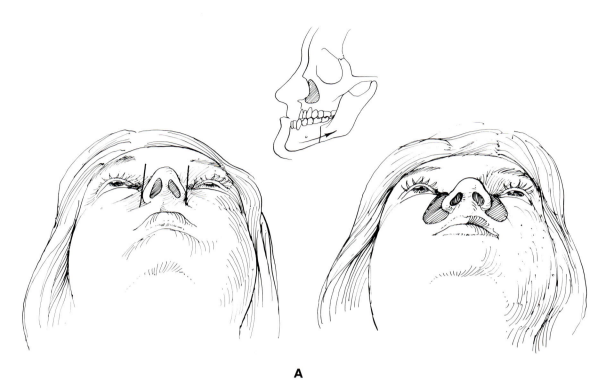

A

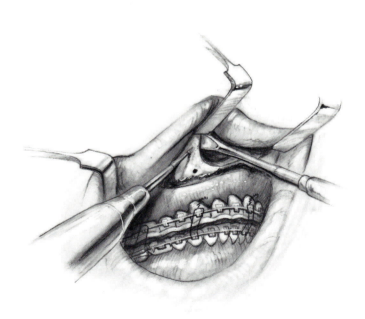

B

PARANASAL AUGMENTATION
Plate 11-1

C. The alloplast is contoured to the desired shape, usually pyramidal, being thickest at its base and tapered to the lateral and superior edges. The implant is inserted and secured to the lateral nasal rim with light-gauge wire. If a porous implant material is utilized it is liberally injected with an antibiotic after insertion just prior to closure.

    If onlay bone grafting is to be done the procedure is identical, and the onlay bone graft is appropriately shaped and secured to the lateral nasal rim. If simultaneous alveolar cleft grafting is being done, as described in detail in Chapter 10, the superior aspect of the alveolar graft is "overpacked" with additional bone layed along the lateral piriform rim to augment the recessive paranasal area.

    After final contouring of the paranasal implants, trial insertion is done, and the patient's face is viewed and palpated to visually and manually evaluate the esthetic result and symmetry.

D. Closure of the incision is done in routine fashion, and tape is placed over the upper lip to maintain pressure on the surgical site for 48 hours postoperatively.

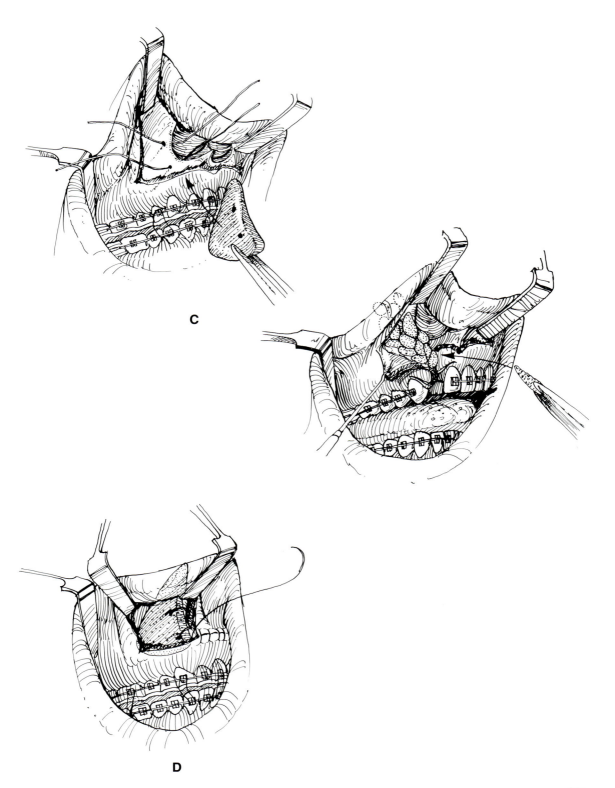

C

D

Malar augmentation

Malar deficiencies occur as unusual isolated idiopathic entities, secondary to ablative surgery, secondary to trauma, and in conjunction with many other severe midfacial abnormalities, such as hemifacial microsomia, craniofacial dysostoses, and Treacher Collins syndrome. Deficiencies in this area can result from osseous or soft-tissue deformities and can be unilateral or bilateral. In many of these conditions malar augmentation, either as the primary procedure done in conjunction with, for example, mandibular osteotomies or as a secondary procedure to the primary midface osteotomies, must be considered. Malar augmentation can provide functional improvement as the result of improved protection of the globe, improved lower eyelid function, and improved facial esthetics.

In malar augmentation both alloplasts and onlay bone-grafting procedures are used. We generally use onlay bone grafts for malar augmentation in cases of severe malar hypoplasia, performed simultaneously with LeFort III midface advancements, as in Crouzon's disease or Apert's syndrome. When secondary augmentation procedures are done we generally use alloplasts because of their simplicity and the predictability of results. The major drawback with the use of some alloplasts in malar augmentation is that a dark discoloration of the soft tissues overlying them occurs if they are placed too superficially or if the overlying tissues are thin.

The three basic approaches to malar augmentation are as follows:
1. Intraoral vestibular approach
2. Infraorbital approach (blepharoplasty)
3. Temporal flap approach

In this section these approaches are discussed and illustrated.

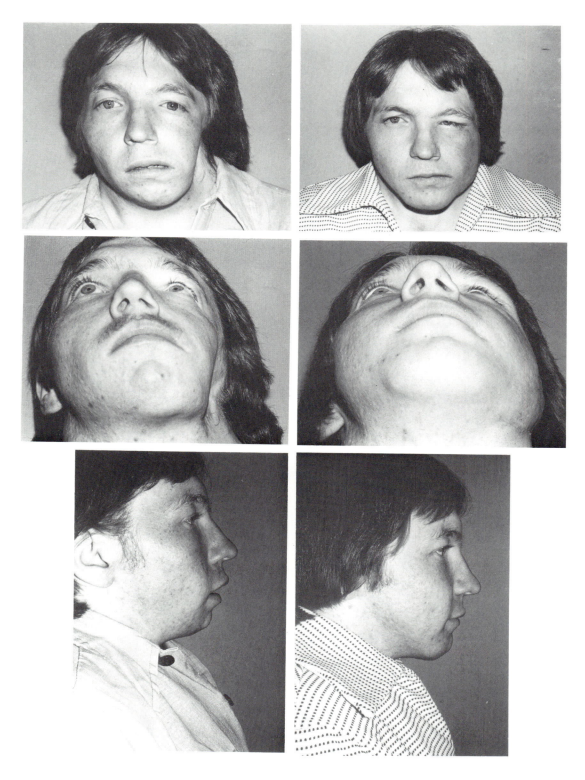

383

INTRAORAL VESTIBULAR APPROACH

Plate 11-2

A. The illustrated case exhibits a mild malar deficiency secondary to a previously untreated displaced malar fracture. No ocular muscle or eye dysfunction exists. The objective of orbitomalar augmentation is primarily to improve facial esthetics.

B. An intraoral incision is made with a diathermy knife in the depth of the maxillary vestibule extending from the midline posteriorly to the zygomaticoalveolar crest area. A subperiosteal dissection is carried superiorly to the inferior orbital rim with preservation of the infraorbital neurovascular bundle. The periosteum around the neurovascular bundle is released rather extensively to avoid undue stretching of it and to permit adequate space for insertion of the implant.

   The infraorbital neurovascular bundle can be freed by carefully incising the periosteum around it and bluntly dissecting the bundle out. The insertion of the septum orbitale is reflected from the orbital rim to provide additional soft-tissue relaxation and the necessary space for stabilization of the implant.

C. Incisions in the periosteum will improve mobility of the soft tissues, decrease soft-tissue tension on the implant, and provide improved surgical visibility. Further this permits relaxation so that the dissection can be carried up along the lateral orbital rim if desired and into the temporal fossa if these areas are indicated for augmentation.

   The infratemporal dissection is most simply done with scissors while palpating the area externally with the other hand.

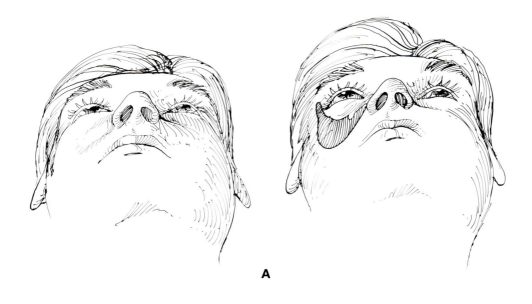

A

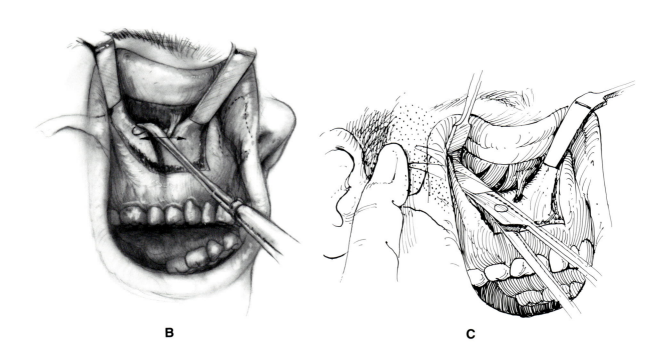

B

C

D. Interosseous holes are placed through the orbital rim and a fine-gauge wire passed through them to properly position and stabilize the implant.

E. Following completion of the soft-tissue dissection an implant is prepared for insertion. In this case the lateral orbital rim and portion of the temporal fossa are to be augmented as well as the malar eminence and infraorbital areas. One piece is prepared for the lateral orbital rim and temporal fossa area and another piece for the remainder of the malar eminence and infraorbital area. A notch is made in the latter implant to fit around the infraorbital nerve.

   The implants are temporarily placed in position to test for fit, and the patient's face is observed and palpated for symmetry of right and left sides. Any adjustments in the implant are made at this time.

F. The implant is positioned and the stabilizing wires secured. If a porous alloplast is utilized appropriate antibiotics are injected into the implant after final placement and the incision closed in two layers. A moderately tight pressure dressing is applied for 48 hours postoperatively.

   When the infraorbital rim is displaced inferiorly, it is important to place the implant so that it extends superiorly to the rim to provide proper lower-lid support and facial symmetry.

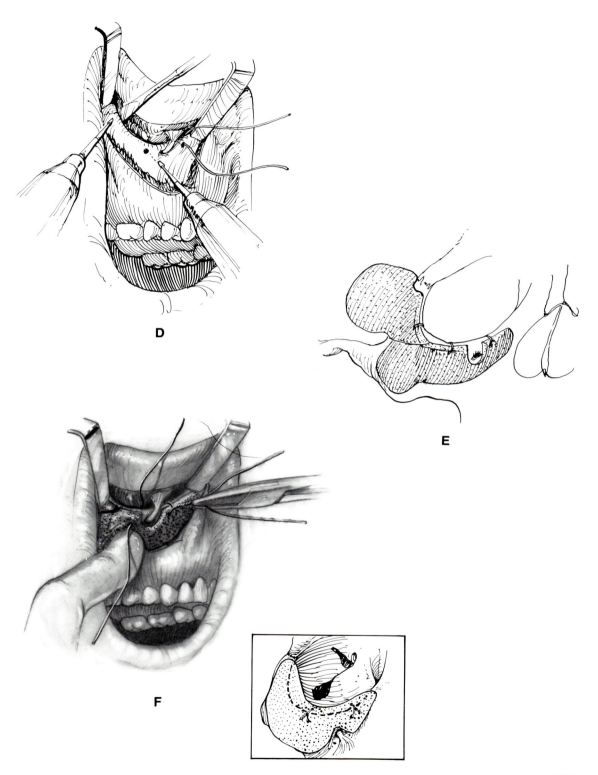

D

E

F

INFRAORBITAL APPROACH (BLEPHAROPLASTY)

Plate 11-3

A. A patient with severe malar deficiency secondary to previous ablative surgery is shown. The globe is protrusive, approximately 6 to 8 mm beyond the infraorbital rim (it is normally about even with the soft tissues overlying the inferior orbital rim). A temporary tarsorraphy is done to protect the globe. An external approach through a blepharoplasty-type incision is made approximately 2 to 3 mm below the lower-lid margin, beginning a few millimeters lateral to the inferior punctum. The natural skin folds are followed in making the incision. Laterally the incision is curved inferiorly at about the lateral canthal area.

B. The initial incision extends only through the skin and into the subcutaneous tissues. The skin and subcutaneous tissues are then undermined inferiorly, above the orbicularis oculi, to a point inferiorly so that the infraorbital rim can be palpated. Appropriate retractors are placed, and the incision is carried through the orbicularis oculi to the inferior orbital rim. Care must be taken when incising onto the inferior orbital rim to avoid cutting through the septum orbitale. This is avoided by appropriate placement of the superior retractor.

INFRAORBITAL APPROACH (BLEPHAROPLASTY)

Plate 11-3

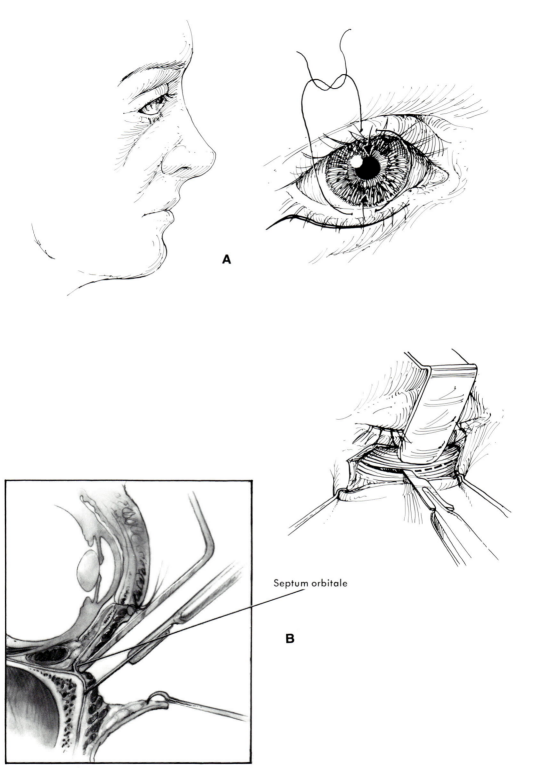

A

Septum orbitale

B

389

C. A subperiosteal dissection extends over the inferior orbital rim onto the orbital floor and down the anterior maxillary wall. Care is exercised to identify and protect the infraorbital neurovascular bundle. The neurovascular bundle is released and dissected out by carefully incising the periosteum around it and bluntly dissecting it out. Extension of the subperiosteal dissection through this incision readily exposes the entire infraorbital rim, malar bone, and lateral orbital rim.

D. The dissection is extended along the lateral orbital rim and can be carried into the temporal fossa if indicated. By making several releasing incisions in the periosteum, as the dissection ascends along the lateral orbital rim, good release of soft tissue is achieved, which facilitates soft-tissue retraction and implant placement.

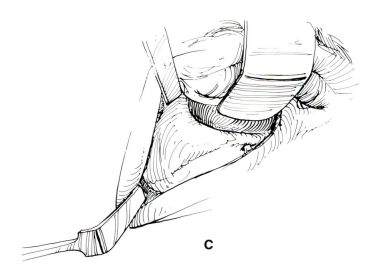

C

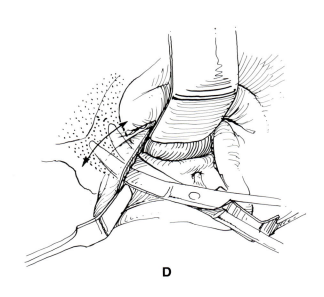

D

E. The implant is appropriately carved (usually in segments if the lateral orbital rim and temporal fossa areas are also to be augmented) and a trial insertion performed. If excessive soft-tissue tension exists during the try in, additional periosteal-releasing incisions are made.

   Interosseous holes through the lateral and inferior orbital rims are placed to secure the implants in place once they are properly shaped and positioned.

F. The implant is positioned and secured to the orbital rim with light-gauge wire. The area is thoroughly irrigated. If a porous implant is used appropriate antibiotics are injected directly into it prior to soft-tissue closure.

   The periosteal layer overlying the alloplast is closed, and then the skin layer is closed. No muscle sutures are placed. A light pressure dressing is applied for 48 hours, and skin sutures are removed in 4 to 5 days.

G. The improved facial appearance and better lower eyelid support are evident.

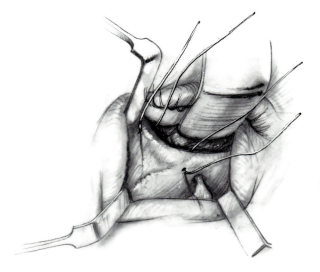

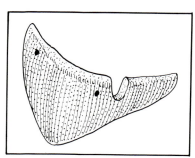

E

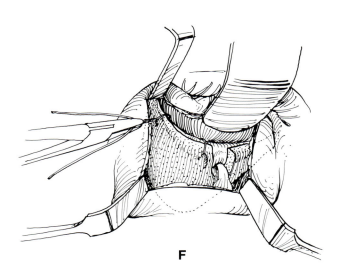

F

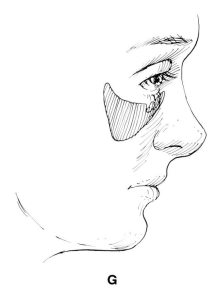

G

393

TEMPORAL FLAP APPROACH

Plate 11-4

A. The temporal flap approach is preferred when more extensive reconstruction of the malar-orbital-frontal area is indicated. Further this can be combined with inferior extension and dissection to afford access to the temporomandibular joint, zygomatic arch, infratemporal fossa, and parotid-masseteric region. Transtemporal extension provides possible access to the entire frontal bone and nasal-orbital-ethmoid areas, as discussed later in this chapter.

The illustrated case demonstrates the temporal approach for access to the right frontal bone, orbit, malar bone, and zygomatic arch.

B. After infiltration with local anesthetic with 1:200,000 epinephrine along the proposed incision line, an incision is made through the skin and subcutaneous tissue down to the periosteum. The incision margins are mobilized and Raney clamps placed for hemostasis. A supraperiosteal incision is begun and carried to the area of the insertion of the temporalis muscle. Here the dissection becomes superficial to the temporalis muscle. The temporal and zygomatic branches of the facial nerve are preserved in this flap. The dissection is carried inferiorly to the area of the zygomatic arch directly on the temporalis muscle. Anterior to the attachment of the temporalis muscle an incision is made through the periosteum to permit exposure of the orbit and malar bone subperiosteally.

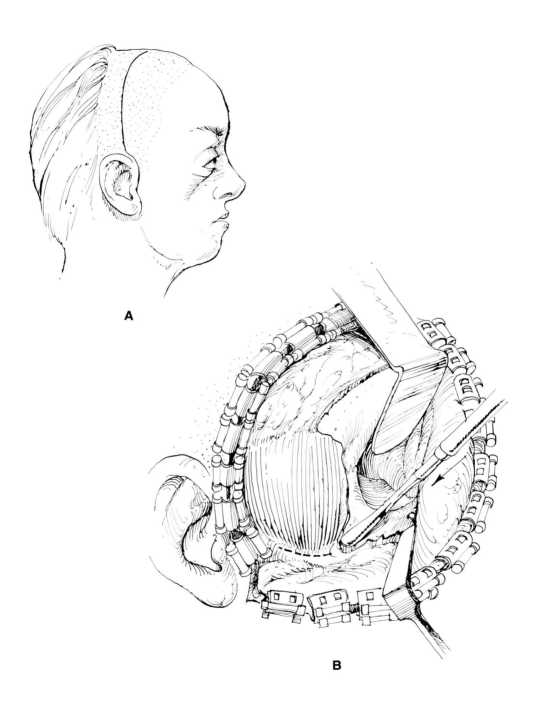

A

B

Plate 11-4

C. With appropriate relaxing incisions the entire superior, lateral, and infraorbital areas as well as the malar eminence are exposed. Appropriately shaped implants are fashioned from bone or an alloplast. In this instance it will constitute an implant that reconstructs the malar bone, infraorbital rim, lateral orbital rim, a portion of the supraorbital rim, and the missing zygomatic arch. The implant is repeatedly fashioned and tried until the fit and desired facial results are achieved. It is then wired in place and the area irrigated with copious amounts of sterile saline solution.

Closure is two layered, and an eye patch and pressure dressing are applied for 48 hours.

D. The improved facial appearance is evident.

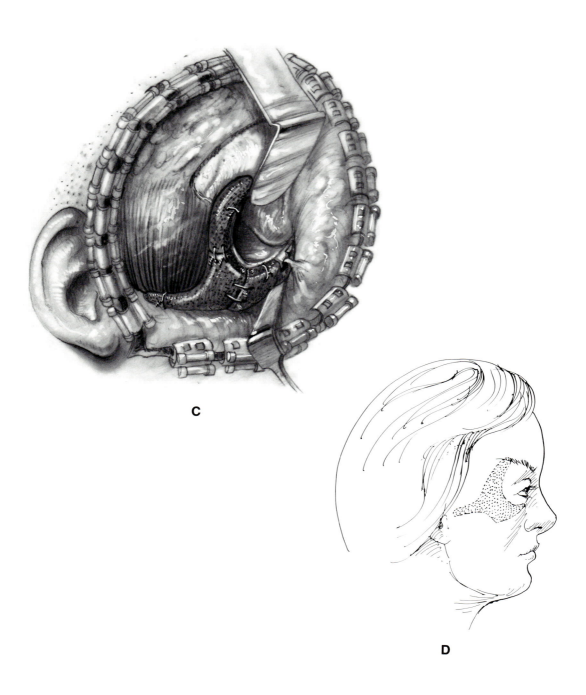

C

D

Nasal augmentation

Nasal deficiencies exist frequently in conjunction with other dentofacial and craniofacial deformities. Anatomically when the nasal bones are hypoplastic with poor anterior and inferior projection, the deformity gives the illusion of an increased intercanthal distance in the frontal view, and in profile the nose has a "skijump" or saddle-nose appearance. Occasionally prominent epicanthal folds are present. Dorsonasal augmentation (1) decreases the relative intraorbital distance, (2) increases the dorsonasal projection, and (3) decreases the nasal tip elevation.

Various techniques have been described and materials recommended for dorsonasal augmentation. Each material, including alloplast, cartilage, and bone, has advantages and disadvantages. Generally we prefer alloplast or cartilage for augmentation of the nasal dorsum. They provide a good, predictable aesthetic result, yet allow normal plasticity of the nose.

Two basic surgical approaches for dorsonasal augmentation that we use are the midcolumellar approach and the intranasal approach. When nasal augmentation is done in conjunction with midfacial or frontal procedures, access to the nose is achieved via a frontal flap or incisions in the glabellar area, because these incisions are already indicated to complete the midface surgery. In this section only the midcolumellar and intranasal approaches are discussed. Dorsonasal augmentation in concert with midface osteotomies via the coronal flap is included in Chapter 12.

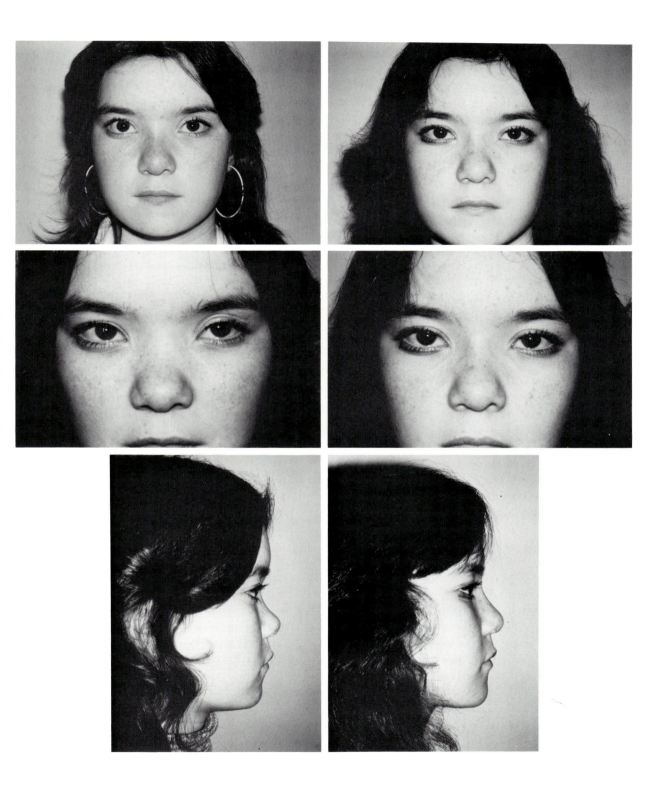

MIDCOLUMELLAR APPROACH

Plate 11-5

A. The illustrated case demonstrates a saddle-nose deformity and bimaxillary protusion. Glabella is retrusive relative to the forehead, and the nasal dorsum is poorly projected. Frontally the nasal dorsum appears flat, creating the illusion that the face is excessively wide in the intercanthal area, although the intercanthal distance is normal. Dorsonasal augmentation will be performed in concert with anterior maxillary and mandibular ostectomies to correct the bimaxillary protrusion.

B. A midcolumellar incision is made after infiltration with local anesthetic and 1:200,000 epinephrine into the columella, nasal dome, and over the dome of the nose. The incision stops short of the nasal tip and is made through the skin and subcutaneous tissues.

C. Iridectomy scissors are used to dissect posteriorly to the cartilaginous nasal septum. Superiorly the dissection is carried between the domes of the alar cartilages. The dissection is then directed superficial to the lateral cartilages onto the dorsal aspect of the nasal bones. A subperiosteal dissection is then carried superiorly over the nasal bone, laterally toward the medial orbital rims, and superiorly onto the glabellar region to provide adequate mobilization of the soft tissues for insertion of the implant. During this dissection care is exercised not to enter the nasal cavity as as to avoid postoperative nasal communication with the implant and probable infection.

MIDCOLUMELLAR APPROACH
Plate 11-5

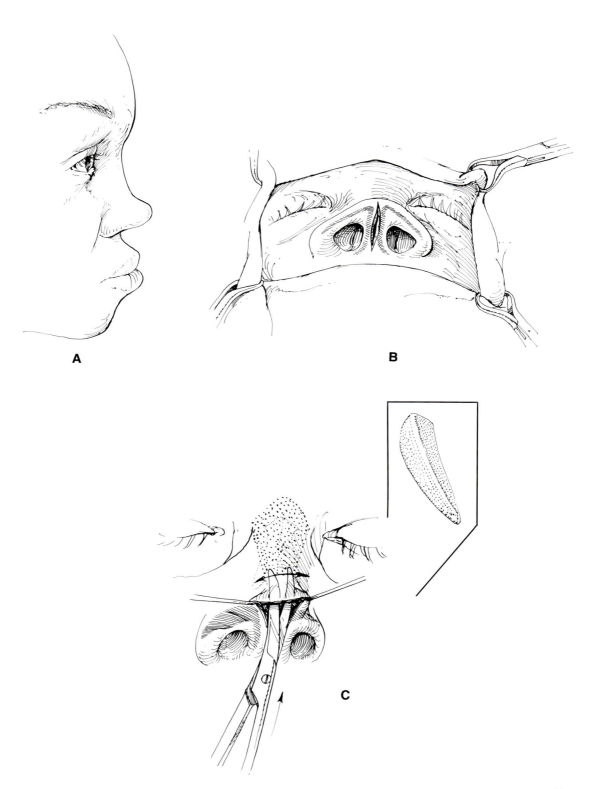

A

B

C

Plate 11-5

D. If the dorsal nasal soft tissues are thin, as they are in most lightskinned patients, the colors of the alloplast must be neutral or it will show through the soft tissues.

   The length of the implant is determined by measuring from the nasofrontal junction to the alar domes. The implant is carved in a pyramidal fashion and slightly hollowed on the undersurface.

E. The implant is inserted in position and the area irrigated with copious amounts of sterile saline solution. If cartilage is used the incision line is sutured at this time; if a porous implant is used it is injected with antibiotics prior to closure.

F. The columellar incision is closed in two layers and a tape pressure dressing applied directly over the implant to minimize edema and hematoma formation and to stabilize the implant. The dressing should be maintained for at least 48 hours.

   The postoperative result reveals improvement in the profile secondary to improved nasal balance as well as chin-lip-nose balance.

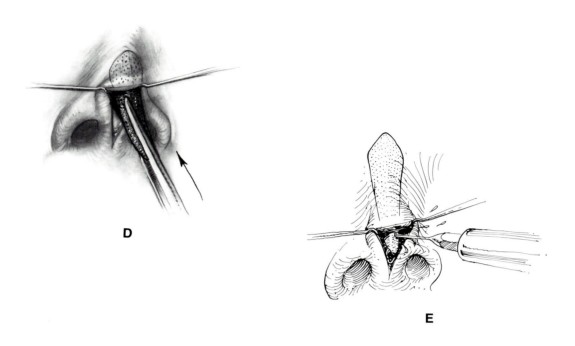

D

E

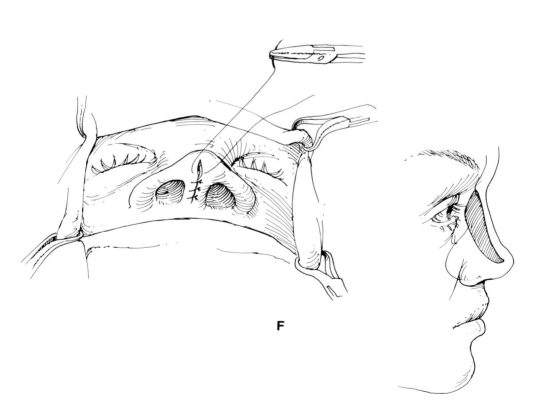

F

INTRANASAL APPROACH

Plate 11-6

A. An intranasal vestibular approach can also be used to augment the nasal dorsum. In one nares an incision is made intranasally anterior to the alar cartilage, beginning at the base of the columella and extending circumferentially halfway around the vestibule.

B. Iridectomy scissors are used to dissect anterior to the alar cartilage, then directed posteriorly between the medial cruz of the alar cartilages and the cartilaginous nasal septum. The dissection is then directed over the lateral cartilages onto the nasal bones to the glabellar area and laterally toward the medial orbital rims.

C. After shaping and placement of the implant the area is irrigated and the incision carefully sutured to prevent leakage of nasal fluids into the surgical site. A pressure dressing is applied as described in Plate 11-5, *F*.

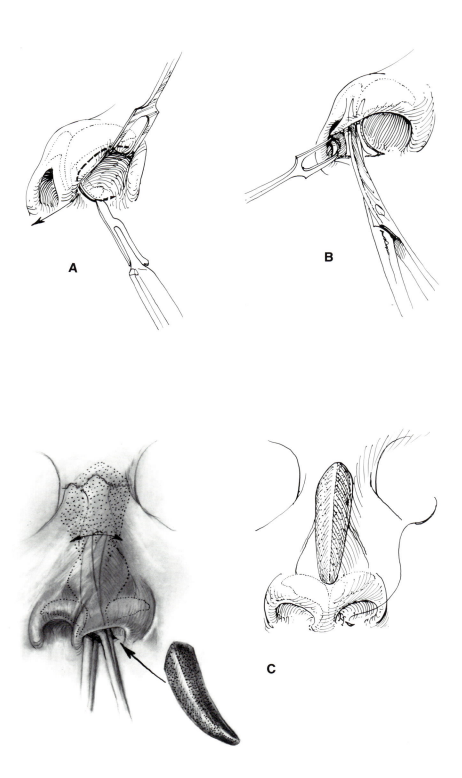

Frontal bone augmentation

Early skeletal release in the infant with craniofacial dysostosis for prevention of frontal and facial bone deformities has been suggested. However, evidence does not exist that this approach is effective in achieving these objectives, because by age 5 years the skull is approximately 90% of its adult dimensions. In the adolescent or adult with frontal bone and supraorbital rim hypoplasia or retrusion the decision must be made as to whether advancement of the frontal bone or augmentation of this area will be done. The latter approach, preferred by us in most instances, is discussed and illustrated in this section.

The choice of materials for frontal augmentation is among autografts, allografts, and alloplasts. On occasion we have used each of these for frontal bone augmentation. During the past 2 years we have primarily utilized alloplasts, because they cause little patient morbidity, can be more readily shaped with improved contour over bone grafts, and appear to be more stable. The specific material may be either a self-curing methylmethacrylate, which can be preformed from a facial moulage and added to at surgery to improve contours and smooth edges, or an implant that can be readily shaped at surgery, such as Proplast.

Finally the timing of frontal bone augmentation must be considered with respect to age of the patient and additional planned or possible craniofacial reconstructive procedures. One approach has been to complete the LeFort II or III midface osteotomies and secondarily perform the augmentation. This is done to reduce the possibility of infection when they are done simultaneously and to optimize the final esthetic result. The other alternative is to simultaneously complete the LeFort III midface advancement and frontal bone augmentation surgery.

Our preferred surgical approach for frontal bone augmentation is described and illustrated.

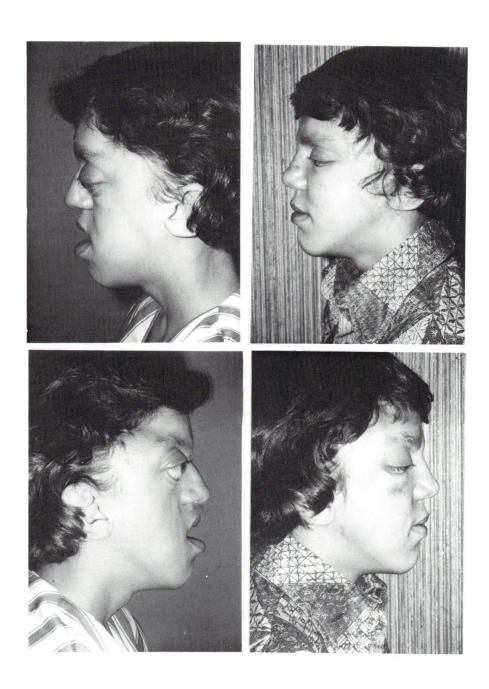

407

FRONTAL BONE AUGMENTATION

Plate 11-7

A. The illustrated case demonstrates craniofacial dysostosis of Crouzon's disease in a 15-year-old girl who is to undergo a LeFort III midface advancement and simultaneous alloplastic augmentation of the frontal bone. Only the frontal augmentation is discussed here. The LeFort III lateral orbital rim cuts extend high (as illustrated in Chapter 12) to produce the desired lateral orbital rim projection and make it essential to augment only the frontal bone–supraorbital rim areas.

   A local anesthetic with a vasoconstrictor is injected along the proposed incision line and the area is irrigated with large amounts of sterile saline solution.

B. A bicoronal flap is raised by making an incision several inches posterior to the hairline from just above the anterior aspect of one ear, transcoronally to the same location on the opposite side. The initial incision is made down to but not through the pericranium. Both edges of tissue from the initial incision are mobilized and clamped with Raney clips for hemostasis.

   This flap is raised supraperiosteally about two thirds of the way to the supraorbital rims. At this point the periosteum is incised and the remainder of the elevation of the bicoronal flap to the orbital, nasal, and ethmoid areas is raised subperiosteally.

C. The supraorbital nerves are dissected out and the bone beneath them removed so they can be preserved as the dissection is carried into the orbits.

   The LeFort III midface advancement is completed in its entirety with all superior osteotomy cuts achieved via the bicoronal flap. Subconjunctional incisions can be added if medial orbital floor exposure is limited.

   The grafts are all wired into place, the mouth secured in intermaxillary fixation, all oral incisions closed, the entire area of the bicoronal flap irrigated with copious amount of sterile saline solution, and the drapes changed in preparation for the frontal bone augmentation.

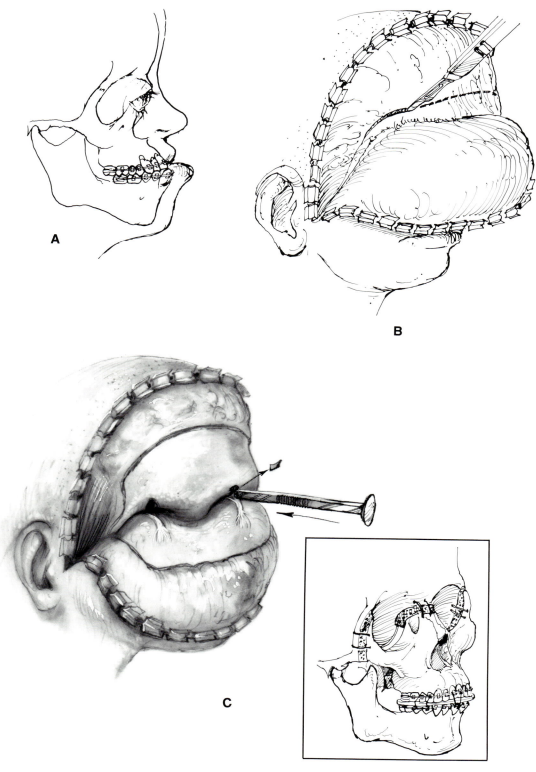

A

B

C

FRONTAL BONE AUGMENTATION

Plate 11-7

D. The absolute amount of supraorbital rim augmentation is such that it will result in projection of the supraorbital rims about 6 to 10 mm anteriorly to the most anterior projection of the globes. The existing relationship between the globes and the supraorbital rims is determined preoperatively by direct measurement.

E. The implant is shaped, added to, or primarily molded, depending on the material being used, so that it is tapered smoothly superiorly and is more concave directly over the bridge of the nose.

   After completion of contouring of the implant holes are drilled through the supraorbital rims to ensure precise placement of the implant and stabilization of it via direct wiring. The implant is then wired in place and the bicoronal flap repositioned temporarily to visualize and palpate it.

   Because the size of the implant is generally considerable, it is usually impossible to reapproximate the edges of the bicoronal flap without relaxation incisions. This is achieved by making multiple transverse incisions through the periosteum in the inferior aspect of the flap after posteriorly undermining the superior aspect of the flap.

F. If bone is to be used we prefer a combined allogenic-autogenous bone graft, because it results in less patient morbidity, appears to undergo less resorptive loss, and heals readily. It is wired in place similarly to an implant. Ideally allogenic cortical onlay grafts are supplemented with autogenous cancellous bone to provide smooth contours and promote rapid osteogenesis.

G. At this time the entire operative field is irrigated with a triple-antibiotic solution and the incision line closed. A large pressure dressing is applied and left in place for 48 hours to prevent hematoma formation and edema.

   The changes in profile relationships of the facial structures with the combined LeFort III midface advancement and frontal bone augmentation are illustrated.

Plate 11-7

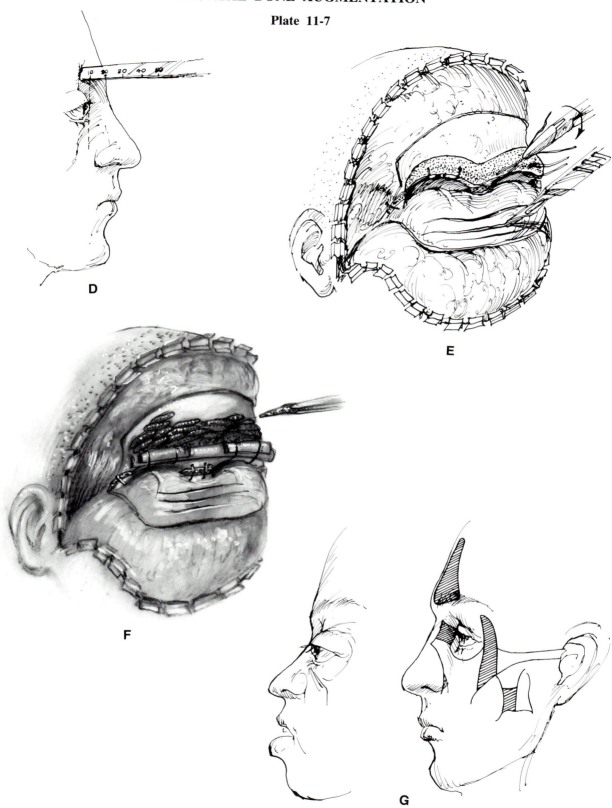

D

E

F

G

CHAPTER 12

Midface osteotomies

Numerous congenital, developmental, and acquired deformities are best treated by a middle third face osteotomy. In the previous chapters the various osteotomies to reposition the maxilla superiorly, posteriorly, anteriorly, and inferiorly and our preferred procedures for augmenting the middle third face structures are described and illustrated. In this chapter extracranial osteotomies for advancing various portions of the middle third face, exclusive of the maxilla, are described and illustrated. Craniofacial procedures such as those utilized for the correction of ocular hypertelorism, which require a combined intracranial-facial approach, are not discussed in this text.

Many middle third face deformities present unique problems with multiple coexisting anomalies of the entire midfacial region. Those engaged in the habilitation of individuals with middle third facial deformities, especially those of congenital origin, must be cognizant that unique ophthalmologic, otolaryngologic, neurologic, dental, speech, and psychological problems coexist with many of these conditions. Moreover, multiple surgical procedures, either per-

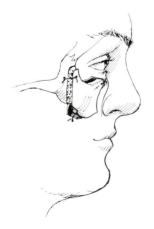

**MALAR BONE
ADVANCEMENT**

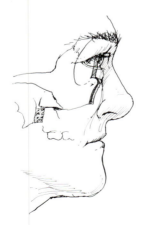

LeFORT II

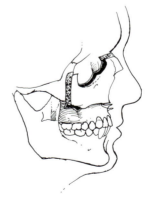

**MODIFIED LeFORT III
(NASOMALAR)**

formed simultaneously or staged, are frequently necessary to achieve optimal treatment results.

A detailed systematic evaluation of facial esthetics in individuals with middle third face deformities is essential to accurately and precisely define the deformity and to plan treatment. This is especially true in deformities of the middle third face because the three-dimensional interrelations of the forehead, nose, globes, infraorbital, malar, and paranasal regions cannot be adequately evaluated by cephalometric examination. Further, *most individuals with middle third facial deformities do not possess stereotyped deformities,* and therefore *the use of ''standard'' operations to correct apparently similar deformities will result in less than optimal results.* In this regard there is often indication for one of the basic middle third face operative procedures described in this chapter, in concert with middle third face augmentation or a mandibular procedure as described in previous chapters.

The development and refinement of middle third face advancement, as described here, has occurred during the last decade. Today it is commonplace that in experienced hands these procedures are performed with good predictability and little patient morbidity. However, in less experienced hands the procedures can have serious and even life-threatening sequelae. Moreover, the relatively small number of cases indicated for these procedures speaks to the issue that they are by and large best performed by individuals with maximum experience.

In this chapter the following techniques are discussed and illustrated: malar bone advancement, LeFort II midfacial advancement, LeFort III midfacial advancement (nasomalar), LeFort III midfacial advancement (malar-maxillary) and LeFort III midfacial advancement.

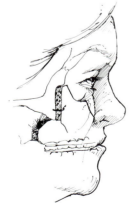

MODIFIED LeFORT III (MALAR-MAXILLARY)

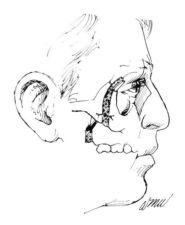

LeFORT III

Malar bone advancement

Malar bone advancement may be indicated in selected cases. When the cheek prominence and inferior orbital rim are hypoplastic, inferiorly located, or retrusive, either unilaterally or bilaterally, the decision must be made as to whether to augment this area or perform malar bone advancement. Augmentation of the malar bone is discussed in Chapter 11.

As with most middle third face deformities, the primary diagnostic criterion for consideration of malar bone advancement is the clinical esthetic evaluation. With regard to considerations for malar bone advancement, two general aspects of this evaluation are important: the globe is used as the stable referent, and the position of the malar bone is not absolute but must be evaluated relatively to the other external facial structures.

In the frontal view with the patient looking straight ahead, normally the lower eyelid touches or slightly covers the inferior limbus of the iris. With malar deficiency or inferiorly positioned infraorbital rim, generally the sclera is exposed to various degrees, between the lower eyelid and limbus. In a normal profile the anteriormost projection of the globe is tangent to or positioned anteriorly to the same extent as the soft tissues overlying the inferior orbital rim. A helpful method for evaluating the interrelationship of the globe to the inferior orbital rim is to examine the patient from the lateral aspect with the clinical Frankfort plane relatively parallel to the floor. When doing so, a line perpendicular to the Frankfort plane will be tangent to the most protrusive aspect of the globe and the soft tissue overlying the inferior orbital rim (± 2 mm). If the rim is more than 5 mm retrusive to this line, malar bone advancement is considered.

When malar deficiency is suspected, the relative profile relationships of the other facial structures must be carefully evaluated. If the chin and nose are relatively prominent, there may be the illusion of malar deficiency when in fact the malar bone is in normal position and the chin and nose are deformed. A careful clinical assessment must be made, because occasionally when the malar bone is advanced in this type of case the eyes may appear enophthalmic, or sunken. On the other hand, if the other external facial features are somewhat weak a slightly retropositioned or hypoplastic malar bone may be in relatively good balance with the other facial features despite its absolute retrusiveness.

Generally augmentation is preferred in the isolated malar bone deformity for several reasons. In congenital deformities the hypoplasia, aplasia, and various anatomic abnormalities (for example, those that exist in Treacher-Collins syndrome) make malar advancement technically very difficult, if not impossible, in most instances. Further, bone grafting is always necessary with advancement, and therefore morbidity accompanies the procedures. Finally, it is generally technically easier to perform more precise surgery with augmentation, thus achieving a superior esthetic and functional result with less extensive surgery.

In selected instances in which the malar bone is not severely hypoplastic or congenitally deformed, malar bone advancement may be indicated. Further, this procedure may be performed in selected instances when this area is deformed secondary to fracture displacement. Although theoretically a bicoronal flap can be used to achieve access for performing malar bone advancement, we believe it provides no benefit, because the blepharoplasty and subciliary incisions leave no visible scar. A subconjunctival incision does not afford the needed access for this surgery, and this is also the case if the surgery is attempted with only an intraoral approach.

The technique we have utilized for malar bone advancement is discussed and illustrated on the following pages.

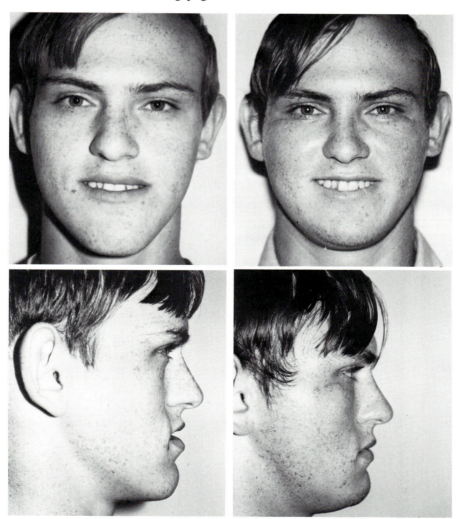

MALAR BONE ADVANCEMENT

Plate 12-1

A. In the illustrated case there is bilateral malar deficiency in a patient with a prominent nose and relatively strong chin. The malar prominence and inferior orbital rim are positioned 7 mm posterior to the anteriormost aspect of the globe. There is no asymmetry in the midfacial region.

   Frontally several millimeters of sclera are exposed beneath the inferior limbus of the iris and the lower eyelid when the patient looks straight ahead.

   In performing unilateral malar bone advancement the objective is to establish symmetry and balance with the normal side. In bilateral malar bone advancement meticulous care must be exercised to maintain the existing facial symmetry. Therefore the patient is draped at surgery with full exposure of the entire upper and middle third face bilaterally, with the oral endotracheal tube exiting inferiorly over the chin.

B. Tarsorrhaphy sutures are placed, and *bilateral subciliary incision lines are marked so that they are symmetric*. For this surgery these incisions extend slightly beyond the lateral canthus area to provide improved access to the inferior orbital rim, floor of the orbit, lateral orbital rim, and malar eminence. The subciliary incision is made through the skin, and the skin and subcutaneous tissues undermined inferiorly above the orbicularis oculi muscle to the level of the inferior orbital rim. With the periorbita and globe retracted superiorly an incision is made through the orbicularis oculi muscle and periosteum on the anterior aspect of the inferior orbital rim as described in greater detail in Chapter 11. The periorbita is reflected from the inferior orbital rim and floor, exposing the lacrimal fossa medially, the inferior orbital fissure posteriorly, and Whitnall's tubercle of the lateral orbital rim.

   The infraorbital neurovascular bundle is identified and partially dissected out to allow the malar bone to be advanced without causing undue tension on the bundle. The dissection is then extended subperiosteally down the lateral aspect of the malar eminence and posterior to the zygomatic buttress while maintaining as much soft-tissue attachment to the malar bone as possible so as to provide adequate vascular supply to the segment after it is mobilized.

416

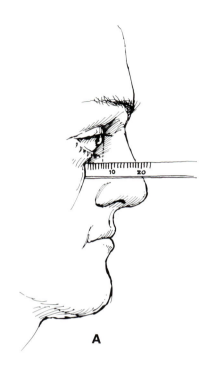

A

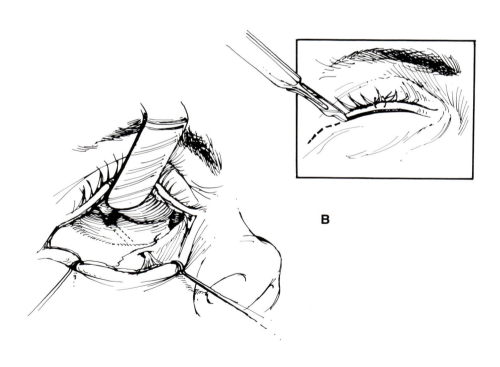

B

MALAR BONE ADVANCEMENT

Plate 12-1

C. Medially the dissection is carried inferiorly toward the nasal piriform aperture. The osteotomy is begun through the medial aspect of the inferior orbital rim just lateral to the lacrimal fossa. This osteotomy is extended inferiorly toward the piriform rim area but approximately 5 to 10 mm lateral to it. This portion of the osteotomy communicates with the maxillary sinus.

D. The osteotomy is then extended posteriorly into the orbital floor, approximately 5 to 10 mm posterior to the inferior orbital rim. A horizontal osteotomy across the orbital floor is completed into the maxillary sinus. The infraorbital neurovascular bundle can usually be identified within its bony canal in the orbital floor through the thin bone overlying it as it transverses anteromedially from the inferior orbital fissure to its exiting foramen. In the area of the infraorbital neurovascular bundle the osteotomy need not be done, as the bone overlying it is very thin and will fracture readily when the malar bone is mobilized.

    The osteotomy is extended laterally and carried superiorly up the lateral orbital wall. This portion of the osteotomy communicates with the temporal fossa. Depending on how much of the lateral orbital rim is indicated for advancement, this cut will be carried to an appropriate level superiorly. Usually it is not necessary to extend this osteotomy above the level of the lateral canthal tendon for malar bone advancement.

E. At its superiormost extent the osteotomy is carried about halfway through the lateral orbital rim and is then directed inferiorly and carried through the posterior aspect of the malar eminence, communicating with the temporal fossa. The area is thoroughly irrigated and suctioned and a moist pack placed.

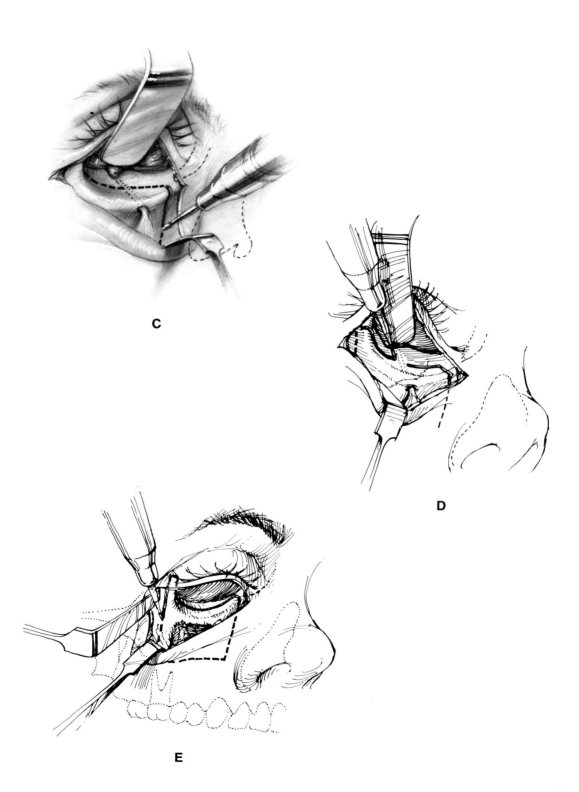

C

D

E

MALAR BONE ADVANCEMENT

Plate 12-1

F. Intraorally a horizontal vestibular incision is made in the depth of the buccal vestibule. The mucoperiosteum is reflected superiorly, anteriorly, and posteriorly only as necessary to expose the inferiormost aspects of the previous osteotomies. This dissection is kept to a minimum in order to maintain as much soft-tissue attachment to the malar segment as possible. A horizontal osteotomy is performed 4 to 5 mm above the apices of the teeth, extending from the inferior component of the vertical anterior osteotomy posteriorly just distal to the zygomatic buttress.

G. To complete the osteotomies a vertical osteotomy is performed with a curved osteotome, extending superiorly from the posterior extent of the horizontal osteotomy superiorly toward the inferior orbital fissure. This cut need not be completed the entire way up to the fissure because some residual bone in this area will readily fracture on mobilization.

All osteotomies are checked for completion with an osteotome.

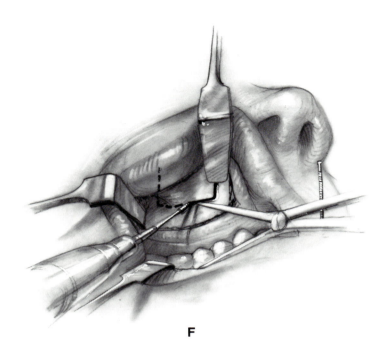

F

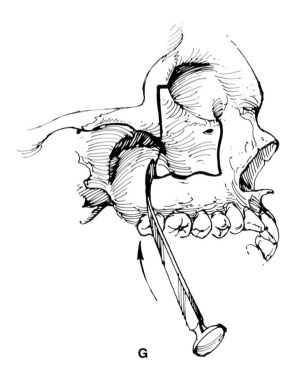

G

MALAR BONE ADVANCEMENT
Plate 12-1

H. Utilizing a Carroll-Girard screw, the malar bone is mobilized and advanced. Placing an osteotome for leverage in the vertical osteotomy of the lateral orbital wall will facilitate mobilization. The segment must be sufficiently mobilized so that it can be held passively in its new position. When the deformity exists bilaterally, the same procedure is performed in an *identical manner* on the other side so that facial symmetry and balance can be maintained.

I. Cortical-cancellous block bone grafts are inserted to provide stability for the advanced segment. *To maintain facial symmetry the osteotomies on the right and left sides as well as the bone grafts must be identical.* The primary stabilizing graft is that placed in the lateral orbital rim area. This graft is secured with two mattress wires. A bone graft is also placed at the medial aspect of the inferior orbital rim to support the projection in that area and is secured with wire. Finally a bone graft is placed and wired interorally at the zygomatic buttress area.

J. The infraorbital area is thoroughly irrigated and suctioned and the incision sutured in a routine fashion, with a deep layer and then closing the overlying skin. It is not necessary to suture the muscle layers of the orbicularis oculi muscle.

   The maxillary sinus is irrigated and suctioned and the intraoral incision closed with a running horizontal mattress suture.

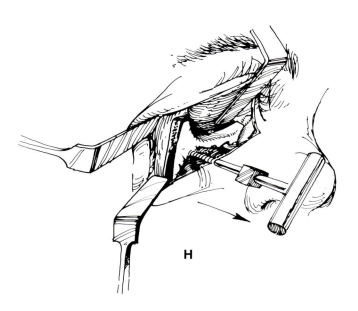

H

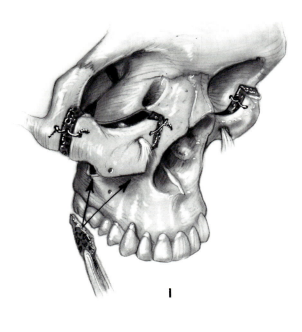

I

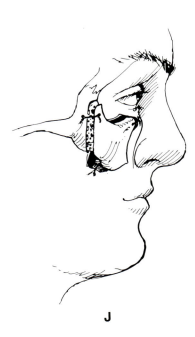

J

LeFort II midfacial advancement

The LeFort II midfacial osteotomies and advancement must be considered in instances when the patient assessment reveals that the nasomaxillary complex is retropositioned, the nose is short, and there is a class III malocclusion. In addition, in unusual instances of nasomaxillary hypoplasia (as in Binder's syndrome), these clinical features exist, but a class I occlusion is generally present.

When these clinical conditions exist the decision as to the preferred operative approach must be carefully evaluated on the basis not only of the existing esthetic and functional deformity but of alternatives such as a high LeFort I advancement and dorsonasal augmentation. If nasal symmetry exists and either asymmetric maxillary advancement or segmentalization of the maxilla is indicated, the latter must be seriously considered as an alternative. Similarly, if the nose is grossly assymetric dorsonasal augmentation must be considered. Cephalometric analysis and dental study model analysis are of little benefit in determining the existing deformity when nasomaxillary deficiency is present. Because nasion is retruded, as is the maxilla, SNA may be normal and SNB excessively large, misleading the surgeon into thinking that mandibular prognathism is present when in fact the deformity exists in the midfacial structures.

When the LeFort II midfacial advancement is to be done, both anteroposterior and vertical (that is, inferior repositioning) movements of the complex must be carefully planned and performed to achieve the desired results. For example, in some cleft patients it may be highly desirable to achieve a major vertical correction (lengthening of the nasomaxillary complex). When this movement is effected the nasal dorsum is usually minimally advanced, whereas the nose and maxilla are lengthened with inferior repositioning of the nasomaxillary complex. The inferior repositioning of the complex autorotates the mandible downward and backward, correcting much of the existing class III malocclusion, therefore requiring minimal anterior repositioning of the nasomaxillary complex. The amount of inferior repositioning indicated for the nasomaxillary complex is dependent on the upper-tooth-to-lip relationship.

There are two basic approaches utilized to gain access to the nasomaxillary complex when performing a LeFort II midfacial advancement: the bicoronal flap and paranasal skin incisions. Because the bicoronal flap is described and illustrated in detail in Chapter 11 and again in the subsequent section on LeFort III midface advancement, the paranasal incision approach is described here.

We generally make the nasoorbital osteotomies posterior to the medial canthal tendons; however, these can be done anteriorly as well (as described in the section on the LeFort III midface advancement). Making these cuts posterior to the medial canthal area decreases potential problems with the lacrimal apparatus, maintains good structure of the lacrimal lakes, and provides a larger bony mass to be advanced.

In this section the basic operative approach we have utilized for the LeFort II midfacial advancement is described and illustrated.

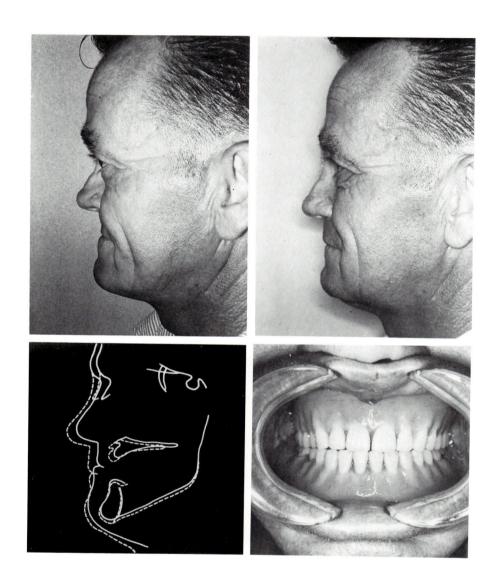

LeFORT II MIDFACIAL ADVANCEMENT

Plate 12-2

A. The illustrated case demonstrates retrusion of the nasomaxillary complex. The dorsum of the nose is poorly projected relative to the globes, the paranasal areas are recessive, and the upper lip is retrusive. The cheeks have good projection relative to the globes. Although the chin appears strong relative to the nose and upper lip, it is assessed to be in normal relationship to the cheeks and forehead.

B. Either of the paranasal incisions illustrated can be used to gain exposure to the entire nasofrontal area. In younger patients the separate bilateral incisions are perhaps more cosmetic, whereas in older patients the natural transverse skin crease in the region of the nasal dorsum is used to connect the two paranasal incisions without additional scar formation.

   Tomographic assessment of the anterior cranial base is essential when performing this procedure and may dictate the level at which the horizontal osteotomy in the glabellar area is to be made. The cribriform plate and anterior cranial fossa may invaginate into the ethmoid areas; however, the anterior cranial base is generally in a relatively normal position in most cases in which a LeFort II midfacial advancement is to be done.

   In some instances the osteotomies are carried anterior and in others posterior to the nasolacrimal sac and medial canthal tendons. When the osteotomies are to be done posterior to the lacrimal fossa the medial canthal tendons can be detached or left intact with apparently little difference in ultimate esthetics. This is discussed in more detail in the subsequent sections on LeFort III midfacial advancement; suffice it here to state that when the major portion of the periorbita is left intact, as it is with the LeFort II approached from the paranasal incisions, the detachment of the medial canthal tendons seems of little consequence with regard to postoperative unfavorable changes in the anatomy in this area. Therefore the soft-tissue dissection illustrated here involves detachment of the medial canthal tendons, exposure of the lacrimal fossa and sac, and performing the osteotomy posterior to the lacrimal sac.

C. The horizontal glabellar osteotomy is generally completed just below the nasofrontal suture. The osteotomy is continued posteriorly into the ethmoid bone and then directed inferiorly, posterior to the lacrimal fossa and sac. The retraction is then done in the orbital floor, and the osteotomy is continued from its inferior aspect anteriorly, completing it through the inferior orbital rim onto the anterior maxillary wall. This same cut is completed on the opposite side.

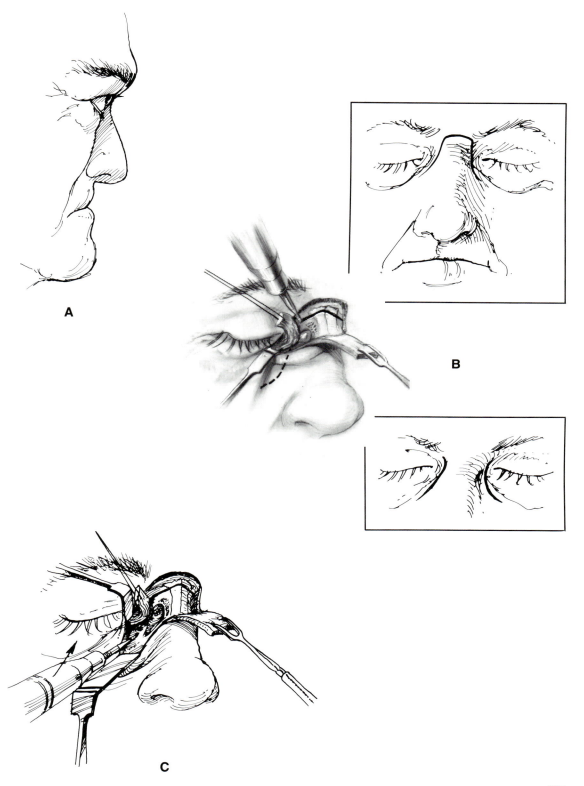

A

B

C

D. The remainder of the osteotomies are completed from an intraoral approach. A circumvestibular incision is made to expose the anterior and lateral maxillary walls. This dissection is extended subperiosteally superiorly until the osteotomy on the anterior maxillary wall is exposed. This osteotomy is then continued downward and backward to the pterygoid plates, staying at least 5 mm above the apices of the maxillary teeth.

E. The pterygomaxillary suture is sectioned with a small curved osteotome as previously described in detail in Chapter 9. Attention is then turned to the horizontal glabellar osteotomy, and an osteotomy through the perpendicular plate of the ethmoid bone and vomer is completed. This cut is made on about a line from the glabellar cut to the posterior maxillary spine.

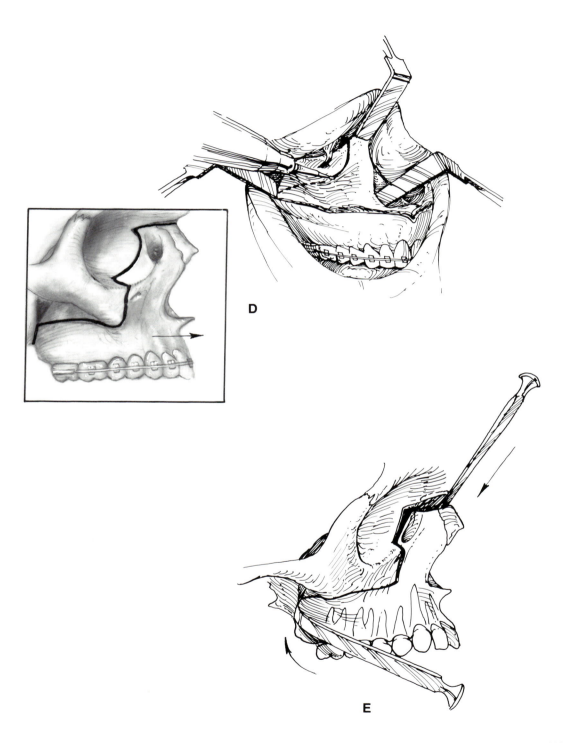

D

E

LeFORT II MIDFACIAL ADVANCEMENT

Plate 12-2

F. Mobilization forceps are utilized to loosen the entire nasomaxillary complex. The initial movement with the mobilization forceps is in an inferior direction. The nasal frontal area is observed closely during the initial phase of mobilization to be certain that the nasomaxillary complex is being mobilized as a single unit. Mobilization is continued until the nasomaxillary complex can be passively placed in the predetermined position. An osteotome can be inserted in the glabellar osteotomy to help lever and mobilize the complex.

G. The teeth are placed in the prefabricated occlusal splint, which overcorrects the occlusion a few millimeters. Intermaxillary fixation is applied, and the nasomaxillary complex is stabilized vertically with infraorbital suspension wiring. Autogenous blocks of cortical-cancellous bone are inserted in the nasofrontal area and wired into position. Cortical-cancellous block grafts are also placed in the pterygomaxillary areas bilaterally, as well as cancellous strips along the lateral maxillary wall and anterior maxillary wall osseous defects. The cancellous bone grafts promote more rapid osseous union of the LeFort II complex.

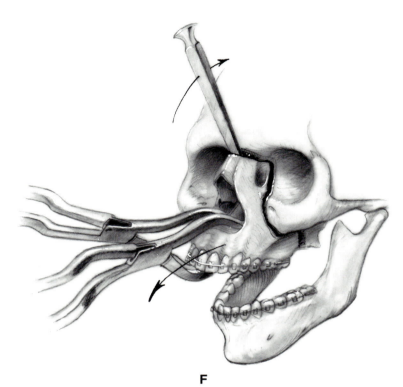

F

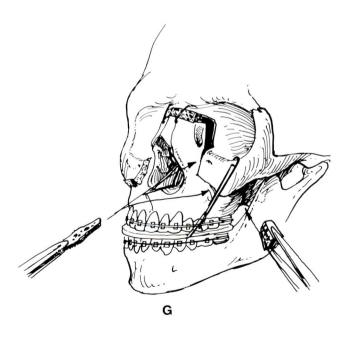

G

LeFORT II MIDFACIAL ADVANCEMENT

Plate 12-2

H. In many cases it may be desirable to lengthen the nasomaxillary complex. This enables the nose to be lengthened surgically and also effects a backward rotation of the mandible, thereby reducing the magnitude of the forward movement of the nasomaxillary complex. In cases where the nasomaxillary complex is primarily being vertically lengthened, bone grafts are necessary in the nasofrontal area and the lateral maxillary area to provide stability. If the nasomaxillary complex is not advanced, grafts are not necessary in the pterygomaxillary suture area.

I. The medial canthal tendons are reattached by placing a nonabsorbable suture, preferably a Burnell-type tendon suture, into each one separately and tying it to the bone on the opposite side. We have found that external pressure is very important in maintaining the repositioned tendons. This is applied by passing two additional nonabsorbable sutures as illustrated and tying them over small cotton rolls. These are left in place for 10 days postoperatively. This provides additional support to the canthal tendons and decreases edema and hematoma formation in this area.

J. Improved esthetic and functional results following the LeFort II midfacial advancement are illustrated.

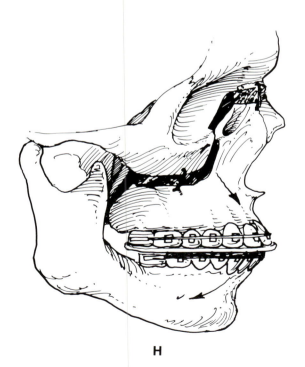

H

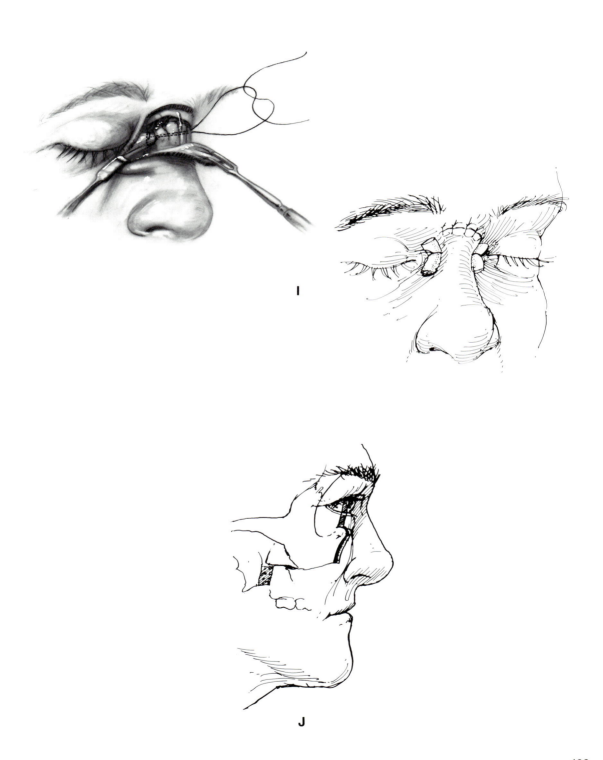

I

J

LeFort III midfacial advancement modified: nasomalar advancement

The indications for use of the LeFort III midfacial advancement are primarily to improve facial esthetics and in some cases to improve nasal airway function. A systematic clinical description is necessary to determine the criteria for use of this surgical approach. The esthetic characteristics inherent in nasomalar deficiency include retruded nasal dorsum, saddle-nose deformity, infraorbital and malar retrusion, and hypoplasia. This causes the eyes to appear relatively protrusive in relation to the inferior orbital rims and nasal dorsum. However, the forehead, supraorbital rims, maxilla, mandible, and occlusal relationships are usually relatively normal.

Cephalometric values and occlusal analysis are basically noncontributory in diagnosis and in planning treatment. The abnormal skeletal structure of the midfacial bones and cranial base that exists in many patients with middle third facial deformities results in deceptive cephalometric values.

The surgical correction of nasomalar retrusion by a modified LeFort III osteotomy, as illustrated here, was first described by us. The nasoorbital osteotomies are performed essentially like those for a standard LeFort III midfacial advancement, and the extraoral access can be achieved through a bicoronal flap, transconjunctival incisions, a glabellar incision or subciliary incisions. The horizontal maxillary osteotomy, from piriform rim to pterygoid plates, is completed through a standard intraoral circumvestibular incision.

After mobilization bone grafts are inserted at the lateral orbital rims and glabellar regions for stabilization. This procedure is technically complex, particularly when the nasal bones are severely hypoplastic, in that it is difficult to mobilize this complex as a single unit. Therefore in instances where the existing deformity suggests this type of midface advancement osteotomy, midface augmentation to the malar-orbital regions and the nasal dorsum must be considered as an alternative.

In this section the advancement of the nasomalar complex, leaving the maxilla stable, is described.

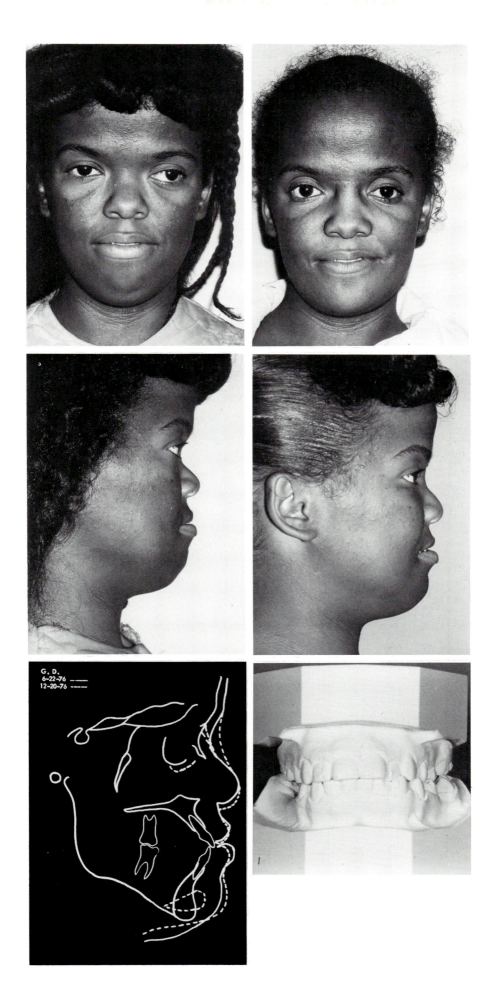

LeFORT III MIDFACIAL ADVANCEMENT MODIFIED: NASOMALAR ADVANCEMENT

Plate 12-3

A. The illustrated case exhibits nasomalar deficiency, which will be corrected with a modified LeFort III midfacial advancement. The objective of this surgical procedure is to advance the nasomalar complex to a normal anatomic relationship with the remainder of the craniofacial complex while keeping the maxilla stable.

B. There are two basic external soft-tissue approaches for correction of this deformity: the bicoronal flap and combined infraorbital subciliary and glabellar incisions. Because the glabellar and subciliary incisions are described in the previous sections on malar bone advancement and LeFort II midfacial advancement, the bicoronal flap approach is illustrated here. This is simply an extension of the temporal flap previously described in detail in Chapter 11.

    The hair is shaved several inches distal to the anterior hairline and the incision outlined about 2 inches posterior to it. Ten milliliters 1:200,000 epinephrine are injected along the proposed incision line, and about 20 ml sterile saline are injected beneath the soft tissues of the forehead below the galea aponeurosis but supraperiosteally. The initial incision is made down to the periosteum. The incision extends from approximately the level of the attachment of the superior helix of the ear transcoronally about 2 inches behind the hairline to the identical location on the opposite side. As the initial incision is made the margins are elevated and Raney clips placed for hemostasis.

C. The bicoronal flap is reflected forward *supraperiosteally,* and an incision is made through the periosteum at approximately two thirds the distance to the superior orbital rims. The flap is then continued downward subperiosteally to the superior orbital rims. The supraorbital neurovascular bundles are released from their bony canals with a small osteotome. This avoids postoperative frontal anesthesia. The flap is then completely rotated inferiorly, exposing the superior orbital rims, nasoethmoid area, lacrimal gland and fossa, and lateral orbital areas.

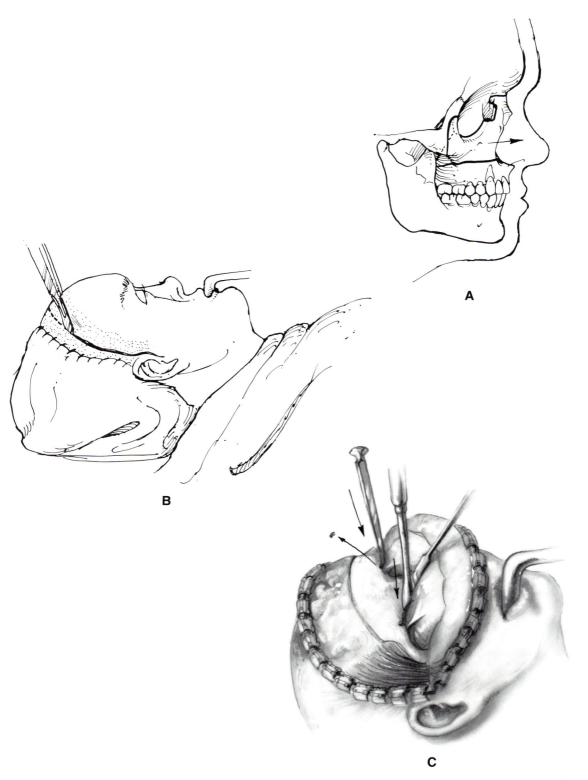

A

B

C

LeFORT III MIDFACIAL ADVANCEMENT MODIFIED:
NASOMALAR ADVANCEMENT
Plate 12-3

D. The soft tissue is dissected from the nasal bones and the frontal processes of the maxilla down toward the inferior aspect of the medial orbital rim. In this instance the attachment of the medial canthal tendons will be maintained and the osteotomies will pass anterior to them. This is done in instances where the intercanthal distance is essentially normal (that is, no telecanthism exists), the lacrimal lakes are normal and symmetric, and the nasal bones are not severely hypoplastic.

The tomographic radiographs are evaluated to determine whether the anterior cranial base extends inferiorly into the ethmoidal area, aiding in the determination of the level at which to perform the horizontal osteotomy in the nasofrontal area. This osteotomy extends laterally slightly into the orbit through the ethmoid bones; then as it extends inferiorly it curves around the medial canthal tendon. Once below the tendon it is curved into the lacrimal fossa. This is done while gently retracting the lacrimal sac to avoid damage to it. The same osteotomies are completed on the opposite side.

LeFORT III MIDFACIAL ADVANCEMENT MODIFIED:
NASOMALAR ADVANCEMENT
Plate 12-3

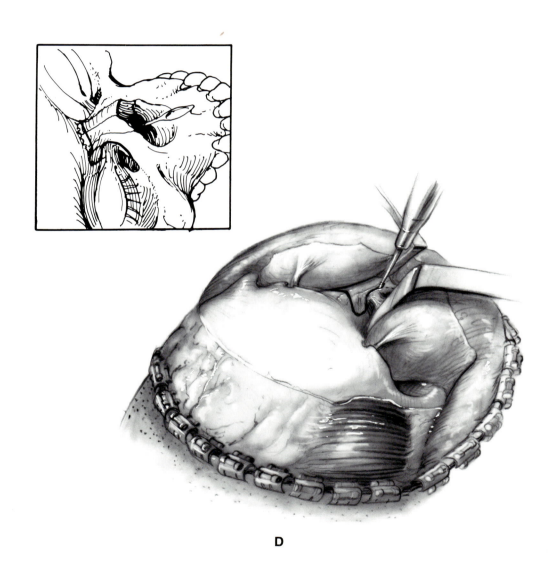

D

439

LeFORT III MIDFACIAL ADVANCEMENT MODIFIED:
NASOMALAR ADVANCEMENT
Plate 12-3

E. When completing the lateral aspect of the coronal flap dissection, when the attachment of the temporalis muscle is reached, the dissection is carried out above the level of the temporalis fascia. The incision through the periosteum is made connecting the coronal periosteal incision to the lateral orbital rim through the periosteum just anterior to the anteriormost attachment of the temporalis muscle. The periosteum is reflected off the lateral orbital rim. The periosteal incision is then continued through the periosteum in the infraorbital rim. The dissection is continued medially on the orbital floor to the area of the lacrimal fossa. The infraorbital neurovascular bundle is dissected out into the soft tissue to decrease the amount of tension on this structure when the nasomalar complex is advanced. If sufficient exposure cannot be achieved medially with the bicoronal flap, subconjunctival incisions or subciliary incisions are made to gain exposure to this area. The conjunctival incision is placed approximately midway between the lower border of the tarsal plate and the fornix. While making this incision traction sutures, inserted through the lower lid, are used to evert the eyelid. After the initial incision is made the ocular conjunctiva, supported by traction sutures, is elevated and retracted upward. The periosteum at the orbital rim is exposed and incised and the lacrimal fossa identified. The conjunctiva can be closed with a running 6-0 nylon suture with the knot placed on the skin to avoid corneal irritation. This suture can be removed in 3 days.

An osteotomy is done through the orbital floor, extending from the inferolateral aspect of the lacrimal fossa, across the orbital floor, approximately 10 mm behind the inferior orbital rim to the anterior aspect of the inferior orbital fissure. In completing the orbital floor osteotomy the infraorbital neurovascular bundle is preserved. Because the floor is usually very thin overlying it and will fracture quite readily, the osteotomy overlying it is not completed through the floor. The osteotomy extends laterally just anterior to the inferior orbital fissure. In severe midfacial hypoplasia this osteotomy may extend into the anterior aspect of the fissure.

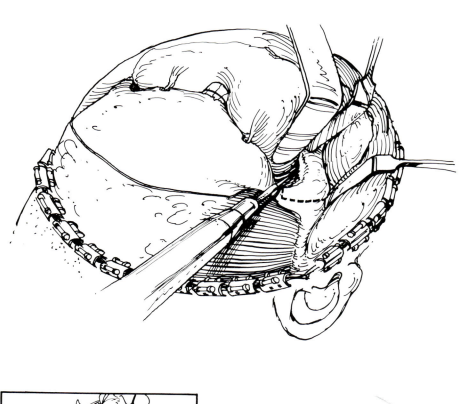

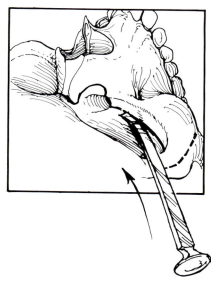

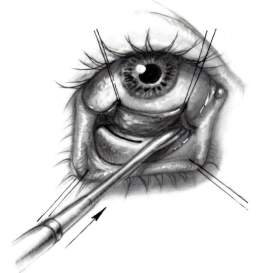

E

LeFORT III MIDFACIAL ADVANCEMENT MODIFIED: NASOMALAR ADVANCEMENT
Plate 12-3

F. The vertical height of the lateral orbital wall cut is dependent on the extent of the deformity in the lateral wall. In this case it will be made about halfway up the lateral orbital rim.

   The osteotomy is then directed vertically in a downward direction through the lateral orbital rim and posterior aspect of the malar eminence, just posterior to the zygomaticomaxillary buttress. The same osteotomies are performed on the opposite side.

G. An intraoral circumvestibular incision is made from one zygomatic buttress to the opposite one. A portion of the anterior and lateral maxillary wall is exposed as well as the piriform rims. However, soft tissue reflection is kept to a minimum in order to maintain good viability of the osseous segments. A periosteal elevator is placed along the lateral nasal wall to protect the nasal mucoperiosteum while the osteotomy is done in this area.

   A horizontal osteotomy is performed along the lateral maxillary wall and extends from the piriform rim posterior to the zygomatic buttress and about 5 mm above the apices. A vertical cut is then made with a curved osteotome, extending from the posterior extent of the horizontal osteotomy superiorly toward the inferior orbital fissure. The same osteotomies are done on the opposite side.

LeFORT III MIDFACIAL ADVANCEMENT MODIFIED:
NASOMALAR ADVANCEMENT
Plate 12-3

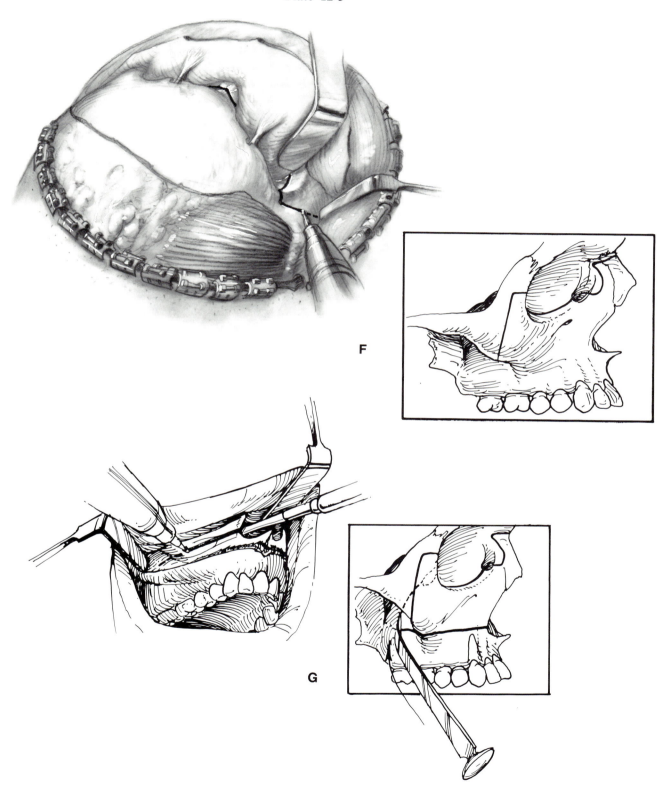

F

G

443

LeFORT III MIDFACIAL ADVANCEMENT MODIFIED: NASOMALAR ADVANCEMENT

Plate 12-3

H. The nasal septum is separated from the maxilla with a nasoseptal osteotome. A thin narrow osteotome is used to section the perpendicular plate of the ethmoid bone and the vomer to the level of the palate. The vertical extent of this osteotomy can be accurately ascertained from the cephalometric radiograph.

I. Interosseous holes are placed in the lateral aspect of the inferior orbital rims, and Carroll-Girard screws are inserted bilaterally to aid in mobilization. In addition osteotomes are inserted into the frontal nasal osteotomy and the vertical lateral orbital rim osteotomies to aid in the mobilization of the nasomaxillary complex. Gentle pressure must be exerted in order to effect mobilization. This must be done carefully because of the small osseous structure in the nasofrontal-ethmoidal area that provides continuity between the left and right malar processes. Following adequate mobilization, the complex is ready for stabilization by bone grafting.

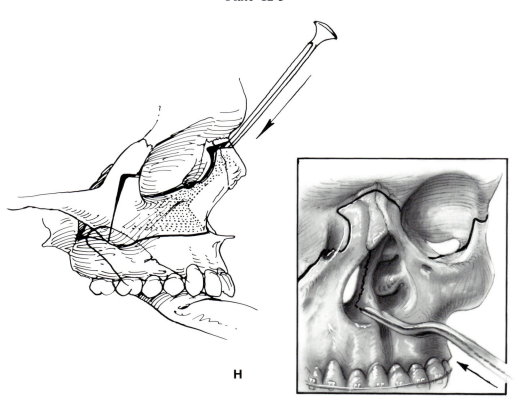

H

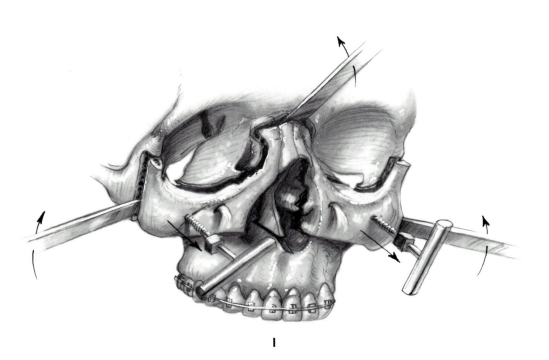

I

LeFORT III MIDFACIAL ADVANCEMENT MODIFIED: NASOMALAR ADVANCEMENT

Plate 12-3

J. Autogenous cortical-cancellous block grafts from the iliac crest are preferred. Bank bone, however, can be used. Bone grafts of appropriate size are sculptured and wired in position in the lateral orbital rim area and also in the nasofrontal area. The bone grafts are secured with interosseous wires. These are most easily stabilized with two separate mattress wires, as illustrated.

   The surgical areas are irrigated and the coronal flap and intraoral incisions closed in a routine fashion. A large pressure dressing is applied over the forehead for 48 hours.

K. Improvement in facial appearance is seen following nasomalar midface advancement.

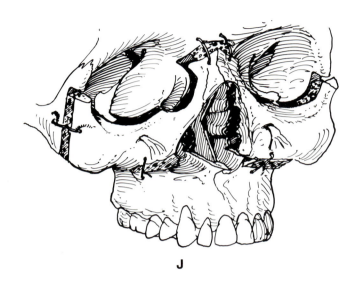

J

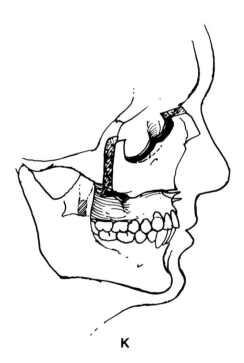

K

LeFort III midfacial advancement modified: malar-maxillary advancement

Like the previously discussed middle third face osteotomies, the malar-maxillary advancement procedure is indicated on the basis of a detailed clinical evaluation of the relationship of the various middle third face structures. This osteotomy would be considered for patients with normal intercanthal distance and lacrimal lakes, normal dorsonasal projection, infraorbital and malar retrusion, and maxillary deficiency, specifically, when in profile a good glabellar projection of the nose exists (that is, in profile it is at least 5 to 10 mm anterior to the most anterior projection of the globe, yet the remainder of the midface is clearly retrusive or deficient. In these cases the use of the standard LeFort III midfacial advancement results in loss of the normal glabellar angle of the nose and a very prominent nose, which often must be secondarily reduced.

Malar-maxillary advancement, when performed in the above circumstances, corrects the existing deformity very nicely and optimizes the balance between the various external structures of the middle third face.

The preferred external approach for this procedure is through two subciliary incisions and an intraoral vestibular incision. The subciliary incisions provide rapid and very adequate exposure of the orbital areas and do not result in noticeable scar formation. Although the bicoronal flap can be used for this procedure, it seems unwarranted and of little or no real advantage.

The mobilization is similar to that for the LeFort II midfacial advancement, as is the bone grafting.

In this section the modified LeFort III malar-maxillary midfacial advancement technique that we have utilized is described and illustrated.

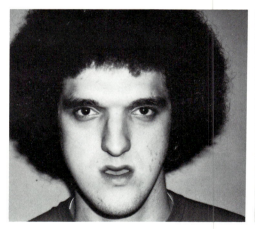 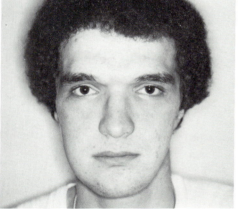

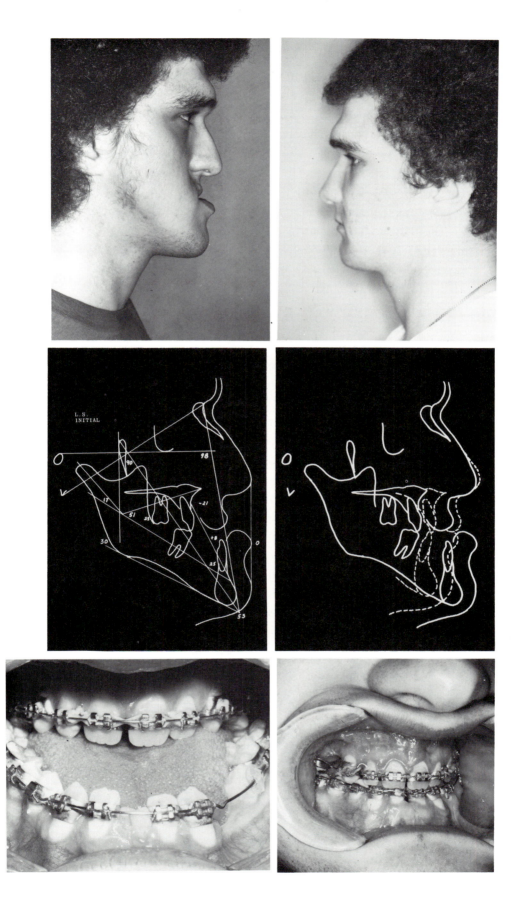

L.S.
INITIAL

LeFORT III MIDFACIAL ADVANCEMENT MODIFIED:
MALAR-MAXILLARY ADVANCEMENT
Plate 12-4

A. The illustrated case demonstrates malar-maxillary deficiency. Clinical examination reveals that the cheeks, infraorbital rims, paranasal areas, and upper lip are retrusive. The globes are in good relationship to the superior orbital rims and nasal dorsum but are protrusive relative to the inferior orbital rims. The chin and nose appear relatively prominent, yet are judged to be normal and in good relationship to the forehead. A class III malocclusions is present. Presurgical orthodontics have been done to level, align, and coordinate the arches in preparation for midfacial advancement surgery.

   The indicated treatment for correction of this dentofacial deformity is a malar-maxillary midfacial advancement. The orbital components of this midface osteotomy are best approached through bilateral subciliary incisions. An intraoral circumvestibular incision is utilized to perform all additional intraoral osteotomies.

B. Subciliary incisions and dissection to the infraorbital rims bilaterally are completed as previously described in detail in Chapter 11. The periorbita is reflected from the orbital floor until the inferior orbital fissure is identified posterolaterally and the lacrimal fossa medially. This dissection is then carried down the anterior maxilla until the infraorbital neurovascular bundle is identified. This dissection is extended inferiorly medial to the neurovascular bundle to the piriform rim of the nose.

   The periosteum is reflected from the lateral orbital rim and lateral aspect of the malar eminence, exposing the anterior aspect of the zygomatic arch.

   A vertical osteotomy is made on the anterior maxillary wall extending from the base of the piriform rim up through the inferior orbital rim, just lateral to the most inferior portion of the lacrimal fossa. The osteotomy is then directed across the orbital floor about 10 mm posterior to the rim and extending toward the anteriormost aspect of the inferior orbital fissure. Care is exercised when crossing the orbital floor so as not to injure the infraorbital neurovascular bundle.

LeFORT III MIDFACIAL ADVANCEMENT MODIFIED: MALAR-MAXILLARY ADVANCEMENT

Plate 12-4

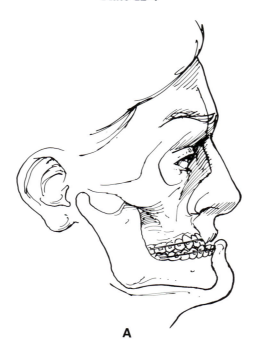

A

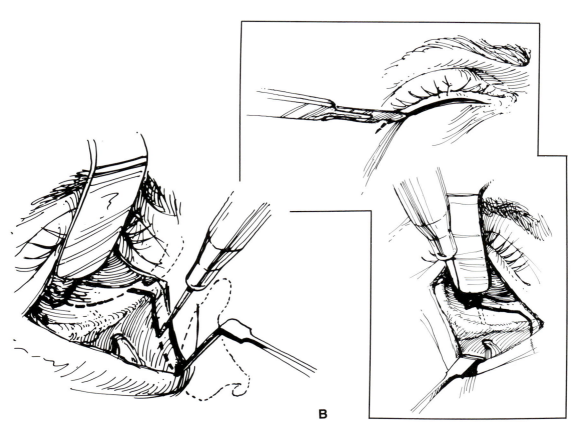

B

451

LeFORT III MIDFACIAL ADVANCEMENT MODIFIED: MALAR-MAXILLARY ADVANCEMENT
Plate 12-4

C. The osteotomy is then directed up the lateral orbital wall approximately 10 mm from the anterior aspect of the lateral orbital rim. The osteotomy is extended vertically to the desired level as determined by the clinical examination. In most cases this osteotomy is extended superiorly just below Whitnall's tubercle.

    The lateral orbital wall osteotomy is extended about halfway through the lateral orbital rim, then directed inferiorly so that it passes along the lateral aspect of the malar eminence and ends just posterior to its buttress to the maxilla. A fine osteotome is used to check for completeness of all the orbital osteotomies. The same osteotomies are performed on the opposite side.

D. Through a circumvestibular intraoral incision the piriform nasal rims are exposed bilaterally and the mucoperiosteum reflected off the lateral nasal walls and floor, exposing the anterior nasal spine and crest. The vertical anterior maxillary osteotomy that has been carried into the piriform aperture from above is identified and checked for completeness through the piriform rim. At this time a nasoseptal osteotome is utilized to separate the nasal septum from the maxilla, because the septum will remain stable with the nasal complex.

E. Next the posterior maxillary osteotomies are completed. The pterygoid plates are separated in the conventional manner, and with the same curved osteotome a cut is extended from the inferiormost aspect of the pterygomaxillary fissure upward toward the inferior orbital fissure. Care is exercised when performing this osteotomy so as not to carry the cut posteriorly or inadvertently drive the osteotome posteriorly into the area of the internal maxillary artery and pterygoid venous plexus.

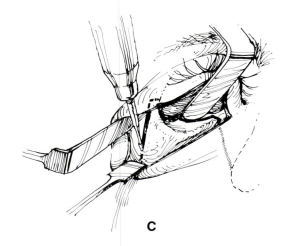

C

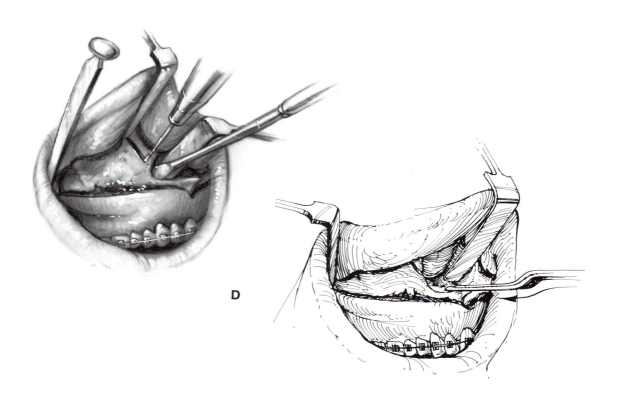

D

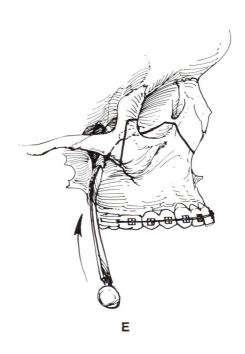

E

LeFORT III MIDFACIAL ADVANCEMENT MODIFIED: MALAR-MAXILLARY ADVANCEMENT

Plate 12-4

F. Mobilization forceps are used to mobilize the malar-maxillary complex. The forceps are first moved downward. As this force is being applied the malar-orbital areas are observed bilaterally to make certain the osteotomy sites are all opening and doing so symmetrically. This is important so as to avoid inadvertent fracturing of one or both malar bones from the maxilla.

Osteotomes inserted bilaterally into the vertical osteotomy of the lateral orbital rim can be used to provide additional force to mobilize the midfacial structures if necessary; however, care must be taken not to apply excessive force or the malar bones can be fractured free of the remainder of the complex.

Following initial freeing of the bones considerable force must be applied in a forward direction to sufficiently mobilize the maxillomalar complex.

G. Following mobilization to the extent that the complex can be passively repositioned anteriorly, the occlusal splint is inserted and intermaxillary fixation applied. These cases should be overcorrected 2 to 3 mm. Autogenous cortical-cancellous block bone grafts are obtained from the ilium and fashioned for insertion into the lateral orbital rim defects and between the pterygoid plates and tuberosities of the maxilla. Bank bone can also be used for these areas.

The bone grafts to be inserted in the pterygoid areas are tapered with the larger end slightly larger than the amount of advancement measured so they can be wedged tightly into place. The lateral orbital rim bone grafts are wired into place with two mattress wires. The defect in the orbital floor is not generally bone grafted. Indeed, if considerable exorbita exists the periorbita may be released to permit release of the periorbital fat. The area of the medial rim cut is packed with cancellous bone to provide a smooth contour and facilitate healing.

In addition to the direct wire fixation of the bone grafts, added vertical stabilization is usually necessary. This can be provided by a head frame, circumzygomatic wires, or transnasal wires.

A transnasal hole is drilled through the stable frontal process of the maxilla on one side to the same place on the opposite side. A wire is passed through this, and then each end is passed into the buccal sulcus and twisted so as to form a small loop in the sulcus. A second wire is passed through this loop to the hole in the splint and tightened.

H. The incisions are closed and intermaxillary fixation maintained for about 6 weeks. On removal the maxilla is tested for stability. If stability has not been achieved, the fixation is reapplied for an additional 2 weeks.

Improved facial esthetics and occlusion are noted.

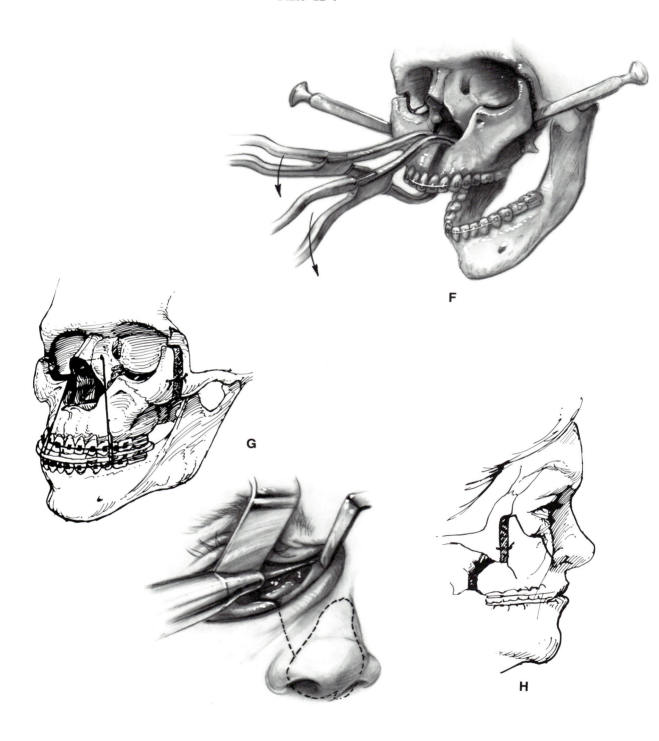

F

G

H

LeFort III midfacial advancement

In the presence of deficiencies involving the nasomalar-maxillary complex, the traditional LeFort III midfacial advancement is generally indicated. These patients have protrusive eyes with or without deficiencies in the supraorbital area. These types of deformities are quite often associated with Crouzon's, Pfeifer's, and Apert's syndromes. However, they can also occur as the result of developmental midfacial hypoplasia and trauma. Cephalometric analysis is usually of little diagnostic benefit for several reasons. Most often there is definite abnormal structure and angulation of the cranial base. Because the midfacial bones are retruded, SNA may be relatively normal and SNB appear excessive when in fact the deformity exists in the midface.

Individuals with total retrusion or hypoplasia of the midface have retrusion of the nose, inferior orbital rims, cheeks, and upper lip relative to the globes. The mandible is usually relatively normal and may be the only normal bone in the face. It will, however, appear relatively prognathic compared with the other facial bones. In syndromes such as Crouzon's, Pfeifer's, and Apert's, often the nasal bones and in particular the infraorbital rim area are extremely hypoplastic and in addition to the LeFort III midface advancement, onlay bone grafts are necessary to provide adequate projection of the cheeks and nasal bones.

Occasionally there will be a differential deficiency relative to the nasomalar complex and the maxilla, with the upper component (nasomalar component) either less or greater in deficiency than the position of the maxilla. Therefore occasionally a LeFort I osteotomy may also need to be incorporated to make the appropriate adjustment for optimal esthetics. Occasionally one side may be more deficient than the other in the maxillomalar area. In such cases the more deficient side can be additionally corrected by simultaneous augmentation with onlay cortical bone grafts or secondarily with alloplastic implants.

Another area of consideration in these patients is the intercanthal distance and level of attachment of the lateral and medial canthal tendons. The traditional approach to this area has been to detach and reattach the tendons as described for the LeFort II procedure. Another approach has been to maintain them and still do the osteotomies posteriorly to them and the lacrimal sac. However, when this is done care must be taken with midface advancement so that the nasofrontal complex is not tipped inferiorly, causing a significant downward curvature of the medial canthal areas. When the medial canthal tendon areas are in an acceptable position prior to surgery, we often prefer to do the osteotomies in this area so as to preserve this relationship by making the medial orbital rim osteotomy anterior to the attachments of the medial canthal tendon. We have found by using this approach that the esthetics and function of the lacrimal lake are better when medial canthal dystopia or telecanthism does not exist. If the medial canthal tendons are detached, it has been our experience that the subsequent esthetics and structural configuration of the medial canthal tendons and lacrimal lakes are often less than optimum. Similar consideration must be made for the deformed lateral canthal area. If the lateral canthal area is relatively normal esthetically (that is, good vertical positioning), the osteotomy is usually done below the level of the canthal tendon. If the entire lateral orbital rim is indicated for advancement, the tendon can be reflected off Whitnall's tubercle without any undue sequelae. If lateral canthal dystopia is present with significant inferior positioning, the entire lateral periorbita is freed and the lateral tendon reattached with a permanent suture at a much higher level on the lateral orbital rim following the stabilization of the advanced nasomalar-maxillary complex. Generally patients undergoing LeFort III midfacial advancement can be intubated nasally and the surgery completed around the nasotracheal tube. If significant nasal obstruction is present because of the close approximation of the posterior aspect of the hard palate to the cervical vertebrae and cranial base, an oral endotracheal tube is used until the midfacial complex is mobilized. Then a nasal endotracheal tube can be inserted and the oral tube removed. It has been our experience that tracheostomies are rarely necessary for airway management of these patients when the oral and nasal airways are appropriately handled.

The traditional LeFort III midfacial advancement that we have utilized for correction of nasomaxillary deficiencies is discussed on the following pages.

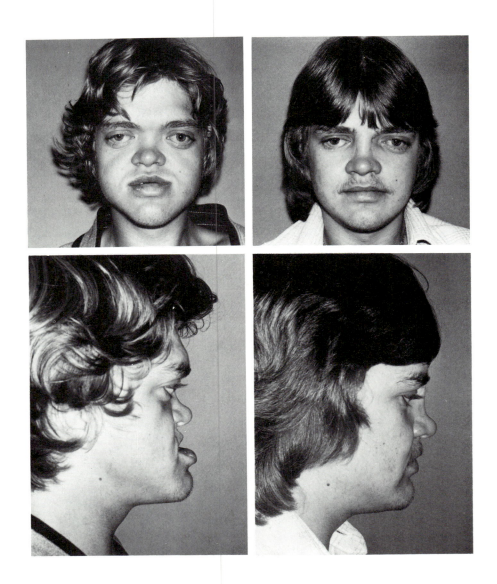

LeFORT III MIDFACIAL ADVANCEMENT

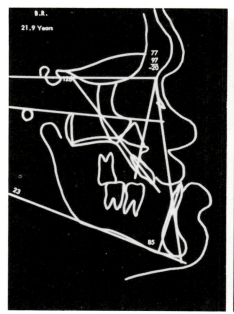
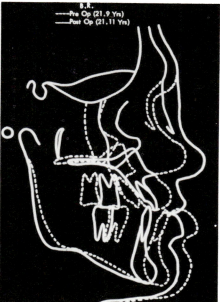

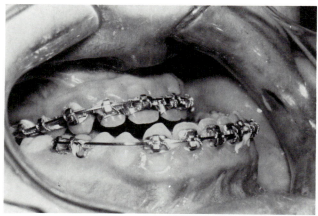

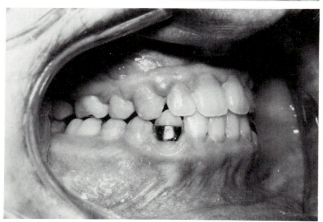

LeFORT III MIDFACIAL ADVANCEMENT
Plate 12-5

A. The illustrated case demonstrates nasomalar-maxillary deficiency secondary to Crouzon's syndrome. The shape of the forehead and supraorbital rims is essentially normal and in satisfactory relationship to the globes. The nasal bones, infraorbital rims, and lateral orbital rim are significantly posterior to the anteriormost projection of the globes. Of importance, this patient has relatively normal intercanthal distance, interpupillary distance, and lacrimal lake anatomy. The mandible appears protrusive; however, it is not. There is a class III malocclusion.

   A LeFort III midfacial advancement is indicated for this patient.

B. The LeFort III midfacial advancement described and illustrated can be approached through two basic external routes: a glabellar incision and bilateral subciliary incisions or the bicoronal flap. The bicoronal flap approach is generally preferred and is utilized in this case. The elevation of this flap has been discussed in detail in this and Chapter 11 and therefore is not presented here.

   The hair is shaved about 6 inches posteriorly, and following a full-face preparation the drapes are sewed to the scalp. Epinephrine and sterile saline are injected supraperiosteally along the proposed incision line. The initial incision is made approximately 2 inches posterior to the hairline. Raney clamps are placed on both edges of the incision line for hemostasis.

   The dissection of the supraorbital areas includes decompression of the supraorbital nerves by removal of the small rim of bone beneath them.

   Following reflection of the bicoronal flap the nasal bones, medial canthal tendons, superior aspect of the lacrimal fossa, lateral orbital rims, and infraorbital rims are exposed sequentially.

LeFORT III MIDFACIAL ADVANCEMENT

Plate 12-5

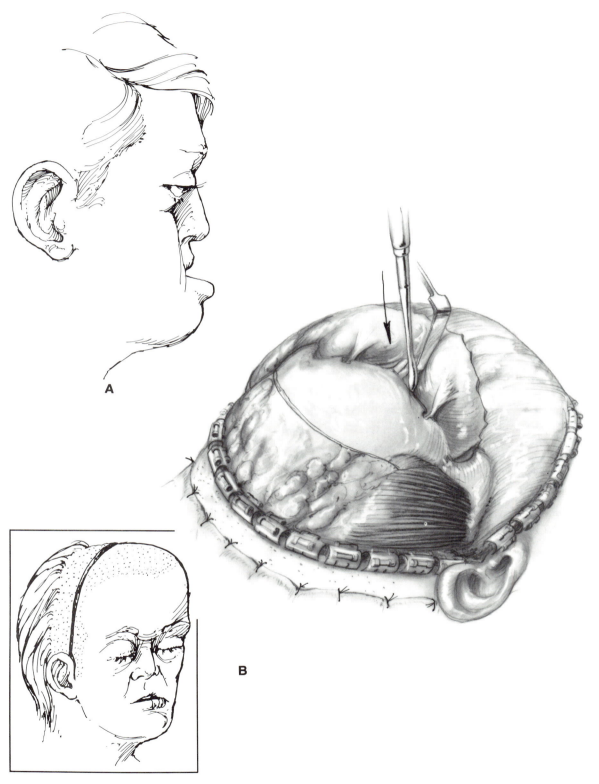

A

B

461

LeFORT III MIDFACIAL ADVANCEMENT
Plate 12-5

C. As the dissection extends inferiorly in the nasoethmoid area, the medial canthal tendons are identified where they attach to the frontal process of the maxilla. They are either reflected off and tagged with suture or left intact. This decision is predicated on those factors discussed at the beginning of this chapter. Below and posterior to this area the lacrimal fossa is exposed with its accompanying lacrimal sac.

The dissection posteriorly into the medial aspect of the orbits need only extend 10 to 15 mm, thus avoiding involvement with the anterior ethmoid artery, which is normally about 20 to 25 mm back in the orbit.

It is generally easiest to begin with the nasoethmoid osteotomies. This osteotomy usually begins just slightly below the nasofrontal suture. Routinely tomographic radiographic examination of the anterior cranial fossa is performed prior to surgery, because abnormal positioning of the cribriform plate and anterior cranial fossa secondary to invagination of the cranial contents inferiorly in this area may exist.

The osteotomies in this region can be done in two basic ways: posterior to the lacrimal fossa and anterior to the attachment of the medial canthal tendon and through the lacrimal fossa. Generally if the intercanthal distance is normal, lacrimal lakes are symmetric, and the bones in this area are not severely hypoplastic, we make this osteotomy anterior to the medial canthal tendons, leaving the tendons attached. Otherwise the osteotomy is made in the more classic fashion, posteriorly in the medial orbit with or without detachment of the tendon. If the midface is to be advanced straight forward without inferior movement in this area, the intercanthal distance is satisfactory, and lacrimal lakes are normal, they can be left attached. However, with any preexisting deformity in this area or planned inferior tipping, they are detached and later reattached.

In this case the latter type of osteotomy is done. The posterior cut was described with the LeFort II midfacial advancement technique discussed earlier in this chapter.

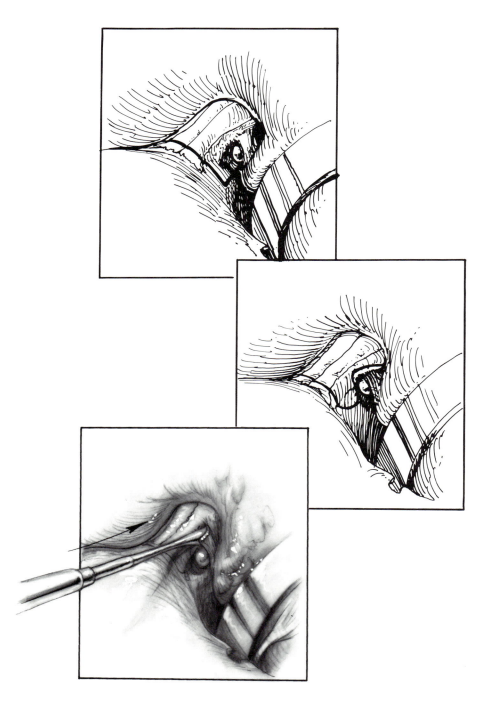

C

LeFORT III MIDFACIAL ADVANCEMENT

Plate 12-5

D. Attention is next directed to exposure of the lateral orbital rim and to the orbital floor. This dissection is carried medially subperiosteally to the inferiormost aspect of the lacrimal fossa.

A horizontal osteotomy is then made across the orbital floor extending from the inferior aspect of the medial orbital osteotomy, approximately 10 mm posteriorly in the orbital floor to the inferior orbital rim, laterally to the anterior aspect of the inferior orbital fissure. When no subconjunctival incisions are made, the medial aspect of this osteotomy is most readily done with a small osteotome. The osteotomy is then extended from the anterior aspect of the inferior orbital fissure laterally and superiorly up the lateral orbital wall.

The superior extent of the lateral orbital rim osteotomy is determined by the degree of lateral orbital rim deficiency. When this is minimal the lateral orbital rim osteotomy is carried only approximately halfway up the lateral orbital rim, is extended in an inferior direction through the posterior aspect of the malar eminence, and then extended inferiorly just posterior to the zygomaticomaxillary buttress.

E. In the illustrated case the lateral orbital rims are quite deficient and require more complete advancement; thus the lateral cut is extended to the superior aspect of the lateral orbital rim. These osteotomies are checked with a fine osteotome for completeness.

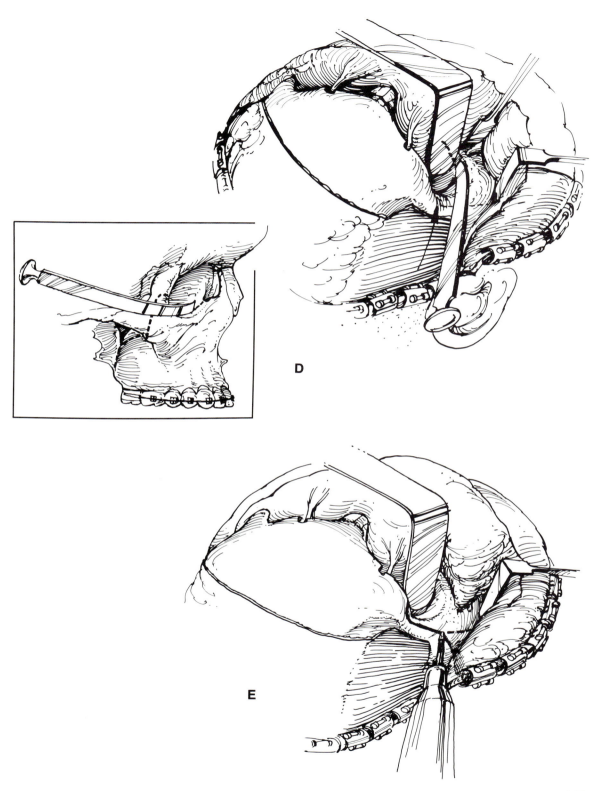

D

E

LeFORT III MIDFACIAL ADVANCEMENT
Plate 12-5

F. At this time the anterior portion of the temporalis muscle is elevated and thereby direct access to the retro-orbital and infratemporal space is gained. This permits the posterior maxillary osteotomy to be completed from the inferior orbital fissure to the pterygomaxillary suture area. This cut can also be approached intraorally as previously described in this chapter. Also the pterygomaxillary suture can be separated through this approach.

G. Access to the pterygomaxillary suture area is gained through an intraoral vertical incision made posterior in the first or second molar area, just behind the buttress of the zygoma. This provides excellent access to the area for completing the separation of the pterygomaxillary suture as well as for inserting the bone graft in this area.

    This incision extends from the attached gingiva superiorly to the depth of the vestibule. A periosteal elevator is used to reflect the mucoperiosteum off the lateral maxillary wall to the pterygoid plates. A small curved osteotome is used to separate the pterygoid plates from the tuberosity of the maxilla. When performing this cut a finger is placed on the palatal aspect in the area of the hamulus to determine that the separation is complete. It is important that the pterygoid plates *not* be fractured so that a bone graft can be wedged tightly in this area.

    Through this intraoral incision the vertical osteotomy can be completed, extending from the superior aspect of the pterygomaxillary junction in an anterosuperior direction toward the inferior orbital fissure area behind the zygomatic buttress. However, when this cut is made intraorally it is a blind cut and therefore is more readily and more safely done from above, as described in Plate 12-5, *F*.

H. The nasal septum is then separated. This osteotomy is completed through the perpendicular plate of the ethmoid bone and vomer with a narrow sharp osteotome to about the region of the posterior aspect of the hard palate. A finger is placed intraorally on the posterior nasal spine area to help with orientation in directing the osteotome inferiorly. This osteotomy is usually done last because of potential bleeding problems.

466

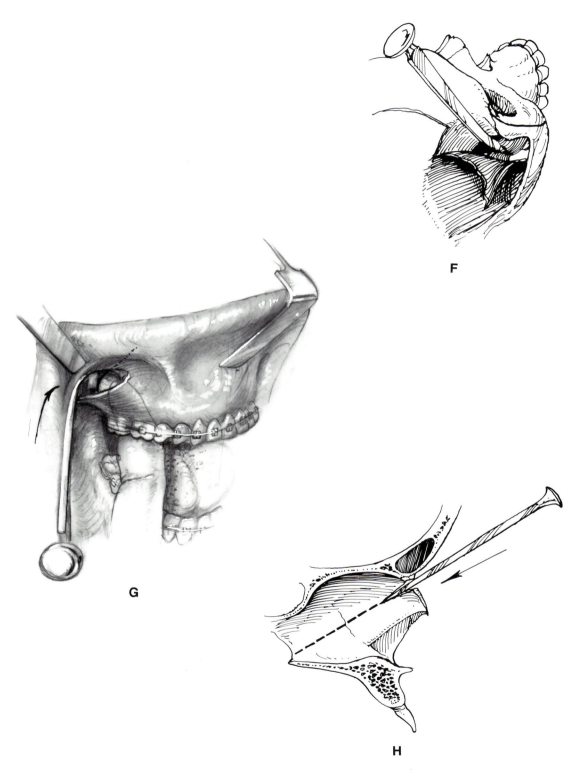

F

G

H

LeFORT III MIDFACIAL ADVANCEMENT
Plate 12-5

I. The midface complex is now ready for mobilization. We have found it advantageous to construct a full-coverage occlusal-palatal acrylic splint, which is inserted prior to utilizing the mobilization forceps. These patients frequently have a component of palatal clefting or a very high arched palate, which can result in inadvertent midpalatal splitting. This splint prevents such splitting. The splint is also designed to overcorrect the maxilla a few millimeters, particularly in the larger advancements.

Osteotomes can also be placed in the lateral orbital rim osteotomy sites to help with leverage in mobilizing the midfacial structures. To begin mobilization, downward and forward pressure is exerted with the mobilization forceps. Following initial mobilization of the bony complex considerable force must be applied to stretch and tear the soft tissues to permit complete mobilization. If considerable tension is required to reposition the midfacial structures forward into the occlusal splint, the relapse is greatly increased. It must be totally mobilized and freed up so that it can be passively placed in its new position.

To achieve this degree of mobilization it is frequently necessary to also utilize the Tessier mobilization forceps. However, when these are used they often comminute the posterior maxilla, which makes it more difficult to firmly wedge a bone graft in this area.

J. Intermaxillary fixation and occlusal splints are used to provide stabilization at the occlusal level. The occlusal splint is constructed so that there is about 4 mm of overcorrection. Bone grafts are fashioned and inserted in the nasofrontal, lateral orbital rim, and pterygomaxillary areas. The grafts to the pterygomaxillary areas are tapered in shape, slightly larger than the intended advancement so that they can be wedged tightly into position.

Definitive stabilization is with external fixation or with the directly wired bone grafts and circumzygomatic suspension wires to the mandible. We have almost exclusively employed the latter with good results. Frequently the infraorbital rims are extremely hypoplastic as well as retrusive, and simultaneous onlay bone grafts are indicated. Cortical bone is best for this purpose.

Intermaxillary fixation is maintained for approximately 6 weeks. Generally class III interarch elastics are utilized for several weeks after removal of the stable intermaxillary fixation to control and maintain the desired occlusion.

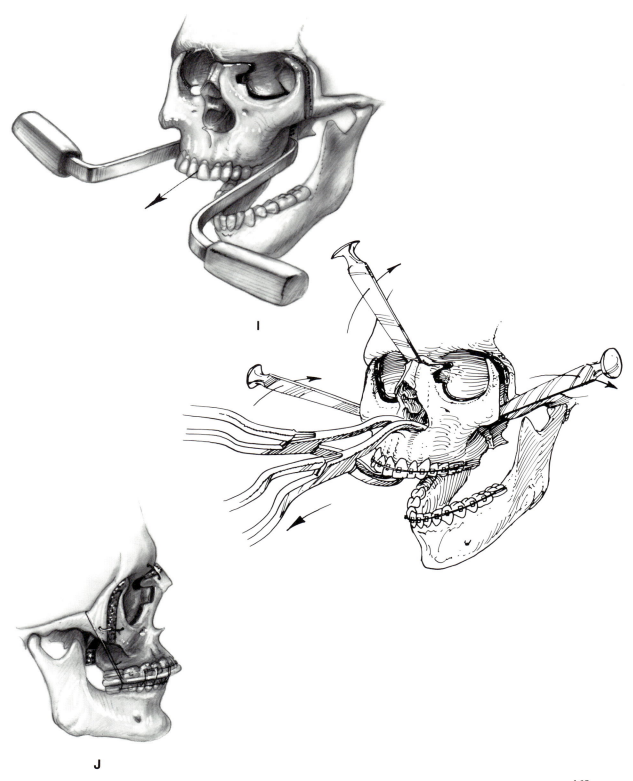

I

J

K. Improved postoperative facial appearance with a good functional result can be seen.

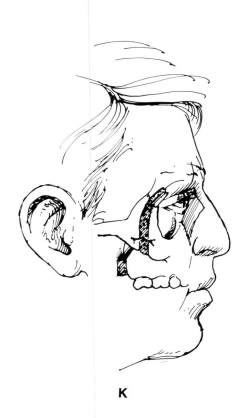

K

Selected references

Chapter 1

Bell, W. H., and Condit, C. L.: Surgical-orthodontic correction of adult bimaxillary protrusion, J. Oral Surg. **28**:578-584, 197.

Bell, W. H., and Dann, J. J.: Correction of dentofacial deformities by surgery in the anterior jaws, Am. J. Orthod. **64**:162-173, 1973.

Bell, W. H., and Levy, B. N.: Revascularization and bone regeneration after anterior mandibular osteotomy, J. Oral Surg. **28**:196-203, 1970.

Booth, D. F., Dietz, V., and Gianelly, A. A.: Correction of class II malocclusion by combined sagittal ramus and subapical body osteotomy, J. Oral Surg. **34**:630-634, 1976.

Fitzpatrick, B.: Total osteotomy of the mandibular alveolus in reconstruction of the occlusion, Oral Surg. **44**:336-346, 1977.

Hofer, O.: Die Vertikale Osteotomies sur Verlangerung des einseitig verkurzten aufsteigen-den Unterkieferastes, A. Stomatol. **34**:826-829, 1936.

Hofer, O.: Operation der prognathie und Microgenie, Dtsch. Zahn. Mund. Kieferheildk. **9**:121-127, 1942.

Hullihen, S. P.: Case of elongation of underjaw and distortion of face and neck, caused by burn, successfully treated, Am. J. Dent. Surg. **9**:157, 1849.

Kent J. N., and Hinds, E. C.: Management of dental facial deformities by anterior alveolar surgery, J. Oral Surg. **29**:13-21, 1971.

Kole, H.: Surgical operations on the alveolar ridge to correct occlusal abnormalities, Oral Surg. **12**:277-288, 1959.

MacIntosh, R. B., and Carlotti, A. E.: Total mandibular alveolar osteotomy in the management of skeletal (infantile) apertognathia, J. Oral Surg. **33**:921-928, 1975.

MacIntosh, R. B.: Total mandibular alveolar osteotomy, J. Maxillofac. Surg. **2**:210-218, 1974.

Neuner, O.: Surgical correction of mandibular prognathism, Oral Surg. **42**:415-429, 1976.

Peterson, L. J.: Posterior mandibular segmental alveolar osteotomy, J. Oral Surg. **36**:454-457, 1978.

Schuchardt, K.: Experiences with the surgical treatment of some deformities of the jaws: prognathia, micrognathia, and open bite. In Wallace, A. B., editor: International Society of Plastic Surgeons, Transactions of Second Congress, London, 1959, Edinburgh, 1961; E. & S. Livingstone.

Chapter 2

Barker, B. C. W., and Davies, P. L.: The applied anatomy of the pterygomandibular space, Br. J. Oral Surg. **10**:43-55, 1972.

Berényl, B.: Open subcondylar osteotomy in the treatment of mandibular deformities, Int. J. Oral Surg. **2**:81-88, 1973.

Byrne, R. P., and Hinds, E. C.: The ramus "C" osteotomy with body sagittal split, J. Oral Surg. **32**:259-263, 1974.

Caldwell, J. B., and Letterman, G. S.: Vertical osteotomy in the mandibular rami for correction of prognathism, J. Oral Surg. **12**:185-202, 1954.

Dal Pont, G.: Retromolar osteotomy for the correction of prognathism, J. Oral Surg. **19**:42-47, 1961.

Epker, B. N.: Modifications in the sagittal osteotomy of the mandible, J. Oral Surg. **35**:157-159, 1977.

Epker, B. N., Wolford, L. M., and Fish, L. C.: Mandibular deficiency syndrome. II. Surgical considerations for mandibular advancement, Oral Surg. **45**:349-363, 1978.

Grammer, F. C., Meyer, M. W., and Richter, K. J.: A radioisotope study of the vascular response to sagittal split osteotomy of the mandibular ramus, J. Oral Surg. **32**:578-582, 1974.

Hawkinson, R. T.: Retrognathism corrected by means of an arcing osteotomy in the ascending ramus, J. Prosthet. Dent. **20**:77-86, 1968.

Hayes, P. A.: Correction of retrognathia by modified "C" osteotomy of the ramus and sagittal osteotomy of the mandibular body, J. Oral Surg. **31:**682-686, 1973.

Herbert, J. M., Kent, J. N., and Hinds, E. C.: Correction of prognathism by an intraoral vertical subcondylar osteotomy, J. Oral Surg. **33:**384-389, 1970.

Hunsuck, E. E.: Modified intraoral sagittal split technique for correction of mandibular prognathism, J. Oral Surg. **26:**250-254, 1968.

Levine, B., and Topazian, D. S.: The intraoral inverted-L double-oblique osteotomy of the mandibular ramus: a new technique for correction of mandibular prognathism, J. Oral Surg. **34:**522-525, 1976.

Massey, G. B., Chase, D. C., Thomas, P. M., and Kohn, M. W.: Intraoral oblique osteotomy of the mandibular ramus, J. Oral Surg. **32:**755-759, 1974.

Obwegeser, H.: Indications for surgical correction of mandibular deformity by sagittal splitting technique, Br. J. Oral Surg. **1:**157-168, 1964.

Obwegeser, H.: The surgical correction of mandibular prognathism and retrognathia with consideration of genioplasty, part 1, Oral Surg. **10:**677-689, 1957.

Reitzik, M., Griffiths, R. R., and Mirels, H.: Surgical anatomy of the ascending ramus of the mandible, Br. J. Oral Surg. **14:**150-55, 1976.

Robinson, M.: Prognathism corrected by open vertical condylotomy, J. So. Calif. Dent. Assn. **24:**22-27, 1956.

Steinhauser, E. W.: Advancement of the mandible by sagittal ramus split and suprahyoid myotomy, J. Oral Surg. **31:**516-521, 1973.

Tamas, F.: The groove of the mandibular neck as a risk factor in vertical osteotomy of the ramus of the mandible, Int. J. Oral Surg. **8:**1-7, 1979.

Trauner, R., and Obwegeser, H.: Surgical correction of mandibular prognathism and retrognathia with consideration of genioplasty, Oral Surg. **10:**677-681, 1957.

Weinstein, I. R.: C-osteotomy for correction of mandibular retrognathia: report of cases, J. Oral Surg. **29:**358-362, 1971.

Wilbanks, J. L.: Correction of mandibular prognathism by a double-oblique intraoral osteotomy: a new technique, Oral Surg. **31:**321-328, 1971.

Winstanley, R. P.: Subcondylar osteotomy of the mandible and the intraoral approach, Br. J. Oral Surg. **6:**134-39, 1968.

Chapter 3

Dingman, R. O.: Surgical correction of mandibular prognathism: an improved method, Am. J. Orthod. **30:**683-687, 1944.

Hovell, J. H.: Surgical treatment of mandibular prognathism, Ann. R. Coll. Surg. Engl. **27:**388-406, 1960.

Plumpton, S.: Surgical correction of unilateral mandibular prognathism by intraoral ostectomy of the symphysis, Br. J. Plast. Surg. **20:**70-73, 1967.

Sowray, J. H., and Haskell, R.: Ostectomy at the mandibular symphysis, Br. J. Oral Surg. **6:**97-103, 1968.

Walker, R. V.: Surgical correction of jaw deformities. In Kruger, G. O., editor: Textbook of oral surgery, ed. 5, St. Louis, 1979, The C. V. Mosby Co.

Whinery, J. G.: Lap joint mandibular ostectomy, J. Oral Surg. **33:**223-224, 1975.

Chapter 4

Bell, W. H.: Correction of the contour deficient chin, J. Oral Surg. **27:**110-114, 1969.

Converse, J. M.: Restoration of facial contour by bone grafts introduced through the oral cavity, Plast. Reconstr. Surg. **6:**295-300, 1950.

Converse, J. M., and Wood-Smith, D.: Horizontal osteotomy of the mandible, Plast. Reconstr. Surg. **34:**464-471, 1964.

Dann, J. J., and Epker, B. N.: Proplast genioplasty: a retrospective study with treatment recommendations, Angle Orthod. **47:**173-185, 1977.

Fitzpatrick, B. N.: Reconstruction of the chin in cosmetic surgery (genioplasty), Oral Surg. **39:**522-527, 1975.

Fitzpatrick, B. N.: Genioplasty with reference to resorption and the hinge sliding osteotomy, Int. J. Oral Surg. **3:**247-251, 1974.

Gonzalez-Ulloa, M., and Stevens, E.: The role of chin correction in profileplasty, Plast. Reconstr. Surg. **41:**477-486.

Hinds, E. C., and Kent, J. N.: Surgical treatment of developmental jaw deformities, St. Louis, 1972, The C. V. Mosby Co.

Hohl, T. H., and Epker, B. N.: Macrogenia: a study of treatment results with surgical recommendation, Oral Surg. **41:**545-567, 1976.

McDonnell, J. P., McNeill, R. W., and West, R. A.: Advancement genioplasty: a retrospective cephalometric analysis of osseous and soft-tissue changes, J. Oral Surg. **35:**640-647, 1977.

Neuner, O.: Correction of mandibular deformities, Oral Surg. **36:**779-789, 1973.

Obwegeser, H.: The surgical correction of mandibular prognathism and retrognathia with considerations of genioplasty, J. Oral Surg. **10:**677-689, 1957.

Chapter 5

Homsy, C. A.: Implant stabilization: chemical and biomechanical considerations, Orthod. Clin. North Am. **4:**295-303, 1974.

Kent, J. N., Homsy, C. A., and Hinds, E. C.: Proplast in dental facial reconstruction, Oral Surg. **39:**347-355, 1975.

Mullison, E. G.: Silicones in head and neck surgery, Arch. Otolaryngol. **5:**481-486, 1972.

Chapter 6

Blair, A. E., and Schneider, E. K.: Intraoral inferior border osteotomy for correction of mandibular asymmetry, J. Oral Surg. **35:**493-496, 1977.

Blomquist, K., and Hogeman, K. E.: Benign unilateral hyperplasia of the mandibular condyle: report of eight cases, Acta Chir. Scand. **126:**414-419, 1963.

Bruce, R. A., and Hayward, J. R.: Condylar hyperplasia and mandibular asymmetry: a review, J. Oral Surg. **26:**281-290, 1968.

Caldwell, J. B.: Surgical management of temporomandibular joint ankylosis in children, Int. J. Oral Surg. **7:**354-359, 1978.

Converse, J. M., Horwitz, S. L., Coccaro, P. J., et al.: The corrective treatment of the skeletal asymmetry in hemifacial microsomia, Plast. Reconst. Surg. **52:**221-229, 1973.

El-Mofty, So: Surgical treatment of ankylosis of the temporomandibular joint, J. Oral Surg. **32:**202-206, 1974.

Hibi, G., Kaneda, T., and Oka, T.: Indications and appreciation of operative procedures for mandibular ankylosis, Int. J. Oral Surg. **7:**333-339, 1978.

Hinds, E. C., Homsy, C. A., and Kent, J. N.: Use of a biocompatible interface for binding tissues and prostheses in temporomandibular joint surgery, Oral Surg. **38:**512-519, 1974.

Hovell, J. H.: Condylar hyperplasia, Br. J. Oral Surg. **1:**105-111, 1963.

Jonck, L. M.: Facial asymmetry and condylar hyperplasia, Oral Surg. **40:**567-573, 1975.

Mavaddat, I.: Intraoral correction of mandibular asymmetry: report of case, J. Oral Surg. **29:**422-425, 1971.

Obwegeser, H. L.: Correction of the skeletal anomalies of oto-mandibular dysostoses, J. Maxillofac. Surg. **2:**73-92, 1974.

Topazian, R. G.: Comparison of gap and interposition arthroplasty in the treatment of temporomandibular joint ankylosis, J. Oral Surg. **24:**405-411, 1966.

Walker, R. V.: Condylar abnormalities. In Hosted, E., and Hansen, E. H., editors: First International Conference in Oral Surgery, Copenhagen 1967, Munksgaard, pp. 81-96.

Ware, W. H.: Growth center transplantation in temporomandibular joint surgery. In Walker, R. V., editor: Transactions of Third International Conference on Oral Surgery, London, 1970, E. & S. Livingstone, pp. 148-157.

Young, A. H.: A follow-up of twelve cases of ankylosis of the mandibular .joint treated by condylectomy, Br. J. Plast. Surg. **16:**75-79, 1963.

Chapter 7

Bell, W. H.: Revascularization and bone healing after anterior maxillary ostectomy, J. Oral Sug. **27:**249, 1969.

Bell, W. H.: Surgical-orthodonic treatment of interincisal diastemas, Am. J. Orthod. **57:**158-164, 1970.

Bell, W. H., and Levy, B. M.: Revascularization and bone healing after posterior maxillary osteotomy, J. Oral Surg. **29:**313, 1971.

Burk, J. L., Provencher, R. F., and McKean, T. W.: Small segment and one tooth ostectomies to correct dentoalveolar deformities, J. Oral Surg. **35:**452-460, 1977.

Clark, D. C.: Immediate closure of labial diastema by frenectomy and maxillary ostectomy, J. Oral Surg. **26:**273-277, 1968.

Cupar, I.: Die chirurgische Behandlung der Form; und Stellungs-veranderungen does Oberkiefers, Osterr. Z. Stomatol. **51:**565, 1954; Bull. Soc. Cons. Acad. R.P.F. Jougosl. **2:**60, 1955.

Epker, B. N.: A modified anterior maxillary ostectomy, J. Maxillofac. Surg. **27:**939, 1969.

Jensen, G., Nelson, R., Pata, M., and Meyer, M.: Quantitation of blood flow following anterior maxillary osteotomy: Wunderer procedure, IADR Abstract No. 921, 1976.

Kole, H.: Surgical operations on the alveolar ridge to correct occlusal abnormalities, Oral Surg. **12:**515-524, 1959.

Kufner, J.: Experience with a modified procedure for correction of open bite, Transactions of the Third International Conference of Oral Surgery, London, 1970, E. & S. Livingston.

Merrill, R. G., and Pedersen, G. W.: Interdental osteotomy for immediate repositioning of dental osseous elements, J. Oral Surg. **34:**118-212, 1976.

Olson, D., Nelson, R., Pata, M., and Meyer, M.: Quantitation of blood flow following anterior maxillary osteotomy: down-fracture technique, IADR Abstract No. 944, 1976.

Peterson, L. F.: Immediate surgical closure of multiple maxillary diastemas, J. Oral Surg. **31:**522-527, 1973.

Sokoloski, P., Nelson, R., Pata, M., and Meyer, M.: Quantitation of blood flow following anterior maxillary osteotomy: Wassmund procedure, IADR Abstract No. 943, 1976.

Wassmund, M.: Lehrbuch der praktischen Chirurgie des Mundes und der Kiefer, Leipzig, 1935, Bd. I. Meusser.

West, R. A., and Epker, B. N.: The posterior maxillary ostectomy: its place in the treatment of dentofacial deformities, J. Oral Surg. 30:562, 1972.

Wolford, L. M., and Epker, B. N.: The combined anterior and posterior maxillary ostectomy: a new technique, J. Oral Surg. 33:842, 1975.

Wunderer, S.: Die Prognathieoperation mittels frontal gestieltem Maxillafragment, Osterr. Z. Stomatol. 59:98, 1962.

Chapter 8

Araujo, A., Schendel, S. A., Wolford, L. M., and Epker, B. N.: Total maxillary advancement with and without bone grafting, J. Oral Surg. 36:849-858, 1978.

Axhausen, G.: Zur Behandlung veralteter disloziert verheilter Oberkieferbruche, Dtsch. Zahn-, Mund-u. Kieferheilkd. 1:334, 1934.

Bell, W. H.: LeFort I osteotomy for correction of maxillary deformities, J. Oral Surg. 33:412-426, 1975.

Bell, W. H., and Epker, B. N.: Surgical-orthodontic expansion of the maxilla, Am. J. Orthod. 70:517-528, 1976.

Burstone, C. J.: Lip posture and its significance in treatment planning, Am. J. Orthod. 53:268-284, 1967.

Cernea, P., et al.: Les osteotomies totales des maxillaires superieurs, Rev. Stomato 1. Chir. Maxillofac. 56:700, 1955.

Dingman, R. O., and Harding, R. L.: The treatment of malunited fractures of the facial bones, Plast. Reconstr. Surg. 7:505, 1951.

Epker, B. N., and Fish, L. C.: The surgical-orthodontic correction of class III skeletal open bite, Am. J. Orthod. 73:601-618, 1978.

Epker, B. N., and Fish, L. C.: Surgical-orthodontic correction of open-bite deformity, Am. J. Orthod. 71:278-299, 1979.

Epker, B. N., Fish, L. C., and Paulus, P. J.: The surgical-orthodontic correction of maxillary deficiency, Oral Surg. 46:171-205, 1978.

Epker, B. N., Friedlander, G., West, R. A., and Wolford, L. M.: The use of freeze-dried bone in middle third face advancements, Oral Surg. 42:278-289, 1976.

Epker, B. N., and Wolford, L. M.: Middle third face ostectomies: their use in the correction of congenital dentofacial and craniofacial deformities, J. Oral Surg. 34:324-342, 1976.

Epker, B. N., and Wolford, L. M.: Reduction chieloplasty: its place in the correction of dentofacial deformities, J. Maxillofac. Surg. 5:134-141, 1977.

Fish, L. C., Wolford, L. M., and Epker, B. N.: Surgical orthodontic correction of vertical maxillary excess, Am. J. Orthod. 73:241-257, 1978.

Gillies, H. D., and Rowe, N. L.: L'osteotomie du maxillaire superieur envisagee essentiellement dans les cas de bec de lievre total, Rev. Stomatol. Chir. Maxillofac. 55:545, 1954.

Gonzales, U. M., and Stevens, E.: Role of chin correction in profile plasty, Plast. Reconstr. Surg. 41:477, 1968.

Hall, H. D., and Roddy, S. C., Jr.: Treatment of maxillary alveolar hyperplasia by total maxillary osteotomy, J. Oral Surg. 33:180-188, 1975.

Hogeman, K. E., and Wilmar, K.: Die Vorverlagerung des Oberkiefers zur Korrektur von Gebissanomalien, Fortschr. Kiefer- Gesichtschir. 12:275-278, 1967.

Hohl, T.: The use of an anatomical articulator in segmental surgery, Am. J. Orthod. 73:428-442, 1978.

Holdaway, R. Cited in Hambleton, R. S.: Soft tissue covering of the skeletal face as related to orthodontic problems, Am. J. Orthod. 50:405-416, 1964.

Hulsey, C. M.: An esthetic evaluation of lip-teeth relationships present in the smile, Am. J. Orthod. 57:132-144, 1970.

Kufner, J.: Experience with a modified procedure for correction of open bite, Transactions of the Third International Conference of Oral Surgeons, London, 1970, E. & S. Livingstone.

Kufner, J: Four-year experience with major maxillary osteotomy for retrusion, J. Oral Surg. 29:549, 1971.

Mohnac, A. M.: Maxillary osteotomy for the correction of malpositioned fractures: report of case, J. Oral Surg. 25:460, 1967.

Obwegeser, H.: Cirurgia del mordex apertus. Rev. Odont. Argentinia 50:429, 1962.

Obwegeser, H. L.: Der offene Biss aus chirurgischer Sicht. Schweitz. Monatsscher. Zahnheilkd. 74:688, 1964.

Obwegeser, H. L.: Treatment of facial deformities in cleft-palate cases by surgical correction of the jaws, Trans. Fourth Int. Congress Plast. Reconstr. Surg. Rome 1967.

Obwegeser, H. L.: Surgical correction of small or retrodisplaced maxillae, Plast. Reconstr. Surg. 43:351, 1969.

Rowe, N. L.: Secondary procedures for the correction

of deformity in the cleft lip and palate patient, Dent. Pract. **5**:112, 1954-55.

Schendel, S. A., Eisenfeld, J. H., Bell, W. H., et al.: The long face syndrome: vertical maxillary excess, Am. J. Orthod. **70**:398-408, 1976.

Schendel, S. A.: Eisenfeld, J., Bell, W., and Epker, B. N.: Superior repositioning of the maxilla: stability and soft tissue osseous relations, Am. J. Orthod. **70**:663-674, 1976.

Schendel, S. A., Oeschager, M., Wolford, L., and Epker, B. N.: Velopharyngeal anatomy and maxillary advancement, J. Maxillofac. Surg. **7**:116-124, 1979.

Stoker, N. G., and Epker, B. N.: The posterior maxillary ostectomy: a retrospective study of treatment results, Int. J. Oral Surg. **3**:153-157, 1974.

Turvey, T. A., and Epker, B. N.: Soft tissue procedures adjunctive to orthognathic surgery for improvement of facial balance, J. Oral Surg. **32**:572-577, 1974.

Wassmund, M.: Lehrbuch der praktischen Chirurgie des Mundes und der Kiefer, Leipzig, 1935, Meusser.

West, R. A., and Epker, B. N.: Posterior maxillary surgery: its place in the treatment of dentofacial deformities, J. Oral Surg. **30**:562, 1972.

West, R. A., and Epker, B. N.: Maxillary alveolar hyperplasia: diagnosis and treatment planning, J. Maxillofac. Surg. **4**:239-249, 1975.

Willmar, K.: On LeFort I osteotomy, Scand. J. Plast. Reconstr. Surg. Suppl. 12, 1974.

Wolford, L. M., and Epker, B. N.: The combined anterior and posterior maxillary ostectomy: a new technique, J. Oral Surg. **33**:842-51, 1975.

Chapter 9

Bell, W. H., and Epker, B. N.: Surgical-orthodontic expansion of the maxilla, Am. J. Orthod. **70**:517-28, 1976.

Bell, W. H., and Turvey, T. A.: Surgical correction of posterior cross-bite, J. Oral Surg. **32**:811, 1974.

Biederman, W.: Rapid correction of class III malocclusion by midpalatal expansion, Am. J. Orthod. **63**:47-55, 1973.

Ellenberg, D. C.: An evaluation of relapse changes following rapid maxillary expansion, Master's Thesis, University of Minnesota Dental School, 1969.

Epker, B. N., Fish, L. C., and Paulus, P. J.: The surgical-orthodontic correction of maxillary deficiency, Oral Surg. **46**:171-205, 1978.

Haas, A. J.: Palatal expansion: just the beginning of dentofacial orthopedics, Am. J. Orthod. **57**:219-255, 1970.

Isaacson, R. J., and Ingram, A. H.: Forces produced by rapid maxillary expansion. II. Forces present during treatment, Angle Orthod. **34**:261-270, 1964.

Kennedy, J., Bell, W. H., Kimbrough, O. L., and James, W. B.: Osteotomy as an adjunct to rapid maxillary expansion, Am. J. Orthod. **70**:123-137, 1976.

Lines, P. A.: Adult rapid maxillary expansion with corticotomy, Am. J. Orthod. **67**:44-56, 1975.

Melsen, B.: A histological study in the influence of sutural morphology and skeletal maturation on rapid palatal expansion in children, Trans. Eur. Orthod. Soc. pp. 499, 1972.

Moss, J. P.: Rapid expansion of the maxillary arch. Part I, J. Pract. Orthod. **2**:165-171, 1968.

Moss, J. P.: Rapid expansion of the maxillary arch. Part II, J. Pract. Orthod. **2**:215-223, 1968.

Timms, D. J.: An occlusal analysis of lateral maxillary expansion with midpalatal suture opening, Dent. Pract. Dent. Res. **18**:435-448, 1969.

Wertz, R. A.: Skeletal and dental changes accompanying rapid midpalatal suture opening, Am. J. Orthod. **58**:41-66, 1970.

West, R. A., and Epker, B. N.: Posterior maxillary surgery: its place in the treatment of dentofacial deformities, J. Oral Surg. **30**:562, 1972.

Chapter 10

Boyne, P. J.: Use of marrow–cancellous bone grafts in maxillary alveolar clefts, J. Dent. Res. **53**:841-47, 1974.

Boyne, P. J., and Sands, N. R.: Combined orthodontic-surgical management of residual palato-alveolar cleft defects, Am. J. Orthodont. **70**:20-37, 1976.

Boyne, P. J., and Sands, N. R.: Secondary bone grafting of residual alveolar and palatal clefts, J. Oral Surg. **30**:87-92, 1972.

Broude, D. J., and Waite, D. E.: Secondary closure of alveolar defects, Oral Surg. **37**:829-840, 1974.

Burston, W. R.: Pre-surgical facial orthopedics in relationship to the overall management of cleft lip and palate conditions, Ann. R. Coll. Surg. Engl. **48**:31-32, 1971.

Dixon, D. A., Edwards, J. R. C., and Newton, I.: Orthodontically induced eruption of the permanent canine combined with alveolar cleft osteoplasty: a new procedure illustrated by a case with stereophotogrammetric reconstructions, J. Maxillofac. Surg. **4**:61-65, 1976.

Epker, B. N., Fish, L. C., and Paulus, P. J.: Surgical orthodontic correction of maxillary deficiency, Oral Surg. **46**:171-205, 1978.

Epstein, L. I., Davis, B. W., and Thompson, L. W.:

Delayed bone grafting in cleft patient, Plast. Reconstr. Surg. **46**:363-68, 1970.

Hogeman, K., Jacobsson, S., and Sarnas, K.: Secondary bone grafting in cleft palate: a followup of 145 patients, Cleft Palate J. **9**:39-42, 1972.

Hotz, M. M.: Pre- and postoperative growth: guidance in cleft lip and palate cases by maxillary orthopedics, Cleft Palate J. **6**:368-372, 1969.

Lynch, J. G., et al.: Cephalometric study of maxillary growth five years after alveolar bone grafting of cleft palate infants, Plast. Reconstr. Surg. **46**:564-567, 1970.

Maisels, D. O.: The timing of various operations required for complete alveolar clefts and this influence on facial growth, Br. J. Plast. Surg. **20**:230-36, 1967.

Perko, M.: Surgical correction of the position of the premaxilla in secondary deformities of cleft lip and palate, Excerpto Medica International Congress Series 174, Rome, 1967.

Wolford, L. M., and Epker, B. N.: Sequencing and timing of treatment in the correction of dentofacial deformities in adult patients with clefts, J.A.D.A. **96**:835-840, 1978.

Chapter 11

Antia, N. H., Daver, B. M., Keswani, M. H., and Buch, V. I.: Prefabricated silicone nasal implants, Plast. Reconstr. Surg. **52**:264-270, 1973.

Beekhuis, G. J.: Silicone rubber implants in nasal reconstructive surgery, Laryngoscope **74**:1405;1419, 1964.

Belinfante, L. S., and Mitchell, D. L.: Use of alloplastic material in the canine fossa-zygomatic area to improve facial esthetics, J. Oral Surg. **35**:121-125, 1977.

Bell, W. H.: Augmentation of the nasomaxillary and nasolabial regions, Oral Surg. **41**:691-697, 1976.

Blinkov, S. M., and Glezer, I. I.: The human brain in figures and tables: a quantitative handbook, New York, 1968, Basic Books, Inc.

Braley, S.: Symposium on synthetics in maxillofacial surgery. II. The silicones in maxillofacial surgery, Laryngoscope **78**:549-557, 1968.

Brown, J. B.: Studies of silicones and Teflon as subcutaneous prostheses, Plast. Reconstr. Surg. **28**:86, 1961.

Brown, J. B., and McDowell, F.: Synthetic implants. In Plastic-surgery of the nose, second revised printing, Springfield, Ill. 1965, Charles C Thomas, Publisher.

Epker, B. N., and Wolford, L. W.: Middle-third facial advancement: treatment considerations in atypical cases, J. Oral Surg. **37**:31-41, 1979.

Epker, B. N., and Wolford, L. W.: Middle-third face osteotomies: their use in the correction of congenital dentofacial and craniofacial deformities, J. Oral. Surg. **34**:324-342, 1976.

Farrell, C. D., and Kent, J. N.: Clinical application of Proplast in oral and maxillofacial surgery, Alpha Omegan, Dec. 1975, pp. 21-26.

Feit, L. J.: Undermining and redraping in rhinoplasty, Trans. Am Acad. Ophtholmol. Otolaryngol. **80**:540-545, 1975.

Fleming, J. P.: Improvement of the face in Crouzon's disease by conservative operations, Plast. Reconstr. Surg. **47**:560-564, 1971.

Flowers, R. S.: Nasal augmentation by the intraoral route, Plast. Reconstr. Surg. **54**:570-578, 1974.

Haake, K.: Clinical evaluation of implanted material used in saddle nose correction, Acta Chir. Plast. **10**:148-156, 1968.

Hellmich, S.: The tolerability of preserved homoplastic cartilage implants in the nose, Z. Laryngol. Rhinol. Otol. **49**:742-749, 1970.

Holmes, E. M.: The correction of nasal skeletal defects, Trans. Am. Acad. Ophthalmol. Otolaryngol. **63**:501-531, 1959.

Janeke, J. B., Komorn, R. M., and Cahn, A. M.: Proplast in cavity obliteration and soft tissue augmentation, Arch. Otolaryngol. **100**:24-27, 1974.

Kent, J. N., Homsy, C. A., and Hinds, E. C.: PROPLAST in dental facial reconstruction, Oral Surg. **39**:347-355, 1975.

Kent, J. N., Homsy, C. A., Gross, B. D., and Hinds, E. C.: Pilot studies of a porous implant in dentistry and oral surgery, J. Oral Surg. **30**:608-616, 1972.

Milward, T. M.: The fate of Silastic and Vitrathene nasal implants, Br. J. Plast. Surg. **25**:276-278, 1972.

Muhlbauer, W. D., Schmidt-Tintemann, U., and Glaser, M.: Long term behavior of preserved homologous rib cartilage in the correction of saddle nose deformity, Br. J. Plast. Surg. **24**:325-333, 1971.

Natvig, P., Sether, L. A., Gingrass, R. P., and Gardner, W. D.: Anatomical details of the osseous-cartilaginous framework of the nose, Plast. Reconstr. Surg. **48**:528-532, 1971.

Ousterhout, D. K., and Zlotolow, I. M.: Methylmethacrylate forehead onlay implant in the treatment of craniofacial deformities such as Crouzon's and Apert's syndromes. Presented at the Fourth Congress, European Association for Maxillofacial Surgery, Venice, Italy, Sept. 1978.

Popisil, O. A., Jackson, I. T., and Moos, K. F.: The use of methylmethacrylate in craniofacial reconstruction. Presented at the Fourth Congress, European Association for Maxillofacial Surgery, Venice, Italy, Sept. 1978.

Chapter 12

Converse, J. M., Horowitz, S. L., Valauri, A. J., and Montandon, D.: The treatment of naso-maxillary hypoplasia: a new pyramidal naso-orbital maxillary osteotomy, Plast. Reconstr. Surg. **45:**527-35, 1970.

Converse, J. M., and Telsey, D.: The tripartite osteotomy of the mid-face for orbital expansion and correction of the deformity in craniostenosis, Br. J. Plast. Surg. **24:**365-374, 1971.

Converse, J. M., and Wood-Smith, D.: An atlas and classification of mid-facial and craniofacial osteotomies, Transactions of the Fifth International Congress on Plastic Surgery, 1971.

Conway, H., Smith, J. W., and Behrman, S. J.: Another method of bringing the midface forward, Plast. Reconstr. Surg. **46:**325-31, 1970.

Epker, B. N., Friedlaender, G., Wolford, L. M., and West, R. A.: The use of freeze-dried bone in middle-third face advancement, Oral Surg. **42:**278-289, 1976.

Epker, B. N., and Wolford, L. M.: Middle-third facial advancement: treatment considerations in atypical cases, J. Oral Surg. **37:**31-41, 1979.

Epker, B. N., and Wolford L. M.: Middle-third facial osteotomies: their use in the correction of congenital dentofacial and craniofacial deformities, J. Oral Surg. **34:**324-342, 1976.

Epker, B. N., and Wolford, L. M.: Middle-third facial osteotomies: their use in the correction of acquired and developmental dento-facial and craniofacial deformities, J. Oral Surg. **33:**491-514, 1975.

Freihofer, H. P. M.: Results after midface osteotomies, J. Maxillofac. Surg. **1:**30-36, 1973.

Gillies, H., and Harrison, S. H.: Operative correction by osteotomy of recessed malar maxillary compound in a case of oxycephaly, Br. J. Plast. Surg. **3:**123-27, 1951.

Henderson, D., and Jackson, I. T.: Naso-maxillary hypoplasia: the LeFort II osteotomy, Br. J. Oral Surg. **11:**77-93, 1973.

Jabaley, M. E., and Edgerton, M. T.: Surgical correction of congenital midface retrusion in the presence of mandibular prognathism, Plast. Reconstr. Surg. **77:**1-8, 1969.

Lewin, M. L., and Argamoso, R. V.: Midface osteotomies for correction of facial deformities (craniofacial dysostosis and maxillary hypoplasia), Trans. Am. Acad. **76:**946-56, 1972.

McCarthy, J. G., Coccaro, P. J., Epstein, F., and Converse, J. M.: Early skeletal release in the infant with craniofacial dysostosis, Plast. Reconstr. Surg. **62:**610-612, 1978.

McCarthy, J. G., Coccaro, P. J., Epstein, F., and Converse, J. M.: Early skeletal release in the infant with craniofacial dysostosis: the role of the sphenozygomatic suture, Plast. Reconstr. Surg. **62:**335-346, 1978.

Murray, J. E., and Swanson, L. T.: Midface osteotomy and advancement for craniosynostosis, Plast. Reconstr. Surg. **41:**299-307, 1968.

Murray, J. E., Swanson, L. T., Cohen, M., and Habul, M. B.: Correction of midfacial deformities, Surg. Clin. North Am. **51:**341-52, 1971.

Obwegeser, H. L.: Surgical correction of small or retrodisplaced maxillae: the dish-faced deformity, Plast. Reconstr. Surg. **43:**351-365, 1969.

Pruzansky, S., Miller, M., and Kammer, J. F.: Ocular defects in craniofacial syndromes. In Goldberg, M. F., editor: Genetic and metabolic eye disease, Boston, 1974, Little, Brown and Co.

Psillakis, J. M., Lapa, F., and spina, V.: Surgical correction of midfacial retrusion (nasomaxillary hypoplasia) in the presence of normal dental occlusion, Plast. Reconstr. Surg. **51:**67-70, 1973.

Sanders, B., Calcaterra, T. C., and Beumer, J. III: Orbital decompression and infraorbital augmentation for correction of exophthalmos secondary to Crouzon disease, J. Oral Surg. **36:**233-237, 1978.

Tessier, P.: Relationship of craniostenoses to craniofacial dysostoses and to faciostenoses: a study with therapeutic implications, plast. Reconstr. Surg. **48:**224-37, 1971.

Tessier, P.: The definitive plastic surgical treatment of the severe facial deformities of craniofacial dysostosis: Crouzon's and Apert's diseases, Plast. Reconstr. Surg. **48:**419-42, 1971.

Tessier, P.: Total osteotomy of the middle third of the face for faciostenosis or for sequelae of LeFort III fractures, Plast. Reconstr. Surg. **48:**533-41, 1971.

Wolfe, S. A.: A rationale for the surgical treatment of exophthalmos and exorbitism, J. Maxillofac. Surg. **5:**249-257, 1977.